The Science of Starving in Victorian Literature, Medicine, and Political Economy

The Science of Starving in Victorian Literature, Medicine, and Political Economy

ANDREW MANGHAM

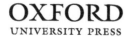

OXFORD
UNIVERSITY PRESS

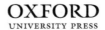

OXFORD
UNIVERSITY PRESS

Great Clarendon Street, Oxford, OX2 6DP,
United Kingdom

Oxford University Press is a department of the University of Oxford.
It furthers the University's objective of excellence in research, scholarship,
and education by publishing worldwide. Oxford is a registered trade mark of
Oxford University Press in the UK and in certain other countries

Published in the United States of America by Oxford University Press
198 Madison Avenue, New York, NY 10016, United States of America

British Library Cataloguing in Publication Data

Data available

Library of Congress Control Number: 2019955920

ISBN 978-0-19-885003-8

Printed and bound in Great Britain by
Clays Ltd, Elcograf S.p.A.

For my parents, Chris and Billy

Acknowledgements

I would like to thank the University of Reading for providing me with the research fellowship which allowed me to work on this project. In particular, I am grateful to Peter Stoneley, Andrew Nash, and Roberta Gilchrist for supporting the fellowship, and to Steven Matthews for encouraging me to apply. I am indebted to Verity Burke and James Green for their assistance. The shape and texture of this book would have been very different were it not for the support of my excellent colleagues in the Centre for Health Humanities at Reading, as well as some members of the Department of English Literature. I have delivered elements of this project at conferences and research seminars too numerous to remember, and I received invaluable feedback and suggestions during those events. Thank you to everyone who listened to my ideas and shared their knowledge. My gratitude also goes to the anonymous reviewers at Oxford University Press; their suggestions were incredibly useful in identifying a couple of errors and oversights. I would like to thank Emma Aston, Rhi Smith, David Nielson, Verity Hunt, Julie Roberts, and Anne-Marie Beller for being excellent friends; Tatiana Kontou and David Tucker were on hand to listen to the ramblings and worries that often accompanies the writing process. And last but not least, I would like to thank my family for their enduring love and patience. I dedicate this book rather fittingly to my parents. My father was a coal miner in the 1980s and, due to the political struggles that shaped the industry at the time, my family experienced long periods of hardship. I don't remember feeling hungry during those periods, which testifies to the sacrifices my parents made, as well as to the wider levels of support and kindness that the people of South Yorkshire showed each other.

Acknowledgements

Contents

Abbreviations

Dickens Journalism   *Dickens's Journalism*, vol. 1: *Sketches by Boz and Other Early Papers, 1833–39*, ed. by Michael Slater (London: J. M. Dent, 1996).

Dickens's Journalism, vol. 2: *'The Amusements of the People' and Other Papers: Reports, Essays and Reviews, 1834–51*, ed. by Michael Slater (London: J. M. Dent, 1996).

Dickens's Journalism, vol. 3: *'Gone Astray' and Other Papers from Household Words, 1851–59*, ed. by Michael Slater (London: J. M. Dent, 1998).

Dickens's Journalism, vol. 4: *'The Uncommercial Traveller' and Other Papers, 1859–70*, ed. by Michael Slater and John Drew (London: J. M. Dent, 2000).

Dickens Letters   *The Letters of Charles Dickens*, vol. 1: *1820–39*, ed. by Madeline House and Graham Storey (Oxford: Clarendon Press, 1965).

The Letters of Charles Dickens, vol. 2: *1840–41*, ed. by Madeline House, Graham Storey, and Kathleen Tillotson (Oxford: Clarendon Press, 1969).

The Letters of Charles Dickens, vol. 3: *1842–43*, ed. by Madeline House, Graham Storey, and Kathleen Tillotson (Oxford: Clarendon Press, 1974).

The Letters of Charles Dickens, vol. 4: *1844–46*, ed. by Kathleen Tillotson and Nina Burgis (Oxford: Clarendon Press, 1977).

The Letters of Charles Dickens, vol. 5: *1847–49*, ed. by Graham Storey, K. J. Fielding, and Anthony Laude (Oxford: Clarendon Press, 1981).

The Letters of Charles Dickens, vol. 6: *1850–52*, ed. by Graham Storey, Kathleen Tillotson, and Nina Burgis (Oxford: Clarendon Press, 1988).

The Letters of Charles Dickens, vol. 7: 1853–55, ed. by Graham Storey, Kathleen Tillotson, and Angus Easson (Oxford: Clarendon Press, 1993).

The Letters of Charles Dickens, vol. 8: 1856–58, ed. by Graham Storey and Kathleen Tillotson (Oxford: Clarendon Press, 1995).

The Letters of Charles Dickens, vol. 9: 1859–61, ed. by Graham Storey, Margaret Brown, and Kathleen Tillotson (Oxford: Clarendon Press, 1997).

The Letters of Charles Dickens, vol. 10: *1862–64*, ed. by Graham Storey, Margaret Brown, and Kathleen Tillotson (Oxford: Clarendon Press, 1998).

The Letters of Charles Dickens, vol. 11: *1865–67*, ed. by Graham Storey, Margaret Brown, and Kathleen Tillotson (Oxford: Clarendon Press, 1999).

The Letters of Charles Dickens, vol. 12: *1868–70*, ed. by Graham Storey, Margaret Brown, and Kathleen Tillotson (Oxford: Clarendon Press, 2002).

Gaskell Letters   *The Letters of Mrs. Gaskell*, ed. by J. A. V. Chapple and Arthur Pollard (Manchester: Manchester University Press, 1997).

Gaskell Letters 2   *Further Letters of Mrs. Gaskell*, ed. by John Chapple and Alan Shelstone (Manchester: Manchester University Press, 2003).

Kingsley, *L&M*   *Charles Kingsley: His Letters and Memories of his Life*, ed. by Frances Kingsley, 2 vols. (London: Macmillan, 1894).

By merely keeping close to facts and not hiding realities under lax generalizations, we shall be led to more humane, as well as truer, conceptions of the proper conditions of industrial life.

J. K. Ingram (1878)[1]

[1] J. K. Ingram, 'Presidential Address', Report of the Forty-Eighth Meeting of the British Association for the Advancement of Science; Held at Dublin in August 1878 (London: John Murray, 1879), pp. 641–58 (p. 650).

Introduction

In 1849, Charles Kingsley wrote a review of Elizabeth Gaskell's *Mary Barton* (1848) for *Fraser's Magazine*. He praised the novel fulsomely, suggesting that its detailed, realistic representation of starvation was its most powerful feature. Do wealthy people, he wondered,

> want to get a detailed insight into the whole 'science of starving'—'clemming' as the poor Manchester men call it? Why people 'clem', and how much they can 'clem' on; what people look like while they are 'clemming' to death, and what they look like after they are 'clemmed' to death, and in what sort of places they lie while they are 'clemming'; and who looks after them, and who—oh, shame unspeakable!—do not look after them while they are 'clemming', and what they feel while they see their wives and their little ones 'clemming' to death round them; and what they feel, and must feel, unless they are more or less than men, after all are 'clemmed' and gone, and buried safe out of sight, never to hunger, and wail and pine, and pray for death any more for ever? Let them read *Mary Barton*.[1]

To nineteenth-century readers the idea of a *science* of starving would probably have brought to mind Malthusian political economy—a way of thinking about hunger as the indication of the wealth of any given nation. By its presence or its absence, starvation, to Malthus and his followers, signified the state of balance between capital and demand; it embodied the successes or failures of domestic production measured against foreign imports; and it evidenced disparities between incomes, rents, and the cost of food. In Malthus's thinking, hunger is the greatest tragedy in human economics: in the worst of times it rises up as a horrible check on those nations whose resources have been overrun by improvident birth rates. Famine was 'the last, the most dreadful resource of nature'. Should practical human measures 'fail in [the] war of extermination' which was required to keep the 'multiplication of the species' in check, 'sickly seasons, epidemics, pestilence and plague [would] advance in terrific array and sweep off their thousands and ten thousands. Should success be still incomplete, gigantic inevitable famine stalks in the rear, and with one mighty blow, levels the population with the

---

[1] [Charles Kingsley], 'Recent novels', *Fraser's Magazine* 39 (1849), pp. 417–32 (p. 430).

The Science of Starving in Victorian Literature, Medicine, and Political Economy. Andrew Mangham,
Oxford University Press (2020). © Andrew Mangham.
DOI: 10.1093/oso/9780198850038.001.0001

food of the world.'[2] Malthus reasoned that we ought to do our best to avoid extreme 'checks' through preventative measures. Marriage among the poor should be discouraged; the Elizabethan Poor Laws, which diminished the will to work, should be abolished; and workhouses should be constructed as places where 'fare would be hard' and occupants would be 'obliged to work'.[3] Thomas Chalmers, author of *The Christian Economy of Large Towns* (1823) agreed. 'Nature', he said, 'when simply left to the development of her own spontaneous principles, will render a better service to humanity than can be done by the legal charity of England; [...] it is better to commit the cause of human want to the safeguards which nature has already instituted'.[4] State interference, in the shape of lenient Poor Laws, simply obstructed the health-giving benefits of what happened when the poor were left to their own devices. It was in moments of hardship, Chalmers added, that people showed their Christian virtues by helping each other and sharing their resources. In spite of such religious applications, the providentialist theory, as discussed by Malthus and Chalmers, was deductive in nature; it based its conclusions on observations of large patterns in social and demographic behaviours and made predictions therefrom. According to some commentators, such as Elizabeth Gaskell's father William Stevenson, it qualified as a bona fide science. In a series of articles written for *Blackwood's Edinburgh Magazine* in 1824 and 1825, Stevenson argued that political economy is 'capable of reaching the dignity of a science'.[5] It stands along chemistry, astronomy, and mathematics as 'perfect, or nearly so', having been 'directed by a careful and legitimate deduction from facts and experience'.[6]

In Kingsley's review of *Mary Barton*, however, Stevenson's daughter's 'science', as it is embodied in her pictures of clemming, is very different to the various foci of political economy. Questions such as 'why do people starve?' and 'how much food would allow them to avoid doing so?' were not all that different to the sorts of enquiries made by political economists, yet the focus on what extreme hunger looks like, how it appears in bodies pre- and post-mortem, and what kind of environments it thrives in brings Gaskell's science closer to the inductive science of medicine than to the deductive sciences of demography and economics. While the links between fiction like Gaskell's and political economy has been the subject

    [2] T. R. Malthus, *An Essay on the Principle of Population*, ed. by Geoffrey Gilbert (1798: Oxford University Press, 2008), p. 61.
    [3] Ibid., pp. 40, 44.
    [4] *The Christian Economy of Large Towns* (Glasgow: Chalmers and Collins, 1823), p. 68. See also Chalmers's *On Political Economy in Connection with the Moral State and Moral Prospects of Society* (New York, NY: Appleton, 1832) and 'Political Economy of a Famine', *North British Review*, 13 (1847), pp. 247–90.
    [5] [William Stevenson], 'The Political Economist I', *Blackwood's Edinburgh Magazine*, 15 (1824), pp. 522–31 (p. 523).
    [6] Ibid., p. 523.

of a number of critical studies,[7] the impact of that other science of starving—the specialist interest in the material aspects of extreme hunger, as developed through physiological research and medical practice—has been almost completely overlooked. In the Foucauldian pattern which has dominated critical approaches to nineteenth-century history and culture, medical and physiological discourses have been grouped with both sanitary reform and political economy to suggest that all such specialisms allowed capitalist values to be disguised, and to operate, as objective research. According to Mary Poovey, 'anatomical analysis [...] began to construct the social in the image of the economic, to the extent that both were subject to the logic of formal and instrumental rationality'.[8] However, physiology and Malthusian theory developed out of significantly different lines of enquiry. The latter followed a method of reasoning laid out in Adam Smith's *Wealth of Nations* (1776) and was, according to John Stuart Mill, reliant upon 'abstract speculation';[9] 'it [was] seldom in [its] power to make experiments':

> In chemistry and natural philosophy, we can not only observe what happens under all the combinations of circumstances which nature brings together, but we may also try an indefinite number of new combinations. This we can seldom do in ethical, and scarcely ever in political science. [...] The consequence of this unavoidable defect in the materials of the induction is, that we can rarely obtain what Bacon has quaintly, but, not unaptly, termed an *experimentium crucis*.[10]

Malthusian political economy could not be expanded by any experimental methodology because its subjects were vast and abstract; its chief discussions concerned topics whose yardsticks were poverty and wealth, life and death. For a range of ethical and logistical reasons, it was impossible to subject such things to experimental conditions. Medical researchers in Britain, Germany, and France, meanwhile, found the educative powers of experimentation extraordinarily powerful during the early years of the nineteenth century. Thanks to the efforts of men like John Hunter, Astley Cooper, Xavier Bichat, and François Magendie, physiology had become, in the words of John V. Pickstone, a science of the

---

[7] See, for example, Ella Dzelzainis, 'Malthus, Women and Fiction', in Robert J. Mayhew (ed.), *Malthus: The Life and Legacies of an Untimely Prophet* (Cambridge, MA and London: Belknapp Harvard, 2014), pp. 155–81.

[8] Mary Poovey, *Making a Social Body: British Cultural Formation, 1830–1864* (Chicago IL and London: Chicago University Press, 1995), p. 20. See also Pamela K. Gilbert, *Cholera and Nation: Doctoring the Social Body in Victorian England* (New York, NY: State University of New York Press, 2008), pp. 4–5.

[9] John Stuart Mill, 'On the Definition of Political Economy; and on the Method of Investigation Proper to It', (1836) in *The Collected Works of John Stuart Mill*, ed. John M. Robson, 33 vols. (Toronto: University of Toronto Press, London: Routledge and Kegan Paul, 1967), vol. 4, pp. 309–39 (p. 329).

[10] Ibid., pp. 327–28.

'functioning of human and animal bodies, established by means of experiment'.[11] The word 'functioning' is important in this context because it illustrates how physiology was interested, first and foremost, in the processes and developments of *life*—phenomena that were believed to lend themselves well, as research subjects, to experimentation and observation. Unlike anatomy, which mapped bodies in the forms of two-dimensional atlases and derived most of its technical knowledge from dissections of the dead, the study of living organisms took *active* processes and the developing natures of vital functions as its key objects of study.

A central focus in the early years of experimental physiology was the digestive system. As Ian Miller has noted in his *Modern History of the Stomach* (2011), the gut and its processes were seen to be the centre of animal vitality: they were 'invariably described as "a focus of vitality—the centre of a department in which the living principle is most abundant and exquisite", the "foundation or root of the complex apparatus", the "great nervous centre of sensorium of organic life" and even as the "great abdominal brain"'.[12] Since the eighteenth century, physiologists had believed that the assimilation of food was nature's central, life-giving enterprise: 'Food utterly symbolized the ambiguous cycles of existence, and the interdependence of all things sublunary'.[13] Through a range of experiments that were intended to supplement the more traditional considerations of case histories and bedside observations, and which will be explored in more detail in Chapter 1, physiologists such as Lazzaro Spallanzani and Hunter painted a picture of starvation that conflicted with Malthusian narratives of famine in two vital ways: firstly, they identified the actual, physical processes involved in starvation—the weakness, the wasting, and the suffering experienced when bodies effectively consume themselves in an effort to stay alive. Although Malthus had disciples such as Harriet Martineau who were keen to demonstrate how his demographic theory played out in individual cases of wrack and ruin,[14] his ideas appear largely to have allowed others to turn a blind eye to what was actually involved in starvation, not solely as a means of excusing themselves from helping the poverty-stricken, but because the actual details of hunger countered a more convenient account of hunger as nature's way of creating balance.

The second and more complex way in which in which scientists and medical men created an opposing idea of starvation to Malthus's consequentialism was in

[11] John V. Pickstone, 'Physiology and Experimental Medicine', in *Companion to the History of Modern Science*, ed. by R. C. Olby, G. N. Cantor, J. R. R. Christie, and M. J. S. Hodge (1990; London: Routledge, 1996), pp. 728–42 (p. 728). Italics in original.

[12] Ian Miller, *A Modern History of the Stomach: Gastric Illness, Medicine and British Society, 1800–1950* (2011; London: Routledge, 2015), p. 14.

[13] Roy Porter, preface to Piero Camporesi, *Il Pane Salvaggio*, trans. as *Bread of Dreams: Food and Fantasy in Early Modern Europe* by David Gentilcore (1980; Chicago IL: University of Chicago Press, 1989), p. 8.

[14] See Harriet Martineau, *Illustrations of Political Economy: Selected Tales*, ed. by Deborah Anna Logan (1832; Ontario: Broadview Press, 2004).

their insistence upon the ambiguity of hunger as a material reality. In the world of human physiology, hunger takes place in the dark, under the skin, and in the obscure territories of the gut. Magendie, an early pioneer of experimental physiology, believed that the nutritive process 'must be regarded as dependent on a special cause, comparable to planetary or molecular attraction in that it was unknown in its nature but manifested in its effects'.[15] In his 1826 *Treatise on Diet*, the physician John Paris used the words 'obscurity' and 'mysterious' to describe the operations of the digestive system: 'No function in the animal economy', he notes, 'presents such elaborate machinery as that of digestion', and 'these are the mysteries which cannot be cleared up until the sealed fountain of vitality is laid open'.[16] Until intracorporeal imaging was developed in the twentieth century, starvation was one of the body's *terra incognita*, an environment governed by laws whose languages were barely understood. In *The Physiology of Common Life* (1859), his major survey of contemporaneous physiological knowledge, George Henry Lewes asked: 'What is this Hunger—what its causes and effects? In one sense we may all be said to know what Hunger is; in another sense no man can enlighten us; we have all felt it, but Science as yet has been unable to furnish any sufficient explanation of it.'[17] Even towards the end of the nineteenth century, after years of laborious research on the subject had been undertaken both in Europe and America, the Edinburgh lecturer A. Lockhart Gillespie admitted that, although 'immense advance [...had] been made since the beginning of the [...] century in the elucidation of physiological problems', we still 'as yet know nothing' about 'the active digestion of nutritive substances'.[18] In more recent times, James Vernon suggests in his cultural history of hunger that 'we need to take seriously the very slipperiness of hunger as a category'.[19] Following Amartya Sen's seminal theory of famine as a failure in 'entitlements' as opposed to global shortages of food,[20] he adds: 'I believe that hunger was never simply a condition grounded in the material reality of the human body [...] hunger has a cultural history that belies its apparently consistent material form.' As a historian of culture, Vernon is 'concerned with elaborating [...hunger's] changing and historically specific meanings'.[21] *The Science of Starving in Victorian Literature, Medicine and Political*

[15] J. M. D. Olmsted, *François Magendie: Pioneer in Experimental Physiology and Scientific Medicine in XIX century France* (New York, NY: Schuman's, 1944), p. 28.

[16] John Paris, *A Treatise on Diet: with a View to Establish, on Practical Grounds, a System of Rules for the Prevention and Cure of the Diseases Incident to a Disordered State of the Digestive Functions* (1826; London: Sherwood, Gilbert and Piper, 1837), pp. 15, 22, 30, 67.

[17] George Henry Lewes, *The Physiology of Common Life*, 2 vols. (London: William Blackwood and Sons, 1859), vol. 1, p. 3.

[18] A. Lockheart Gillespie, *The Natural History of Digestion* (London: Walter Scott, 1898), pp. 14–15.

[19] James Vernon, *Hunger: A Modern History* (Cambridge, MS and London: Belknap Press of Harvard University Press, 2007), p. 8.

[20] Amartya Sen, *Poverty and Famines: An Essay on Entitlement and Deprivation* (Oxford: Oxford University Press, 1981).

[21] Vernon, *Hunger*, pp. 8–9.

Economy follows this line of thinking in a number of ways, particularly on the links forged between hunger's 'historically specific meanings' and the way 'the struggle to define and regulate hunger produce[s] its own networks of power, its own political constituencies, its own understanding of the responsibilities of governments, and its own forms of statecraft'.[22] Where I part company with Vernon's thesis is around his idea that the 'slipperiness' of hunger, as a cultural history, belies its material form. The history of starvation as a physiological and medical phenomenon shows, in fact, how definitions of hunger as shifting, obscure, and intransigent rely quite heavily on the body as a material thing.

In the nineteenth century, the man whose research most overtly illustrated the slipperiness of hunger was, ironically, the same man who got closest to witnessing and interacting with the actual processes of digestion. The American surgeon William Beaumont's *Experiments and Observations on the Gastric Juice, and the Physiology of Digestion* (1833) was based on the hundreds of tests he performed on a man named Alexis St. Martin. On 6 June 1822, while he was working as a salesman, St. Martin was accidentally shot with a musket ball. He was eighteen years old at the time and was placed under the care of Beaumont for the treatment of a gastric fistula. The young man's wound consisted of a hole 'the size of a man's hand' in the side of his abdomen, from which protruded a portion of the lung and stomach.[23] The surgeon managed to restore the lung but was unable to close the hole out of which came 'pouring [...] the food [St. Martin] had taken for his breakfast'.[24] After numerous failed attempts to mend the wound, the hole began to heal, extraordinarily, without closing: by 1824 St. Martin 'had perfectly recovered his natural health and strength; the aperture remained; and the surrounding wound was firmly cicatrized to its edges'.[25] He went on to marry and have several children; he 'enjoyed *general* good health, and [even] suffered much less predisposition to disease than is common to men of his age and circumstances in life'.[26] With his strong constitution and a window to the workings of his stomach, St. Martin offered a unique research opportunity for medical experts such as Beaumont. According to physiologist Andrew Combe:

Two or three other cases have [...] occurred in which the cavity of the stomach was laid open by external wounds, but in none except that of Alexis St. Martin, observed by Dr. Beaumont, did perfect recovery take place while the opening remained unclosed. In all of them, death occurred in a longer or shorter time, without affording any opportunity of observing the phenomena of really *healthy* digestion.[27]

[22] Ibid., p. 8.
[23] William Beaumont, *Experiments and Observations on the Gastric Juice, and the Physiology of Digestion*, ed. by Andrew Combe (1833; Edinburgh, Maclachlan and Stewart, 1838), p. 8.
[24] Ibid.   [25] Ibid., pp. 17–18.   [26] Ibid., p. 21.
[27] Andrew Combe, Preface to Beaumont, *Experiments and Observations*, p. vi. Italics in original.

Beaumont invited St. Martin to work as his domestic servant and, over an eight-year period, the former performed around 240 controlled investigations on the latter's digestive system. Although Beaumont called these investigations 'experiments', they mostly consisted of observations such as the following:

EXPERIMENT 43.
At 1 o'clock P. M. [...] dined on *broiled veal* and *bread,* and drank half a pint of *water.* Digestion completed in four and a half hours.[28]

Beaumont did, however, experiment with different foods and tested St. Martin's digestion in a range of situations, such as before and after exercise, in different weather conditions, and so on. 'Having no theory to support, and no favourite point to establish', writes Combe, 'Beaumont [told] plainly what he saw, and [left] every one to draw his own inferences.'[29] Yet Beaumont did come up with a hypothesis. Hunger is not, as some had suggested, caused by 'the friction of the internal coats of the empty stomach', nor is it, as Magendie had claimed, 'the action of the nervous system' with 'no other seat than the system itself, and [with] no other causes than the general laws of organization'.[30] Beaumont said: 'my impression is that the sensation of hunger is produced by a *distention* of the gastric vessels, or that apparatus, whether vascular or glandular, which secretes the gastric juice; and is believed to be the effect of repletion by this fluid'.[31] When the stomach receives food, it secretes gastric fluid through its follicles. When it receives no food, the follicles do not secrete their fluid, and the gastric juices build up. George Henry Lewes states 'there are several analogies which give colour to this explanation. Thus, milk is slowly accumulated in the breast, and the sense of fullness, if unrelieved, soon passes into that of pain.'[32] A similar theory had been suggested by Leeds surgeon Charles Thackrah in 1824: 'During digestion', he argued, the gastric juice 'is mixed with the food; but after the cessation of this process, the juice is accumulated on the sensible surface of the stomach, which it particularly irritates'.[33] 'Ingenious as the idea is', Lewes writes, 'closer scrutiny causes us to reject it'.[34] The same argument would suggest that 'tears must be accumulated in advance, because they gush forth so copiously on the first stimulus of grief'.[35] Furthermore, it is a 'physiological fact, that when food is injected into the veins or the intestines [thus bypassing the stomach], the sensation of Hunger disappears, although the stomach is as empty as it was before';[36] indeed, Beaumont himself had kept St. Martin alive during the early stages of his recovery

---

[28] Beaumont, *Experiments and Observations*, p. 195.   [29] Ibid., vii.
[30] From Magendie's *Summary of Physiology,* quoted in Beaumont, *Experiments and Observations,* p. 46.
[31] Ibid., p. 47.   [32] Lewes, *Physiology of Common Life,* vol. 1, p. 29.
[33] Charles Turner Thackrah, *Lectures on Digestion and Diet* (London: Longman, et al, 1824), p. 34.
[34] Lewes, *Physiology of Common Life,* vol. 1, p. 29.   [35] Ibid., p. 30.   [36] Ibid.

by injecting food *per anum*. Whether its results were correct or incorrect, Beaumont's research showed that hunger was difficult to observe and to make concrete conclusions about. What is telling about Lewes's refutation of Beaumont's theory is the way it does not seek to offer an alternative to the latter's science, but rather advocates 'closer scrutiny' of the same; a better understanding of the body, it was suggested, complicates (rather than confirms) the hypothesis. Such a material focus was central to the creation of starvation as a slippery category. In the hands of some converts to the providentialist way of looking at hunger, the usefulness of starvation, as a natural correction or 'Act of God', was gospel—its harrowing prognostications were carved in stone. Yet under physiology and medicine, hunger evolved into a topic in which little seemed able to be taken for granted. In a study of the representation of hunger and famine in the Victorian periodical, Charlotte Boyce draws upon Peter J. Gurney's idea that 'the struggle over the representation of scarcity was particularly acute during this crucial period', concluding that 'anxiously repeated poetical and iconographical depictions' attest to 'the idea that hunger's gnawing reality resists representation [...] as the printed page inevitably supplants the attenuating bodies of English and Irish sufferers with an intricate web of visual and textual signifiers'.[37] What nineteenth-century medical theory shows us is that the attenuating bodies of the starving were already an intricate web of visual and textual signifiers: the burden of representation reflected a burden of specialist interpretation—a burden which, I argue, became an alternative way of thinking creatively, critically, and politically about extreme poverty.

In his *Introduction to the Study of Experimental Medicine* (1865), Claude Bernard characterizes medical research as follows:

> Our experimenter puts questions to nature; but [...] as soon as she speaks, he must hold his peace; he must note her answer, hear her out and in every case accept her decision. [...] An experimenter must not hold to his idea, except as a means of inviting an answer from nature. But he must submit his idea to nature and be ready to abandon, to alter or supplant it, in accordance with what he learns from observing the phenomena which he has inducted.[38]

Bernard's *Introduction* was the century's most detailed study of the philosophy of science as it relates to medical research and practice. It stated that 'experimental reasoning is the only reasoning that naturalists and physicians can use in seeking

[37] See Peter J. Gurney, '"Rejoicing in Potatoes": The Politics of Consumption in England During the "Hungry Forties"', *Past and Present*, 203 (2009), 99–136 (p. 101); Charlotte Boyce, 'Representing the "Hungry Forties" in Image and Verse: The Politics of Hunger in Early-Victorian Illustrated Periodicals', *Victorian Literature and Culture*, 40 (2012), pp. 421–49 (p. 445).

[38] Claude Bernard, *Introduction à l'Étude de la Médecine Expérimentale*, trans. by Henry Copley Greene as *An Introduction to the Study of Experimental Medicine* (1865; New York, Dover Publishing, 1957), pp. 22–3.

the truth and approaching it as nearly as possible'.[39] David Carroll, Suzy Anger, and Jonathan Smith have said, in different contexts, that the nineteenth century was an age in which scientific methodologies, alongside other hermeneutic enterprises, were tested in varying ways and in different contexts by scientists, philosophers, religious figures, and writers of fiction.[40] Bernard's experimentalism learned a great deal from the preceding generation of physiologists whose work had been synonymous with questions about the efficacy of the experimental method as an approach to research. He was a student of the pioneering Magendie, a man who had 'set himself up as a prophet of experimental physiology',[41] and who has often been identified as the French Hunter. John Hunter himself had demonstrated, through a range of experiments (to be discussed in Chapter 1), how physiology was the stuff of complex, shifting, and often invisible matter. Understanding the vital principle, he argued, involved observing the circulations, generations, and wastes of the body. But observation was not all-powerful. Hunter believed, like many of his contemporaries, in vitality as a 'mysterious, non-mechanical life-force whose energies animated the living world' and 'whose self-activating powers were [not] comprehensible via the laws of motion'.[42] Such a sceptical view sprung up, as Catherine Packham has argued, in response to empiricist failures in medicine (such as the mechanical theories of the seventeenth century) which had attempted 'to explain the actions and functioning of living bodies' using laws of mechanics.[43] Hunter's more complicated notion of the body suggested, by contrast, that corporeality is comprised of a thousand different stories, many of them difficult to read, but each full of information that can be subjected to experimental trials.

In her 1993 study of self-starvation, Maud Ellmann discusses Franz Kafka's story 'The Hunger Artist' (1922):

> The unnamed hero locks himself into a cage to starve for the amusement of the populace. It is the public gaze that keeps him visible, however ruthlessly he wills his flesh to disappear, and it is only when he is deprived of this surveillance that he dies. The moral seems to be that it is not by food that we survive but by the gaze of others; and it is impossible to live by hunger unless we can be seen or represented doing so.

[39] Ibid., p. 31.

[40] See David Carroll, *George Eliot and the Conflict of Interpretations: A Reading of the Novels* (Cambridge: Cambridge University Press, 1992), p. 35; Suzy Anger, *Victorian Interpretation* (Ithaca, NY and London: Cornell University Press, 2005), pp. 1–21; and Jonathan Smith, *Fact and Feeling: Baconian Science and the Nineteenth-Century Literary Imagination* (Madison, WI: University of Wisconsin Press, 1994), pp. 11–44.

[41] Pickstone, 'Physiology and Experimental Physiology', p. 728.

[42] Catherine Packham, *Eighteenth-Century Vitalism* (Basingstoke: Palgrave Macmillan, 2012), p. 2.

[43] Ibid., pp. 1–2. See also Kenneth J. Carpenter, *Protein and Energy: A Study of Changing Ideas of Nutrition* (Cambridge: Cambridge University Press, 1994), pp. 5–7.

> Self-starvation is above all a performance. [...] Anorectics are 'starving for attention': they are *making a spectacle of themselves*, in every sense. [...] Even though the anorectic body seems to represent a radical negation of the other, it still depends upon the other as spectator in order to be *read* as representative of anything at all.[44]

Terms such as 'voluntarily' are decidedly problematic in discussions of self-starvation, but if we acknowledge, for now, that there are differences between those who starve *voluntarily* (anorectics, hunger-strikers) and those who do so *involuntarily* (victims of famine and extreme poverty), we can also concede that both groups have in common a certain textuality. In Ellmann's phrase, 'the starving body is itself a text, the living dossier of its discontents, for the injustices of power are encoded in the savage hieroglyphics of its sufferings.'[45] Her theoretical position insists, I would argue rightly, that all forms of starvation are a response to (or a result of) unjust, often hegemonic (as in cases of anorexia) forms of power. Yet, by looking at the science of starvation, as it emerged in medicine and physiology, we see hunger's (il)legibility to be powerful, not because it is a spectacle or a performance, but because it is written in *matter* that demands and challenges interpretation. The physiology of hunger distinguishes itself from the knee-jerk reactions of providentialist political economy through the readability of its material codes. 'To give materiality its due', observe Diana Coole and Samantha Frost in *New Materialisms* (2010), is to be 'alert to the myriad ways in which matter is both self-constituting and invested with—and reconfigured by—intersubjective interventions.'[46] While nineteenth-century physiologists moved away from the vagueness of eighteenth-century vitalist principles, they retained, as we have seen, the identification of certain aspects of life, including nutrition's materiality, as difficult to isolate, categorize, and make complete sense of. In the context provided by what Thomas Carlyle famously termed the 'Condition of England' question, medical and physiological experts asked with more urgency, and in more detail, what differentiated 'normal', 'everyday' hunger from starvation, and how the latter could be distinguished from 'secondary conditions' such as exhaustion and fever. Such onerous tasks were no easier for them than they had been for their eighteenth-century counterparts, and interpretive struggles translated, as we see in the extract I quoted from Claude Bernard, into recognitions of the dangers, to paraphrase Coole and Frost, of investment (or intrusion) of intersubjective intervention. It was recognized by students of the human body that the science of starving needed

---

[44] Maud Ellmann, *The Hunger Artists: Starving, Writing, and Imprisonment* (Cambridge, MA: Harvard University Press, 1993), p. 17. Italics in original.

[45] Ibid., pp. 16–17.

[46] Diana Coole and Samantha Frost, *New Materialisms: Ontology, Agency, and Politics* (Durham, NC: Duke University Press, 2010), p. 7.

to understand its evidence as phenomena that misleads, is often unforthcoming with its answers, and is beset with opportunities for erroneous thinking.

Joseph Childers's excellent study *Novel Possibilities* (1995) argues that nineteenth-century developments in sanitary science sought to 'resolv[e] the problems of the lower classes—both the problems the lower classes possess and the problems they pose for the middle and upper classes' by recognizing the need for a ' "better and scientific" attention to the mechanisms by which the poor are observed and their destitution alleviated.'[47] It is demonstrated, in the same work, that sanitarians and novelists had a common wish to reconstruct social questions in such 'better and scientific' terms. The languages of physiology and medicine, I argue—tied, in varying ways, to experimental ventures in research and eagle-eyed observation in treatment—became vital to the provision of better and more scientific understandings of poverty. They confirmed Marx's and Engels's view that 'man's ideas, views and conceptions, in one word, man's consciousness, changes with every change in the conditions of his material existence.'[48] Indeed, biological science provided a material basis upon which man's ideas, views, conceptions, and consciousness could be better examined; it shed light on the historical materialism which consisted of 'the real individuals, their actions, and their material conditions of life.'[49]

Like sanitary reform, the collection of novels written, roughly, between 1845 and 1865, and now known as social-problem fictions, explored states of scarcity with a level of complexity that learned a great deal from science's understanding of the powers and limitations of the empirical method. While the view of the period's fiction as developing a mode of realism that alarmed readers out of their indifference to poverty has become commonplace, such assertions have not gone far enough in questioning exactly *where* the idea of a radical, confrontational, and self-critical realism comes from. What I argue here is that novels written by Charles Kingsley, Elizabeth Gaskell, and Charles Dickens during these years developed what Terry Eagleton has called 'somatic (bodily) or anthropological realism': a creative materialism that 'takes seriously what is most palpable about men and women—their animality, their practical activity and corporeal constitution.'[50] Corporeal materialism involves appropriating ways of seeing that are developed through the biological sciences, both as a means of dissecting, and ultimately refuting, conservative ideas that emerged, in large part, out of Malthus's theory, and of becoming a method of scrutinizing how we talk about, and represent, poor

[47] Joseph W. Childers, *Novel Possibilities: Fiction and the Formation of Early Victorian Culture* (Philadelphia: University of Pennsylvania Press, 1995), p. 73.

[48] Karl Marx and Friedrich Engels, *The Communist Manifesto*, ed. by Gareth Stedman Jones (1848; London: Penguin, 2002), p. 241.

[49] Karl Marx and Friedrich Engels, *The German Ideology* (1846), in *Writings of the Young Marx on Philosophy and Society*, trans. and ed. by Loyd D. Easton and Kurt H. Guddat (1967; Indianapolis, IN: Hackett, 1997), p. 408.

[50] Terry Eagleton, *Materialism* (New Haven and London: Yale University Press, 2016), p. 35.

social conditions. Following George Levine's influential account of realism as 'self-conscious about the nature of [the] medium',[51] a number of studies have sought to highlight self-reflexivity as a key feature of the social-problem novel. Catherine Gallagher has offered the best evidence, arguing that these works 'found themselves uncovering the tense structure of their own form, making the always unsettled assumptions of the novel the objects of their scrutiny'.[52] These are texts, adds Carolyn Lesjak, that 'question [...] *how* one represents labor as much as *what* one represents'.[53] What my book argues is that the self-reflexive realism of the social-problem novel owes much to the scientific, social, and philosophical impact of medicine and physiology.

As Kingsley notes in his review of *Mary Barton*, Gaskell tells us everything we need to know about clemming (the dialectal term derived from the Old English *clemen*, meaning *pinched*) in modern times. What he does not mention, but which is critical, is the way Gaskell explores political and rhetorical uses of *clemming* as a metonym for broken social order. In radical and socialist contexts, Gaskell shows, *clemming* and *starving* had become bywords for crimes inflicted by the bourgeois on the working population. In *On Cases of Death by Starvation* (1844), the naturalist, lecturer, and radical author Johann Lhotsky lifted a definition of famishment from the pages of the *Dictionnaire des Sciences Médicales* (1812–22):

> If hunger is prolonged, it is accompanied by a flattening of the abdomen, and a general weakness and lassitude; the respiration and circulation decrease, as well as the animal heat, but the cutaneous and pulmonary absorptions are increased— all which is followed by a change in the nature of the different secretions and excretions. The urine becomes unnatural, acrimonious, acid, and oft-times converted by the cold into a jelly. The saliva flows in much greater abundance than usual, at least for some time. [...] Then follow convulsions, fainting, delusion of the senses, spasms and attacks of furor [...Finally] spasms and fainting follow, which are concluded by death.[54]

Alongside this insistently materialist account of hunger, Lhotsky provided a number of political comments on the more abstract question of how somatic pathology works as a symbol of social injustice. He and his readers live in 'the acme of a *Social Disorganization*, which must have reached its uttermost pitch

---

[51] George Levine, *The Realistic Imagination: English Fiction from Frankenstein to Lady Chatterley* (Chicago, IL: Chicago University Press, 1981), p. 4.

[52] Catherine Gallagher, *The Industrial Reformation of English Fiction 1832–1867* (Chicago, IL: Chicago University Press, 1985), p. xii.

[53] Carolyn Lesjak, *Working Fictions: A Genealogy of the Victorian Novel* (Durham, NC and London: Duke University Press, 2006), p. 11. Italics in original.

[54] [Johann Lhotsky], *On Cases of Death by Starvation, and Extreme Distress among the Humbler Classes* (London: John Ollivier, 1844), pp. 2–3.

before it could burst forth into such hideous and abominable symptoms'.[55] Such pessimistic symbolism was nothing new, but there was something unique about the way Lhostky moved from radical anger to the language of medicine: the symptoms of societal degeneracy burst out, he says, like skin lesions and manifest as individuals experiencing the reality of starvation. He also criticizes the political economists who had failed to understand the true meaning of hunger because they had been unable see it as an 'event' with real consequences: on Malthus's theory that 'over-population will find its own level [and] that it will open its own safety-valves', he reminds his readers that 'the chief safety-valve', is nothing short of 'death, drear horrible death'.[56] Drawing on Theodor Adorno's ideas on the holocaust, Eagleton suggests that the Irish Famine 'threaten[s] the death of the signifier' in cultural commentary; it 'threatens to burst through the bounds of representation as surely as Auschwitz did', and it 'strains at the limits of the artic-ulable, and is truly in this sense the Irish Auschwitz. In both cases, there would be something trivializing or dangerously familiarizing about the very act of repre-sentation itself.'[57] Gallagher has similarly suggested that the body in Victorian social discourses was 'unavailable as a metaphor of order and harmony' and was 'equally untranscendable and unperfectable'.[58] Exploring the broader topic of working-class hunger, Lhotsky falls foul of the danger identified by Eagleton. However well-intentioned his argument, he refurbishes starvation as an attack on the politics of the ruling class; his approach is every bit as problematic, if we are to judge it on its truthfulness, as those arguments which leapt upon political econ-omy as a justification for the early century's legislative attacks on the working classes. In the chapters that follow I broadly agree with Eagleton's perception of famine as an event that 'strains at the limits of the articulable', yet I disagree with his claim that texts of the period were necessarily silent on these limits. In explor-ing the 'dark territories' of the body in their empiricist studies of starvation, physiology and medicine developed an epistemological toolkit and a vocabulary through which hunger could be recast as subject and archetype of a more com-plex and critically powerful mode of discussing poverty. Unlike Lhotsky's *On Cases of Death by Starvation*, for example, works of fiction like *Mary Barton* showed an alertness to the possible uses and abuses of the topic. Through the appropriation of images and methodologies developed by experts in science, the novel self-consciously explored the varying ways in which the 'reality' of starving could be challenged and reshaped by the feelings of individuals and social

[55] Ibid., p. 6. Italics in original.   [56] Ibid., pp. 6-7.
[57] Terry Eagleton, *Heathcliff and the Great Hunger: Studies in Irish Culture* (London and New York, NY: Verso, 1995), pp. 11, 12, 13.
[58] Catherine Gallagher, 'The Body Versus the Social Body in the Works of Thomas Malthus and Henry Mayhew', in *The Making of the Modern Body: Sexuality and Society in the Nineteenth Century*, ed. by Catherine Gallagher and Thomas Laqueur (Berkeley, Los Angeles, CA and London: University of California Press, 1987), pp. 83-106 (p. 90).

groups.[59] The construction of starvation as material was a complex and thought-ful means of allowing literature such as Gaskell's to engage with contemporaneous historical events with a view to highlighting the strengths and weaknesses of epistemological and political commitments to certain ways of seeing.

Despite their telling differences, Kingsley, Gaskell, and Dickens were each committed to portraying the emotional, private, and moral aspects of the social debate; they were involved in what Vernon has termed 'the humanitarian discovery of hunger' which, from the 1840s, 'connected people emotionally with the suffering of the hungry and refuted the Malthusian model of causation'.[60] Vernon attributes this humanitarian discovery to 'novel forms of news reporting', and overlooks the rich and dynamic interchange that took place between the period's fiction and biological science.[61] What the authors of social-problem fiction found at this time, perhaps surprisingly, was that the humanitarian aspects of the hunger question were not only linked to, but were also given a new role by interpretations of starvation as a material phenomenon. Studies of hunger in literature and history have tended to concentrate on the symbolic potential of privation. Most famously, Sandra M. Gilbert and Susan Gubar discussed 'the genesis of hunger' as a feminine symbol of intellectual frustration in the work of Charlotte Brontë.[62] Since then, Gail Turley Houston has explored hunger as a metaphor that represents 'the emptiness in the Victorian upper-class woman's life',[63] while, more recently, Michel Delville and Andrew Norris have suggested that while 'studying hunger and disgust requires special attention not only to the workings of human consciousness but also to the organic circuitry beneath our skin', a 'fuller apprehension of the political status and agency of [the] starving subject' necessitates the perception of 'the starving self as an unstable and incomplete being, hesitating between identification and alienation, incorporation and rejection, nature and culture, intimacy and extimacy, pleasure and disgust'.[64] Hunger's 'flight into figuration' is an extraordinary power which allows hunger to emerge as a 'political crux, a point at which the subject is traversed by multiple crises—moral, social, libidinal, intellectual, environmental and, probably sooner than we think, existential'.[65] While starvation did emerge in the late eighteenth and early nineteenth centuries

[59] Ellmann notes: 'It is only in a unified collective, like [...] the workers in a factory, or a social class which has matured into a "class unto itself," that the experience of hunger sheds its intonations of submission and clarifies itself as solidarity or insurrection'. *The Hunger Artists*, p. 6.

[60] Vernon, *Hunger*, p. 16.   [61] Ibid.

[62] Sandra M. Gilbert and Susan Gubar, *The Madwoman in the Attic: The Woman Writer and the Nineteenth-Century Literary Imagination* (New Haven, CT and London: Yale University Press, 1979), pp. 372–98.

[63] Gail Turley Houston, *Consuming Fictions: Gender, Class, and Hunger in Dickens's Novels* (Carbondale and Edwardsville, IL: Southern Illinois University Press, 1994), p. xii.

[64] Michel Delville and Andrew Norris, *The Politics of Hunger and Disgust: Perspectives on the Dark Grotesque* (London: Routledge, 2017), pp. 6, 1.

[65] Ibid., p. 15.

as a political and conceptual crux with all of the linguistic and figurative power ascribed to it by Delville and Norris, my study shows how this developed out of the complexities of its material forms rather than by any transcendence of the body. If the physiological and realist texts I deal with in this study teach us anything, it is that 'conceptual force and complexity' and 'corporeality' were not mutually exclusive forces.

Contrary to a perception of the social-problem novel which has dominated scholarship for a number of years, then, I do not see the genre and its obvious sentimentalism as opposing forces. To counter Raymond Williams's influential view, the power of the former is *not* weakened by the inevitable encroachments of the latter.[66] Drawing on the work of Nancy Armstrong, Carolyn Lesjak argues that Gaskell's interest in domestic detail allows her to construct a way of writing that is both realistic and sentimental:

> For want of a better term, Gaskell's "sentimental realism" allows her both to feel for the workers and their plight and to detail their workday existence, both in the domestic and the political realm. Contra Williams, it is not a question of Gaskell's sentimentalism jeopardizing her realism or vice versa or of the two being at odds with one another but rather of each mode enabling the other.[67]

In Chapter 3, I suggest that domestic details, like corporeal details, are drawn with a materialistic interest that comes from the example of physiological approaches to poverty. For complex historical reasons that I discuss in Chapter 1, it is essential that we locate the interdisciplinary roots of social-problem realism in order to distinguish it from the forms of reasoning, like those used by politicians committed to a conservative interpretation of political economy, which it saw as too simplistic. By contrast, physiology and medicine provided examples of how emotion and feeling were not the *result* of a realist view, but rather part of the descriptive language used in realism. In a science article that appeared in Dickens's journal *All the Year Round* it was suggested that a German textbook on hunger, *Die Nahrungs und Genussmittelkunde*, was all the more interesting because it had

> a pathetic interest thrown own over it from the fact that it was written in years of hunger, cold, and misery, that in closing the preface to the first part, the author says he is on the brink of the grave, and may not survive to complete what he has so laboriously commenced.[68]

[66] See Raymond Williams, *Culture and Society* (1958; London: Penguin, 1984), pp. 99–119.
[67] Lesjak, *Working Fictions*, 34. See also Nancy Armstrong, *Desire and Domestic Fiction: A Political History of the Novel* (Oxford: Oxford University Press, 1987).
[68] Unsigned, 'Metamorphosis of Food', *All the Year Round*, 5 (1861), pp. 6–9 (p. 6) .

There is implied here a connection between truthfulness, or authenticity, and pathetic interest. Similarly, in Kingsley's review of *Mary Barton*, it is noticed that Gaskell's ability to comprehend the emotional sides of the topic comprises a significant and vital part of the latter's realist aesthetics. In addition to outlining 'what people look like while they are "clemming" to death, and what they look like after they are "clemmed"', the novel details the way people *feel* when they (or their loved ones) starve. This is not just a means of providing a fuller picture of poverty, or of making realism subservient to emotion, but also an indication of the way in which the inescapability of subjectivity, as embodied in feeling, formed a crucial consideration for the materialist realism of the social-problem novel.

*   *   *

My aim in this study is not to offer an account of the strengths and weaknesses of the British State's strategies for understanding social problems, or to see the novel as an enlightened comment on such manoeuvres; there are numerous studies which have undertaken this work through a range of specific approaches.[69] Rather, my argument is that the social novels of Kingsley, Gaskell, and Dickens promoted the development of knowledge and sympathy not through a subordination of 'material facts' to 'the unsounded truths of the spirit', but through an emphasis, informed by science, on the material sufferings of the starving and, more importantly, on detailed analysis of what it means to go hungry and to observe and to write about it in a way that seeks to be truthful. In giving Kingsley, Gaskell, and Dickens a long chapter of their own, I have sought to avoid homogenizing their work under the 'social-problem novel' banner. Although I get a lot of use out of that term in some broader discussions, I would not wish to claim that there was any unified mission across the different fictions I discuss. Looking at them separately allows me to consider the varying influences that social and scientific contexts had upon each author. Gaskell's writing from inside the heart of industrial Manchester, with strong Unitarian influences, meant that her work emerged from a different, though not entirely unrelated, context to Kingsley's early, left-leaning devotions to Christian Socialism and the theologian F. D. Maurice. Dickens's encounters with social reformers and his enthusiasm for Carlyle gave his work a satirical sting that is notably absent from the works of Kingsley and Gaskell. Yet there is overlap between each of these writers' influences as well. All three authors knew (or at least met) each other, and the successes of each suggest

---

[69] See Childers, *Novel Possibilities*; Mary Poovey, *Making a Social Body; Victorian Literature and the Victorian State: Character and Governance in a Liberal Society* (Baltimore, MD and London: Johns Hopkins University Press, 2004); Pamela K. Gilbert, *Mapping the Victorian Social Body* (New York, NY: State University of New York Press, 2004), Pamela K. Gilbert, *The Citizen's Body: Desire, Health and the Social in Victorian England* (Columbus, OH.: Ohio State University Press, 2007); Gilbert, *Cholera and Nation*; Eileen Cleere, *The Sanitary Arts: Aesthetic Culture and the Victorian Cleanliness Campaigns* (Columbus, OH: Ohio State University Press, 2014).

it is unlikely that they did not know each other's written work: the stormy relationship between Gaskell and Dickens has been well-documented by biographers;
Gaskell admired Kingsley and sought him out on a couple of occasions; Kingsley
reported finding Dickens 'a genial lovable man, with an eye like a hawk. Not high
bred but excellent company, and very sensible.'[70] Dickens was married in the
church where Charles Kingsley's father was rector,[71] and he owned a volume of
the author's poems at the time of his death.[72] Like Dickens, Kingsley admired
Carlyle; as did Gaskell, who also liked F. D. Maurice. All three authors had some
correspondence with Edwin Chadwick, the man who both authored the New
Poor Law (1834) and became a key player in debates over the understanding of
starvation in mid-century Britain.

Despite differences and varying levels of inconsistencies in their politics, the
three authors shared an antipathy towards Malthusianism. In recent years, there
has been a sensible drift in scholarly research towards a more balanced understanding of Malthus's influence, and, in particular, the well-intentioned objectives
of *The Principle of Population* (1798). Gallagher has observed, for instance, that
political economists 'were motivated by [...] a genuine desire to understand the
phenomena they observed.'[73] In the preface to *The Popularization of Malthus in
Early Nineteenth Century England* (2006), James P. Huzel writes that when he first
encountered Malthus as a 'young and admittedly idealistic graduate student' he
had been 'deeply hostile,'[74] yet acquaintance with the later Malthus taught him
that most antagonistic responses to Malthusianism are based on misreadings.
Early critics attacked Malthus 'not on what he said but for public opinions his
writings supposedly encouraged.'[75] Yet it is naïve to suggest, as Robert J. Mayhew
does, that Malthus's theory was 'the "first" inconvenient truth';[76] history shows it
to have been neither inconvenient nor truthful. Certainly during the Irish Famine,
the consequentialist message of Malthusianism offered a very convenient fudge
for both the English government and the wealthy landowners who proclaimed a
problem in the habits of the Irish working class in order to obscure a fuller view
of the questionable ethics underpinning the storing of corn for export and the

---

[70] Quoted in Susan Chitty, *The Beast and the Monk: A Life of Charles Kingsley* (London: Hodder
and Stoughton, 1974), p. 174.

[71] Una Pope-Hennessy, *Charles Dickens* (1945; London: Reprint Society, 1947), p. 68.

[72] See J. H. Stonehouse, *Catalogue of the Library of Charles Dickens from Gadshill* (London:
Fountain Press, 1935), p. 68.

[73] Catherine Gallagher, *The Body Economic: Life, Death, and Sensation in Political Economy and the
Victorian Novel* (Princeton, NJ: Princeton University Press, 2006), p. 3.

[74] James P. Huzel, *The Popularization of Malthus in Early Nineteenth Century England* (Aldershot:
Ashgate, 2006), p. xi. A similar reassessment is offered by Niall O'Flaherty's 'Malthus and the "End of
Poverty"', in *New Perspectives on Malthus*, ed. by Robert J. Mayhew (Cambridge: Cambridge University
Press, 2016), pp. 74–104.

[75] Huzel, *Popularization*, p. 8.

[76] Robert J. Mayhew, *Malthus: The Life and Legacies of an Untimely Prophet* (Cambridge, MA and
London: Belknapp Harvard, 2014), p. 4, 65, 66.

taking of land belonging to poor families. What is more, Malthus's theory was only ever a theory, never a truth. With the development of artificial fertilizers, foreign imports, and industrial-scale farming, population figures did not outrun food resources as Malthus predicted. In physiology and literature, as we shall see, the nineteenth century saw not only alternative ways of thinking about hunger, but also demonstrations of the ways in which appropriations of politico-economic theories, like those committed during the Irish Famine, had made simplistic and dangerous interpretations both appealing and dogmatic. As Amartya Sen concludes in his powerful *Poverty and Famines* (1981), in political economy 'the mesmerizing simplicity of focusing on the ratio of food to population has persistently played an obscuring role'. The truth, he suggests, is that 'the concept of nutritional requirement is a rather loose one [and] there is no particular reason to suppose that the concept of poverty must itself be clear-cut and sharp'.[77]

In Chapter 1, I begin by underscoring how, contrary to views like those expressed in Terry Eagleton's influential *Heathcliff and the Great Hunger* (1995), political economy was not 'a gross, materialist language, heavy with biological ballast',[78] but a set of abstractions based on moral judgement and laissez-faire approaches to wealth and well-being. While I do not disagree with Eagleton's sense of Ireland, especially during the famine years of the 1840s, as stubbornly material, I take issue with the claim that political economy was a material science which offset the realities of Ireland against an English ideal of abstract subjectivity. What my study argues is that the materialities of medicine and physiology offered a language through which stories like those relating to the Irish Hunger offered a powerful challenge to the simplifying abstractions of conservative political economy which, as part of a wider commitment to laissez faire, developed into a dogmatic form of thinking in which the poor were to blame for their problems, and were better left to learn the harsh lessons of nature. Looking at the major works that pioneered dietetics, gut physiology, and hunger therapeutics, in Chapter 1 I set out how scientists, surgeons, and doctors offered an alternative narrative of hunger as unnecessary, unjust, and unnatural. Comparing understandings of famine and sickness during the Irish Hunger with the ill-assumed confidence of statisticians, Chapter 1 also studies how science developed a critically sophisticated, multi-textured mode of exploring the meanings, languages, and aftermaths of hunger.

My second chapter considers the conflict-laden work of Charles Kingsley. A man of the cloth like Malthus, Kingsley was also an avid follower of the scientific developments I outline in Chapter 1. In 1842 he urged one of his correspondents to 'study medicine...I am studying it'.[79] In the three social novels, *Yeast* (1848),

---

[77] Sen, *Poverty and Famines*, pp. 8, 13.
[78] Terry Eagleton, *Heathcliff and the Great Hunger*, p. 8.
[79] Kingsley, *L&M*, vol. 1, p. 64.

Alton Locke (1850), and *Two Years Ago* (1857), we see the fruits of these labours, particularly in how the languages and methods of biology offered the author a means of challenging the view of starvation as an inevitable and necessary evil. In his portrayals of radical characters, Kingsley also discusses how scientific ideas precluded the political reformation of starvation as a stick with which to beat the well-to-do. Famous for locking horns with John Henry Newman on the abstract question of what constitutes truth, Kingsley argues a case for seeing topics such as the physiology of hunger not as an enemy of providentialist or radical thinking, but as the means of creating a more critical and intelligent understanding of poverty.

Elizabeth Gaskell's novels *Mary Barton* (1848), *North and South* (1854–55), and *Sylvia's Lovers* (1863) form the primary focus of my third chapter. These works, I argue, confirm Kingsley's suspicion that a material view of starvation—and poverty more generally—offers a reason*able* and reason*ing* interpretation of the Condition of England question. Starvation, or 'clemming', refuses to be integrated, in Gaskell's fictional world, into a catch-all economic or demographic theory. Instead, it is a phenomenon that paradoxically demands confrontation while evading perception through both the anatomies of workers and their surroundings. In line with the interlinking findings of biological scientists and Unitarian thinkers, Gaskell broaches the intricate, emotional questions of reform by recasting them as flesh-and-blood issues perceived through the eyes of her heroines, asking for the sort of careful consideration, advocated by science, that explored the strengths and weaknesses of such subjective interpretations.

My fourth and final chapter illustrates how Charles Dickens found the materiality of starvation to be a powerful method for addressing the social injustices that famously angered him. Less balanced than Gaskell, and less conflicted than Kingsley, he pulled no punches when it came to the 'Parrots of Society', those subscribers to hypocritical, dogmatic interpretations of political economy whose efforts to deal with social problems became, he believed, abortive subscriptions to a malicious way of thinking. I claim that we need to understand these red-hot polemics as a response to, and an appropriation of, the scientific registers of men such as Thomas Southwood Smith and the specialist respondents to the Tooting Disaster of 1848–9, where 126 schoolboys died from famine-related cholera. Dickens found in science a type of materialism that allowed him to formulate his challenges to the shallow cant of reformers and politicians as an attack on their perceived stupidity: more than the other authors I explore in this work, Dickens was able to use the science of starving as a means of marrying a radical position to a more thoughtful and compassionate one.

1

Starvation Science and Political Economy

As ulcers, which first appear in isolate spots upon the body, enlarge
until, touching each other, they become confluent, so had the famine,
limited in its earlier stages to certain localities, now spread itself over
the entire country.

John O' Rourke, *The Great Irish Famine* (1874)[1]

Irish Hunger

Anthony Trollope's *Castle Richmond* (1860) is one of only a few Victorian novels
set within the Irish Famine. Generally sympathetic towards both the Poor Laws
instituted in Ireland and the view that 'Famine is the consequence of God's mercy
rather than his wrath',[2] the text's rich descriptions highlight how famine is, paradoxically, both easily identified and difficult to know. The narrator states on a
number of occasions that the famished people of Ireland developed a certain look
during the crisis:

In those days there was a form of face which came upon the sufferers when their
state of misery was far advanced, and which was a sure sign that their last stage
of misery was nearly run. The mouth would fall and seem to hang, the lips at the
two ends of the mouth would be dragged down, and the lower parts of the
cheeks would fall as though they had been dragged and pulled. There were no
signs of acute agony when this phasis of countenance was to be seen, none of the
horrid symptoms of gnawing hunger by which one generally supposes that famine
is accompanied. The look is one of apathy, desolation, and death. When custom
had made these signs easily legible, the poor doomed wretch was known with
certainty. 'It's no use in life meddling with him; he's gone,' said a lady to me in
the far west of the south of Ireland, while the poor boy, whose doom was thus

---

[1] John O'Rourke, *The Great Irish Famine* (1874; Dublin: Veritas, 1989), p. 177.
[2] Terry Eagleton, *Heathcliff and the Great Hunger: Studies in Irish Culture* (London and New York,
NY: Verso, 1995), p. 15.

The Science of Starving in Victorian Literature, Medicine, and Political Economy. Andrew Mangham,
Oxford University Press (2020). © Andrew Mangham.
DOI: 10.1093/oso/9780198850038.001.0001

spoken, stood by listening. [...] And then she pointed out to me the signs on the lad's face, and I found that her reading was correct.[3]

Easily legible signs and confident readings are reflected in the prose's level of detail: the symptoms are so uniform that the author feels confident enough to lay them out in a novel that, like most of his work, aimed for a high standard of verisimilitude. Yet, as one might expect with any description of starvation, the writing is interesting for its identification of what is deficient: when the look of hunger is present there is an absence of the more 'horrid symptoms' and it is this lack, combined with the inconsistency between signs and absences, that leads to a statement ('one generally supposes') that is out of sequence with the confident knowledge characterizing the rest of the passage. In another passage, the text's hero, Herbert Fitzgerald, reflects on the harshest measures of the Poor Law when he encounters a famished family:

Mike was [the] husband, and [...] having become a cripple through rheumatism, he had not been able to work on the roads. In this condition he and his should of course have gone into the poor-house. [...] But then, as long as a man found work out of the poor-house [which Mike manages to do, though the wages are terrible], his wife and children would not be admitted into it. They would not be admitted if the fact of the working husband was known. The rule in itself was salutary [...] But in some cases, such as this, it pressed very cruelly. Exceptions were of course made in such cases, if they were known: but then it was so hard to know them![4]

This last sentence exposes a tension between rule and exception, and the failure of perception that the law contrarily encourages and comes into conflict with. The idea of a one-solution-fits-all approach, as embodied in the New Poor Law, implies that the mechanisms of civic order—the government boards and parish committees—have an omniscient view of everything; the fact that they do not allows individual cases to slip through the net; these people are unknown, essentially, by the very measures that claimed to know them better than they knew themselves. What is important about *Castle Richmond*, and social-problem literature more generally, is the way it uses descriptions of bodies and environments as a means of exploring the implications of failures of knowledge. *Castle Richmond* supports Terry Eagleton's theory that 'nature in Ireland is too stubbornly social and material a category, too much a matter of rent, conacre, pigs and potatoes for

---

[3] Anthony Trollope, *Castle Richmond*, ed. by Mary Hamer (1860; Oxford: Oxford University Press, 1989), pp. 369–70.
[4] Ibid., p. 372.

it to be distanced, stylized and subjectivated'.[5] Nature, in Trollope's novel, is also a matter of filth, excrement, putrefaction, and physical suffering:

> [Herbert] stood for a time looking round him till he could see through the gloom that there was a bundle of straw lying in the dark corner beyond the hearth, and that the straw was huddled up, as though there were something lying under it. Seeing this he left the bridle of his horse, and stepping across the cabin moved the straw with the handle of his whip. As he did so he turned his back from the wall in which the small window-hole had been pierced, so that a gleam of light fell upon the bundle at his feet, and he could see that the body of a child was lying there, stripped of every vestige of clothing.
>
> For a minute or two he said nothing—hardly, indeed, knowing how to speak, and looking from the corpselike woman back to the lifelike corpse, and then from the corpse back to the woman, as though he expected that she would say something unasked. But she did not say a word, though she so turned her head that her eyes rested on him.
>
> He knelt down and put his hand upon the body, and found that it was not yet stone cold. The child apparently had been about four years old.[6]

The image of starving mother and child was a common focus in texts describing the Famine; 'the spectacle of such vulnerable victims functioned', according to Charlotte Boyce, 'as a ready stimulus to pity'.[7] More often than not, it was a trope that drew upon a traditional, spiritual iconography of Madonna and Child to symbolize the Christian values which, according to a large number of social reformers, were essential to any successful discussion of poverty. Yet, Trollope's child is not the holy cherub of Renaissance art: she is famished, probably pestilential, and so dirty that Fitzgerald chooses to uncover her remains with a riding whip rather than touch her with his bare hands. The infant does not ascend immediately to heaven, as Victorian fictional children often do when they die, but is weighed down by her own corporeality: 'lifelike', in the dirt, and barely cold. Fitzgerald, a well-to-do and well-intentioned outsider, finds himself in a world full of signs yet bereft of language: the child's starvation can be read easily enough, but cannot, it seems, be articulated. This is a scene which embodies how nineteenth-century starvation developed into a discussion of knowing. The novel's realism and confidence in the signs of starving speaks boldly about the will to understand hunger; yet the silence between characters and the range of unasked and

---

⁵ Eagleton, *Heathcliff and the Great Hunger*, p. 8.   ⁶ Trollope, *Castle Richmond*, pp. 370–1.
⁷ Charlotte Boyce, 'Representing the "Hungry Forties" in Image and Verse: The Politics of Hunger in Early-Victorian Illustrated Periodicals', *Victorian Literature and Culture*, 40 (2012), pp. 421–49 (p. 434).

unanswered questions announces, with equal boldness, the limits of what we *do* know and what we *can* know about hunger.

God's Will in Ireland

It was the great misfortune of the people of Ireland that the British relief efforts during the Hunger of the 1840s were managed by the government secretary Charles Trevelyan, a man firmly prejudiced against the Irish character: 'the great evil with which we have to contend', he wrote to Colonel Jones in 1846, is 'not the physical evil of the famine, but the moral evil of the selfish, perverse and turbulent character of the people'.[8] Head of the Treasury, Trevelyan was a man whose thought was shaped by a rigid evangelicalism. He invented, 'in accordance with the principles of *laissez-faire*', the phrase '"the operation of natural causes", to which he considered Ireland should be left'.[9] As Eric B. Ross notes: 'Malthusian theory was quickly brought into play [in Ireland] in order to attribute the ensuing famine and death, not to colonial underdevelopment, but to over-population'.[10] Trevelyan had been educated at the East India College at Haileybury, 'where he had been greatly influenced by [Malthus's] lectures'.[11] In 1846, he wrote to Lord Monteagle, a County Limerick landowner, that the Great Hunger was 'altogether beyond the power of man' and 'the cure has [to be] applied by the direct stroke of an all wise Providence'.[12] In *The Irish Crisis* (1848), a long essay originally published in the *Edinburgh Review*, he added: 'posterity will trace up to [the] famine the commencement of a salutary revolution in the habits of a nation long singularly unfortunate, and will acknowledge on this, as on many other occasions, Supreme Wisdom has educated permanent good out of transient evil'.[13] According to Trevelyan, the intervention of Supreme Wisdom justified the lack of any serious interference from his office: 'British policy in Ireland attempted to render an errant Irish population fit for the systematicity of modern life, and fit for the stern judgement of a Protestant God'.[14] Historians tend to agree that the strategy proved to be a disastrous way of tackling the need for relief: the famine lead to a million

---

[8] Quoted in Cecil Woodham-Smith, *The Great Hunger: Ireland 1845–1849* (1962; London: Penguin, 1991), p. 156.

[9] Woodham-Smith, *Great Hunger*, p. 374.

[10] Eric B. Ross, *The Malthus Factor: Poverty, Politics and Population in Capitalist Development* (New York, NY: Zed Books, 1998), p. 29.

[11] Ibid., p. 46.

[12] Charles Trevelyan, letter to Lord Monteagle, 9 October 1846, in *The Irish Famine*, ed. by Colm Tóibín and Diarmaid Ferriter (London: Profile, 2002), pp. 71–2 (p. 72).

[13] Charles Trevelyan, *The Irish Crisis* (London: Longman et al., 1848), p. 1.

[14] Gordon Bigelow, *Fiction, Famine, and the Rise of Economics in Victorian Britain and Ireland* (Cambridge: Cambridge University Press, 2003), p. 117.

deaths, and a similar number of individuals leaving Ireland for good.[15] But even more damaging was the view that the Hunger ought to be viewed as a 'salutary revolution'. In 1848, the term 'revolution' had a particular and urgent resonance, yet it is the word 'salutary' that reveals the most about Trevelyan's social prejudices and preconceived notions. Meaning that which produces overall benefit, 'salutary' originates from the Latin 'salutaris', meaning 'health', and it has, therefore, ancient associations with anything that is health-giving and wholesome. As crop failures may be identified as Acts of God, they must, according to Trevelyan's way of thinking, be beneficial to the Irish people in the long run. The English minister Charles Vansittart agreed. Like the Abbé Ranvier in Zola's *Germinal* (1885), he exploited 'dreadful misery and the bitter resentment of hunger, and [brought] to his task all the armour of a missionary preaching to savages for the greater glory of his faith'.[16] Famine, Vansittart catechized, ought to be viewed 'in the light it was designed by God—as a visitation—a chastisement of [...] national sins and crimes—for the grasping, gambling, monopolising, covetous spirit, which of late has engrossed the minds of all ranks and classes of men'.[17] The 'hand of God' doles out salutary lessons first, and wrathful punishments second: while starvation and famine were 'doubtless designed by God to rebuke us for our worldliness and impiety', they were intended 'to bring us nearer to Him, and make us feel and acknowledge our insufficiency, and dependence upon Him, the Author and Preserver of our lives'.[18] An anonymous correspondent to the London *Times* similarly argued that 'if the potato famine in Ireland were to continue five years longer, it would prove a greater blessing to the country than any that has ever been devised by parliamentary commissions from the Union'.[19] In 1846, Trevelyan shut down the relief scheme which had been instituted by Robert Peel in the preceding year: 'The only way to prevent the people from becoming habitually dependent on Government', he said, 'is to bring the operations to a close'. The fact that a new crop of potatoes failed, he added, 'only makes it more necessary'.[20]

---

[15] There is a vast amount of historical scholarship on the Irish Hunger which regrettably I do not have room to discuss at length in these pages. Woodham-Smith's *Great Hunger* is the most succinct, and most measured, account. See also Austin Bourke, *The Visitation of God: The Potato and the Great Irish Famine* (Dublin: Lilliput Press, 1993); Cormac Ó Gráda, *Black '47 and Beyond: The Great Irish Famine in History, Economy and Memory* (Princeton, NJ and London: Princeton University Press, 1999); Cormac Ó Gráda, *Famine: A Short History* (Princeton, NJ and London: Princeton University Press, 2009); Cormac Ó Gráda, *Ireland before and after the Famine: Explorations in Economic History* (Manchester: Manchester University press, 1993).

[16] Emile Zola, *Germinal*, trans. by Leonard Tancock (1885; London: Penguin, 1987), p. 373.

[17] Charles Vansittart, *A Sermon on Famine: The Expediency of a Public Fast, and the Duty of Personal Abstinence in the Present Time of Dearth* (London: James Burns, 1847), p. 9.

[18] Ibid., pp 30, 23.

[19] 'B.', letter to the editor, *The Times*, 1 September 1846, in Tóibín and Ferriter, *The Irish Famine*, pp. 179–80 (p. 180).

[20] Charles Trevelyan, letter to Randolph Routh, 17 July 1846. On 4 August Routh wrote to Trevelyan: 'You cannot answer the cry of want by a quotation from political economy' (quoted in Woodham-Smith, *Great Hunger*, pp. 89, 91).

Between approximately 1740 and 1850, such associations between famine and divine providence were challenged by corporeal accounts of starvation which, like Trollope's realism in *Castle Richmond*, showed that there was little about the phenomenon which could be seen as healthy or salubrious. To those acquainted with the realities of the famine, such as Cork magistrate N. M. Cummin, the spectacle of what actually happens to the body when people starve hinders any belief in God as having sent such horrors as a blessing. In a letter to the Duke of Wellington he noted that:

> The scenes that presented themselves [are] such as no tongue or pen can convey the slightest idea of. In the first [hovel], six famished and ghastly skeletons, to all appearance dead, were huddled in a corner on some filthy straw, their sole covering what seemed a ragged horse-cloth and their wretched legs hanging about, naked above the knees. I approached in horror, and found by a low moaning that they were alive, they were in fever—four children, a woman, and what had once been a man. It is impossible to go through the details, suffice to say, that in a few minutes I was surrounded by at least 200 such phantoms, such frightful spectres as no words can describe. By far the greatest number were delirious either from hunger or from fever. The demoniac yells are still ringing in my ears, and their horrible images are fixed upon my brain.[21]

Cummin's Dantean netherworld seems almost as fantastic as *The Times* correspondent's idea of the famine as a gift from heaven; his account of 'what had once been a man' implies that starvation converts the living into a revenant. The tone of his letter then shifts in order to focus on grisly materials:

> The same morning the police opened a house in the adjoining lands, which was observed shut for many days, and two frozen corpses were found lying upon the mud floor *half devoured by rats*. A mother, herself in fever, was seen the same day to drag out the corpse of her child, a girl about twelve perfectly naked; and leave it half covered with stones. In another house [...] the dispensary doctor found seven wretches lying, unable to move, under the same cloak—one had been dead for many hours but the others were unable to move either themselves or the corpse.[22]

The hellish scenes of the former passage have given way to the corpses, in this one, of the real world—frozen to mud floors, buried beneath stones, unable to move under the weight of their starving physicality. As Piero Camporesi has

---

[21] N. M. Cummin, letter to Duke of Wellington, December 1846, quoted in R. Arthur Arnold, *The History of the Cotton Famine* (London: Saunders et al., 1864), pp. 17–18.
[22] Cummin, letter to Wellington, p. 18. Italics in original.

observed, nothing reminds us of our own flesh and blood more than the fact that, to other living creatures such as the rats mentioned by Cummin, we are ourselves considered a source of food.[23] Overall, what appears to be figured in Cummin's response is a conflict between the interpretation of starvation as determined by, and therefore symbolic of, forces beyond human control, and an understanding of the same problem using a language tuned into both the materiality of bodies and environments and the tangibility of solutions. Vansittart's suggestion that he and his contemporaries should turn to God, observe a national day of fasting, and encourage 'a *rigid personal self-denying course of action in our households*', was not, at least, the 'donothingism' that Thomas Carlyle had identified as 'so ingrained in our Practice', and so wrongheaded, that it only added to the miseries of the poor.[24] Yet Vansittart's providentialism was, like the Dantean section of Cummin's letter, a remnant of the past; it was uncharacteristic of the more secular approaches to the problems of hunger that were developing at the time, though it did not, as Trevelyan's record shows, represent a way of thinking that lacked force in the nineteenth century. Indeed, Malthus's essay had invested the providential view with new energy by effectively repackaging convenient and conservative opinions as a 'scientific' principle which appealed to common sense.

Salutary Starvation

In 1800 Edmund Burke published *Thoughts and Details on Scarcity*, arguing that the ebb and flow of wealth was a natural law comparable to the will of God.[25] In a prescient justification of Trevelyan's opinions during the Irish crisis, Burke advised his readers 'manfully to resist [...] to supply the poor those necessaries which it has pleased the Divine Providence for a while to with-hold from them'.[26] It was an injunction that suited the spirit of a period in which Malthus's view of 'moral evil [as] absolutely necessary for the production of moral excellence' had been taken to heart.[27] There developed, according to Boyd Hilton, a popular view that God had created a natural system in which starvation was not a direct mani-festation of his wrath, but 'the "probable" and predictable consequence of specific

[23] Piero Camporesi, *Il Pane Salvaggio*, trans. as *Bread of Dreams: Food and Fantasy in Early Modern Europe* by David Gentilcore (1980; Chicago IL: University of Chicago Press, 1989), pp. 27–9.
[24] Vansittart, *Sermon on Famine*, p. 14. Italics in original; Thomas Carlyle, *Chartism* (London: James Fraser, 1840), p. 64.
[25] Tim Fulford, 'Apocalyptic Economics and Prophetic Politics: Radical and Romantic Responses to Malthus and Burke', *Studies in Romanticism*, 40:3 (2001), pp. 345–68 (p. 352).
[26] Edmund Burke, *Thoughts and Details on Scarcity* (1800), quoted in Fulford, 'Apocalyptic Economics', p. 19.
[27] T. R. Malthus, *An Essay on the Principle of Population [1798 edition]*, ed. by Geoffrey Gilbert (1798; London: Penguin, 2008), p. 151. See D. L. LeMahieu, 'Malthus and the Theology of Scarcity', *Journal of the History of Ideas*, 40:3 (1979), pp. 467–74.

wrong behaviour' which had violated the laws of his well-designed, self-sustaining system.[28] D. L. LeMahieu illustrates that Malthus went to some lengths to 'reconcile the chilling implications of his population theory with the goodness and benevolence of God'.[29] He (Malthus) argued, for example, that:

> Every express command given to man by his Creator is given in subordination to those great and uniform laws of nature which he ha[s] previously established; [...] it becomes our positive duty as reasonable creatures, and with a view of executing the commands of our Creator, to inquire into the laws which he has established for the multiplication of the species.[30]

Those selected by nature to pay the extreme price 'should be left [to] the punishment of severe want'; 'he should be taught to know that the laws of nature, which are the laws of God [have] doomed him and his family to starve for disobeying their repeated admonitions'.[31]

In his 1816 refutation of Malthus's theory, James Grahame accused the former of perceiving 'famine, disease, and war, as *benevolent remedies* by which nature has enabled human beings to correct the disorders that would arise from that redundance of population which the unrestrained operation of her laws would create'.[32] In the 1817 edition of his *Essay*, Malthus rejected the claim as absurd and reminded his readers that he had always advocated the use of preventative checks as a means of avoiding the more devastating, positive checks of war, pestilence, and famine.[33] This was certainly the lesson that Harriet Martineau took from his treatise, as is made apparent in her highly popular *Illustrations of Political Economy* (1832). Like *Castle Richmond*, Martineau's collection of short stories portrayed the evils of hunger in great detail:

> Ye little know what it is to lie down at night cold and aching, and to toss about unable to sleep, when sleep seems the one thing that would give ye ease, since ye cannot have food. Ye little think what sleep is when it comes,—how horrible fancies are ever rising up to steal away the sweetness of rest—how all that ye see and all that ye touch turns to food, and turns back again before ye can get it into your mouth; or, worse still, to fancy ye are driven by some evil power to strangle

---

[28] Boyd Hilton, *The Age of Atonement: The Influence of Evangelicalism on Social and Economic Thought 1785–1865* (Oxford: Oxford University Press, 1988), p. 15.

[29] LeMahieu, 'Malthus and the Theology of Scarcity', p. 467.

[30] T. R. Malthus, *An Essay on the Principle of Population [1806 edition]*, ed. by Patricia James, 2 vols (1806; Cambridge: Cambridge University Press, 1989), vol. 2, p. 205.

[31] T. R. Malthus, *Essay* [1803 edition], James (ed.), vol. 2, p. 140.

[32] James Grahame, *An Inquiry into the Principle of Population* (1816), cited in *Population: Contemporary Responses to Thomas Malthus*, ed. by Andrew Pyle (Bristol: Thoemmes Press, 1994), p. 224. Italics in original.

[33] See Pyle (ed.), *Population*, pp. 224–45.

and devour whatever is most precious to you. Ye little think what it is to wake with a parched mouth and hands clenched, so that they are like an infant's all the day after, and the limbs trembling and the sight dim, as if fifty years had come over ye in a night.[34]

Contrary to *Castle Richmond*, however, there is not a similar level of physical detail to that we see in writings such as Cummin's, where frozen bodies get half-devoured by rats. Despite references to material symptoms, in fact, we see in Martineau a preoccupation with 'horrible fancies', strange desires, and the inability to do what ought to come naturally (sleep, for instance). Martineau's perception of hunger actually has more in common with that other Malthusian, Ebeneezer Scrooge's concept of dyspepsia.[35] Jacob Marley's ghost, he says, 'may be an undigested bit of beef, a blot of mustard, a crumb of cheese, a fragment of an underdone potato'. Fancying himself an empiricist, Scrooge adds: 'You see this toothpick? [...] I have but to swallow this, and be for the rest of my days persecuted by a legion of goblins, all of my creation.'[36] Like Martineau, he links the question of what goes on in the stomach with the representation of what goes on, more abstractly, in the mind. The reason for this, I argue, is that a more material or physiological focus, like Trollope's and Cummin's, would belie the notion that, in overpopulated nations, starvation is salutary. Such a notion relied, as we saw in the thinking of Trevelyan, upon the ignoring of tangible evidences and the prioritizing of abstract, often unsupported theory. 'Natural laws', insisted Martineau, 'regulate the production of life [...] The imprudent must see their children pine in hunger, or waste under disease till they are ready to be carried off by the first attack of illness.'[37] Although her focus might seem to be physical in nature, it is worth remembering Martineau's conception of 'waste' here so that we might compare it to the physiological understandings of the same subject later. Similarly, we will also need to return to Martineau's euphemistic idiom 'carried off' when we turn to the more determinist arguments of Herbert Spencer.

In the meantime, we shall follow up on how Martineau's Malthusian text reveals that the 1798 *Essay* suggested that God's systems of natural balance were, in Malthus's own words, 'a blessing' and 'a gift'. Some 'evil[s] in the world', he

[34] Harriet Martineau, *Illustrations of Political Economy: Selected Tales*, ed. by Deborah Anna Logan (1832; Ontario: Broadview Press, 2004), p. 100.

[35] For an excellent overview of dyspepsia in the literature and medicine of the nineteenth century, see Emilie Taylor-Brown, 'Being "Hangry": Gastrointestinal Health and Emotional Well-Being in the Long Nineteenth Century', in *Gut Feeling and Digestive Health in Nineteenth-Century Literature, History and Culture*, ed. by Manon Mathias and Alison M. Moore (Cham, Switzerland: Palgrave Macmillan, 2018), pp. 109–32.

[36] Charles Dickens, *A Christmas Carol* (1844), in *Christmas Books*, ed. by Ruth Glancy (Oxford: Oxford University Press, 1988), pp. 1–90 (p. 19).

[37] Martineau, *Illustrations*, pp. 84–5.

added, were 'absolutely necessary'.[38] In a system wonderfully balanced by divine forces, how could any part be out of place or, worse still, evil? 'Nothing', Malthus wrote,

> can appear more *consonant to our reason*, that those beings which come out of the creative process of the world in lovely and beautiful forms, should be crowned with immortality; while those which come out mis-shapen, those whose minds are not suited to a purer and happier state of existence, should perish, and be condemned to mix again with their original clay.[39]

Nothing can be more consonant to our reason—or, in other words, nothing could be more rational or natural than a process which rewards the prudent and punishes the reckless. In a later edition of the *Essay*, in which Malthus reinforced his claim that the old Poor Laws should be abolished, he argued that the poverty-stricken should have no '*right* to support'. Instead, it was only correct that they should feel the hardships that had been brought on by their own behaviours:

> This poverty ha[s] arisen entirely from their own ignorance of imprudence; and it would be perfectly clear, from the manner in which it had come upon them, that if their plea were admitted and they were not suffered to feel the particular evils resulting from their conduct, the whole society would shortly be involved in the same degree of wretchedness.[40]

This time he carefully avoided words like 'should' in order to counter the claim that he had been preaching a fire-and-brimstone sort of gospel. William Hazlitt suggested, for instance, that Malthus's 'name hangs suspended over [the] heads [of the poor], *in terrorem*, like some baleful meteor'.[41] Although suggestions that he 'deployed his "positive checks" with an almost apocalyptic venom'[42] are clearly exaggerated, the *Essay on Population* 'echoed the language of divine mandate'[43] by suggesting that it was natural, and within the fine balance set by God, that starvation occurs. As Mary Poovey explains, the 'belief [was] that God is lawful' and 'nature is lawful too. [...] By this interpretation, the apparent evil of the principle of population actually "produced a great overbalance of good," because the

---

[38] Malthus, *Essay* [1798], p. 157.   [39] Ibid., p. 156. Italics added.

[40] Malthus, *Essay* [1806], p. 212. Italics in original.

[41] William Hazlitt, *A Reply to the Essay on Population by the Rev. T. R. Malthus*, in *The Complete Works of William Hazlitt*, ed. by P. P. Howe, 21 vols (1807; London and Toronto: J. M. Dent, 1830), vol. 1, pp. 177–364 (p. 181).

[42] Arnold, *Famine*, pp. 37–8. See also Fulford, 'Apocalyptic Economics'.

[43] Alison Bashford and Joyce E. Chaplin, 'Malthus and the New World', in Robert J. Mayhew (ed.), *New Perspectives on Malthus* (Cambridge: Cambridge University Press, 2016), pp. 105–27 (p. 112).

"strong excitements" occasioned by seeing this principle at work create both labour and self-control'.[44]

That ideas on the providential law of starvation continued to exert considerable influence in the nineteenth century is illustrated by the interpretations of the sufferings of the Irish people as consummate with the lessons of nature. In 'A Theory of Population' (1852), an article written for the *Westminster Review*, Herbert Spencer suggested that the crisis in Ireland was an illustration of the universal law of improvement:

By daily-accumulating experience [one] becomes impressed with the inherent tendency of things towards good—sees going on universally a patient self-rectification. [One] finds that the *vis medicatrix naturæ*—or rather the process which we describe by that expression—is not limited to the cure of wounds and diseases, but pervades creation. From the lowly fungus which, under varying circumstances, assumes varying forms of organization, up to the tree that grows obliquely, if it cannot otherwise get to the light—from the highest human faculty which increases or dwindles according to the demands made on it, down to the polype that changes its skin into stomach and its stomach into skin when turned inside out—[one] everywhere sees at work an essential beneficence.[45]

This law of essential beneficence was a presumption maintained, as Jessica Straley notes, throughout Spencer's career: 'progress, whether biological, psychological, or sociological takes the same direction from simplicity to complexity'.[46] Writing in the wake of the Irish Hunger, Spencer saw Ireland as confirmation of his theory that those laws which applied to the adaptive techniques of fungi and polyps also pertained to human populations:

The effect of pressure of population, in increasing the ability to maintain life, and decreasing the ability to multiply, is not a uniform effect, but an average one. In this case, as in all others, Nature secures each step in advance by a succession of trials, which are perpetually repeated, and cannot fail to be repeated, until success is achieved. All mankind in turn subject themselves more or less to the discipline described; they either may or may not advance under it; but, in the nature of things, only those who *do* advance under it eventually survive. For, necessarily, families and races whom this increasing difficulty of getting a

---

[44] Mary Poovey, *A History of the Modern Fact: Problems of Knowledge in the Sciences of Wealth and Society* (Chicago, IL and London: Chicago University Press, 1998), p. 288.

[45] [Herbert Spencer], 'A Theory of Population, deduced from the General Law of Animal Fertility', *Westminster Review*, 57 (1852), pp. 468–501 (p. 469).

[46] Jessica Straley, 'Of Beasts and Boys: Kingsley, Spencer, and the Theory of Recapitulation', *Victorian Studies*, 49:4 (1997), pp. 583–609 (p. 590).

living which excess of fertility entails, does not stimulate to improvements in production—that is, to greater mental activity—are on the high toad to extinction; and must ultimately be supplanted by those whom the pressure does so stimu-late. This truth we have recently seen exemplified in Ireland. And here, indeed, without further illustration, it will be seen that the premature death, under all its forms, and from all its causes, cannot fail to work in the same direction. For as those prematurely carried off must, in the average of cases, be those in whom the power of self-preservation is the least, it unavoidably follows, that those left behind to continue the race must be those in whom the power of self-preservation is the greatest—must be the select of their generation. So that, whether the dan-gers to existence be of the kind produced by excess of fertility, or of any other kind, it is clear, that by the ceaseless exercise of their faculties needed to con-tend with them, and by the death of all men who fail to contend with them successfully, there is ensured a constant progress towards a higher degree of skill, intelligence, and self-regulation—a better co-ordination of actions—a more complete life.[47]

Philip Abrams wrote about Spencer that 'he had turned the Invisible Hand into an Invisible Fist'. The philosopher's social theory drew upon the work of Malthus in order to say, about the socially dependent, that 'the whole effort of nature is to get rid of such, to clear the world of them, and make room for better [...] If they are not sufficiently complete to live, they die, and it is best they should die.'[48] In addition to highlighting the links between Spencer's idea that the Irish Hunger confirmed how 'nature's violence had always been [...] a powerful force in the species' education',[49] the long passage I quoted above offers an example of the kind of language that developed around starvation, and the kinds of value-laded judgements implicit in such writing. Notice, for example, how positive Spencer is in describing the effects of nature's laws: this is how 'success in achieved'; it is an 'advance', 'a progress towards a higher degree', a 'better coordination', and a 'more complete life'. Famine, in this context, is a 'trial' through which Nature secures advance. Indeed, the use of that one word 'trial' exemplifies how Spencer's argu-ment is also reliant on the same euphemisms we saw in Martineau's *Illustrations of Political Economy*: those who are not 'the select of their generation', for whom 'self-preservation is not the greatest' concern, will find themselves simply 'carried off'. What such sanitized references to starvation allowed commentators such as Martineau and Spencer (following Malthus) to do was transfer the onus of responsibility for hunger onto the individuals themselves; these were the people

---

[47] Spencer, 'Theory of Population', pp. 499–500.
[48] Herbert Spencer, *The Study of Sociology* (1873), quoted in Philip Abrams, *The Origins of British Sociology: 1834–1914* (Chicago and London: Chicago University Press, 1968), pp. 76, 74.
[49] Straley, 'Beasts and Boys', p. 591.

who had not shown themselves to be 'select of their generation' and had unwittingly put themselves forward, to avoid euphemisms, to die.

Material Starvation

As I noted in the Introduction to this work, modern scholars have tended to identify Malthusianism as a result of the empiricist tradition which, according to Foucault's *The Order of Things* (1966), provided certain underlying epistemological assumptions that determined what was acceptable for all scientific discourses. In such a framework, biological science may be mentioned in the same breath as political economy. Catherine Gallagher argues, for instance, that Malthus 'linked political economy to the life science of the early nineteenth century by concentrating on Man in nature, and on natural, corporeal Man'; for him, 'the blooming body' was 'about to divide into two feebler bodies that are always on the verge of becoming four starving bodies'.[50] Gallagher notes also that, for Malthus, 'concrete bodies, and not abstract units of labour, are the measure of value'.[51] Malthus himself perceived the moral elements of his theory to 'awaken inert, chaotic matter, into spirit; to sublimate the dust of the earth into soul; to elicit an ethereal spark from the clod of clay'.[52] His perception of the human body worked with ideas drawn from the vitalist tradition of eighteenth-century medicine, which believed that the spiritual and moral business of the soul was housed, or weighed down, by the workings of the 'mortal tabernacle'.[53] Contrary to many vitalists, nonetheless, Malthus's *Essay on Population* has very little to say about actual matter such as blood, bones, tissues, and waste. This omission might not seem like much of an oversight given that Malthus was a preacher, not a physician; yet, it is important that we distinguish Malthus's broad accounts of the workings of reproduction, disease, and famine (which were largely abstract in nature) from the developing 'life sciences' of the eighteenth century, especially medicine and physiology, which created a completely different and conflicting view of hunger using an approach to bodies that was committed to challenging the abstractness of traditional interpretations.

[50] Catherine Gallagher, *The Body Economic: Life, Death, and Sensation in Political Economy and the Victorian Novel* (Princeton, NJ: Princeton University Press, 2006), pp. 4, 39. See also Maureen N. McLane, *Romanticism and the Human Sciences* (Cambridge: Cambridge University Press, 2000), p. 112.

[51] Catherine Gallagher, 'The Body Versus the Social Body in the Works of Thomas Malthus and Henry Mayhew', in *The Making of the Modern Body: Sexuality and Society in the Nineteenth Century*, ed. by Catherine Gallagher and Thomas Laqueur (Berkeley, Los Angeles, CA. and London: University of California Press, 1987), pp. 83–106 (p. 96).

[52] Malthus, *Essay* [1798], p. 143.

[53] George Cheyne, *The English Malady: or, a Treatise of Nervous Diseases of all Kinds* (London: G. Strahan, 1733), p. 362. On the influence of medical vitalism on political economy, especially Adam Smith, see Catherine Packham, *Eighteenth-Century Vitalism: Bodies, Culture, Politics* (Basingstoke: Palgrave Macmillan, 2012), pp. 83–108.

In 1733, for instance, George Cheyne, surgeon and fellow of the Royal College of Physicians at Edinburgh, published the work for which he is best remembered—*The English Malady*. Addressing the Englishman's reputed proneness to nervous disorder, the treatise drew upon the author's own experiences, as well as the research he had undertaken for the earlier *Essay on Health and Long Life* (1725), to suggest that 'the whole life of Physick, and the Wisdom of animal Life, consists in adjusting Diet and Medicines to the Habit and the Distempers'.[54] Cheyne's experiences of growing 'excessively fat, short-breath'd, *Lethargic* and *Listless*', combined with his '*Head-ach, Giddiness, Watchings, Lowness*, and *Melancholy*', were linked to his love of 'Dineing and Supping in *Taverns*, and in the Houses of my Acquaintances of *Taste* and *Delicacy*'.[55] A vegetable and milk diet had, he says, nursed him back to health, but he was wary of interfering with the diets of his patients unless they could be linked directly to the cause of sickness, or when, in cases of chronic illness, other measures had failed.[56] If excessive consumption could thus be linked to nervous maladies, it followed that the sick patient was likely to be the author of his or her own wretchedness: 'it is the miserable *Man* himself that creates his Miseries and begets his Torture'.[57] Cheyne has 'thus [been] thought of as recasting traditional Christian bodily anxieties into physiological and medical mediums'.[58]

Anita Guerrini has demonstrated, moreover, that 'Cheyne criticised theories that did not conform to the true and certain laws of physics and geometry [...] He emphasized the substructure of matter as the key to physiology',[59] which is borne out in *The English Malady*:

The Human Body is a Machin of an infinite Number and Variety of different Channels and Pipes, filled with various and different Liquors and Fluids, perpetually running, glideing, or creeping forward, or returning backward, in a constant *Circle*, and fending out little Branches and Outlets, to moisten, nourish, and repair the Experiences of Living. [...] The Intelligent Principle, or *Soul*, resides somewhere in the Brain, where all the Nerves, or Instruments of Sensation terminate, like a *Musician* in a finely fram'd and well-tun'd Organ-Case; [...] these Nerves are like *Keys*, which, being struck on or touch'd, convey the Sound and Harmony to this sentient Principle, or *Musician*.[60]

This understanding of the body as a complex machine, with an infinite number and variety of different channels, suggests that illness has more to do with structural

---

[54] Cheyne, *English Malady*, p. viii.   [55] Ibid., pp. 326, 329.
[56] Ibid., pp. vi–vii.   [57] Ibid., p. 29.
[58] Roy Porter, *Flesh in the Age of Reason: How the Enlightenment Transformed the Way We See Our Bodies and Souls* (2003; London: Penguin, 2004), p. 238.
[59] Anita Guerrini, *Obesity and Depression in the Enlightenment: The Life and Times of George Cheyne* (Norman, OK: University of Oklahoma Press, 2000), p. 64.
[60] Cheyne, *English Malady*, pp. 4–5.

imbalance, or upset, than divine or natural providence. In his preface, Cheyne dismissed the benighted idea of nervous distemper as '*Witchcraft, Enchantment, Sorcery* and *Possession*'—calling it a 'constant Resource of Ignorance'.[61] Also disdained, more importantly, were the dogmatists—the '*Unthinking*' and the '*Philomaths*, who, without Experiment or Observation, want only to shew away' new ideas and 'wound in the Dark' with their own dated opinions.[62] Despite such efforts, 'the *Laws of Nature*, and the immutable *Relations of Things*, are too stubborn to bend to such *Gentlemen*'.[63] In the term 'immutable relations of things', it may appear that the key word is 'relations', but it was just as possible that 'things' was intended for emphasis; tangible matter is what Cheyne sees as challenging the abstractions of philomaths (*philomath* is intended to be derogatory here, implying the love of knowledge for knowledge's sake, rather than the love of truth). Cheyne had made his own deductions from 'the best and soundest *Natural Philosophy*; and [...] by the plainest Reasoning, drawn from these *Causes* and this *Philosophy*, a *Method of Cure* and a *Course of Medicine* specifically obviating these Causes, confirmed by long Experience and repeated Observations'.[64] Life sciences required what Lorraine Daston and Peter Galison have identified as 'sharp and sustained observation [...] The eyes of both body and mind [must converge] to discover a reality otherwise hidden to each alone.'[65] 'Where the *Philosopher* ends', Cheyne says, 'the *Physician* begins':

> If I could choose, I should name only those for my *Judges*, who to a competent Knowledge of the *Laws of Nature* and *Mechanism*, have join'd an Acquaintance with the best *Natural Philosophy*, the latest *Discoveries in* Natural History, *and the Powers* and *Virtues* of *Medicines*, and have been long conversant in the Practice of *Physick* and Attendance on the Sick and Diseased.[66]

It is out of Cheyne's belief in the material basis of pathology, and his insistence on the empiricist mode, that his theories of 'diætetick management', waste, and 'animal oeconomy' develop:

> Both the *End* and *Rule*, the *Design* and *Measure* of Eating and Drinking, could not be no other but the supply of the Waste of *Action* and *Living*. The *Friction* and *Collision* that necessarily follows upon the *Interpretability* of Matter, the Communication of Motion, and the Impressions of the Bodies that Surround us, must necessarily rub off, and wear out some Parts from our bodily Machin. The necessary *Collisions* that are made in our Juices, in breaking and subtilizing their

---

[61] Ibid., p. x.   [62] Ibid., pp. xii–xiii.
[63] Ibid., p. xii.   [64] Ibid., p. x.
[65] Lorraine Daston and Peter Galison, *Objectivity* (New York, NY: Zone Books, 2007), p. 58.
[66] Cheyne, *English Malady*, p. xiv.

Parts, to render them fit for the Animal *Functions*: the various *Secretions* of what is not proper to be retained, or what is necessary for the Preservation of the Individual, make a continual *Waste* of our Substance. To supply all which, it was absolutely necessary, that a due and equal Proportion or Proper Nourishment should be design'd us. There is also established by the Rules of the *Animal OEconomy*, a Balance between the Forces of Elasticity of the Solids, or the moving Organs and Channels, and the Resistance of the Fluids mov'd in them [...] And whenever any of these *Rules* are long and notable transgress'd [...] the Individual must suffer Diseases, Pains, and Miseries.[67]

It stood to reason that, as water gradually erodes a stone, the flow and ebb of corporeal fluid wears away the solid forms of the body. Food, according to Cheyne, is what repairs the waste.

Half a century later, the celebrity surgeon and physiologist John Hunter defined 'pathology, or the physiology of disease' as a '*perversion of the natural actions of the animal œconomy*'.[68] In his *General Anatomy Applied to Physiology and Medicine* (1800), Xavier Bichat stressed the need for

analyzing with precision the properties of living bodies, in showing that every physiological phenomenon is ultimately referable to these properties considered in their natural state; that every pathological phenomenon derives from them augmentation, diminution, or alteration; that every therapeutic phenomenon has for its principle the restoration of the part to the natural type, from which it has been changed.[69]

In the developing research climate of eighteenth- and early nineteenth-century medicine, matter was the foundation of life, and pathological states represented a *deviation* from the processes that were synonymous with health. In considering the '*Interpretability* of Matter', especially the balance between food and waste, physiologists broke ranks with the traditional assumption that pathology, especially when connected to diet, was a sort of judgement against the individual. Theories on the corporeality of waste, in particular, allowed an alternative narrative to that which would be updated, by political economists, to suit the capitalist energies of the Victorian age. The diseases and famines that providentialist theory

---

[67] Cheyne, *English Malady*, pp. 29–30. Cheyne was not the first to use the term *animal oeconomy*. James Keill suggested that the 'Animal Body is a pure Machine, and all its Actions from which Life and Health do flow are the necessary Consequences of its Oeconomy': *Essays on Several Parts of the Animal Oeconomy* (London: George Strahan, 1717), p. vi.

[68] John Hunter, *Lectures on the Principles of Surgery* (1786–87; Philadelphia: Haswell et al, 1839), p. 10. Italics in original.

[69] Xavier Bichat, *Anatomie Générale: appliquée à la Physiologie et à la Médecine*, trans. as *General Anatomy, applied to Physiology and Medicine* by George Hayward (Boston, MS: Richardson and Lord, 1822), pp. vii–viii.

perceived to be *enactments* of natural law were repositioned as *violations* of the same; they came to be seen, as Stephen J. Cross notes in his research on John Hunter, as 'a malfunction, [...] a pathological modification of the normal (healthy) actions of organs and parts'.[70]

This is a conclusion that could only be reached after meticulous research into the anatomy of digestion and hunger, and the discussion of certain methodological points which the new science of physiology posed. Lazzaro Spallanzani, a Catholic priest and hobbying physiologist, came to investigate the subject of digestion 'with such thoroughness', according to one late-Victorian historian, 'as practically to begin a new epoch in the history of the subject'.[71] His *Dissertations Relative to the Natural History of Animals and Vegetables* (1780) reported a number of experiments he had conducted on the gastric juices of both himself and a range of animals. He had been inspired by the French physicist René Antoine Ferchault de Réaumur to induce different creatures to swallow a small sponge attached to piece of string.[72] Thus obtaining a sample of their digestive juices, Spallanzani introduced the fluids to various substances and watched the gastric process in action.[73] While we may 'draw very plausible inferences concerning human digestion from observations of this numerous class', Spallanzani noted, 'especially from birds of prey, the cat and dog, which resemble us so much in the structure of the stomach', what was really required was a series of accurate experiments on humans:

> In the writings of the ancient and modern physicians no topic is more frequently discussed, yet there is little else besides supposition: direct experiments made upon Man are entirely wanting, and their researches are illuminated only by the twilight of conjecture, and supported by precarious hypotheses. If therefore it was necessary on other occasions to have recourse to experiment, on the present it was absolutely indispensable. Upon reflection it appeared that the principal experiments were reducible to two heads, viz. to procure human gastric fluid, in order to examine it in the manner that of animals have been examined; and to swallow tubes full of various vegetable and animal substances, in order to see what changes they undergo in the stomach.[74]

In considering human digestion as a subject in physiological research, Spallanzani leads not with a sermon about excess and moderation, as one might expect, but

[70] Stephen J. Cross, 'John Hunter, the Animal Oeconomy and Late Eighteenth-Century Physiological Discourse', *Studies in History of Biology*, 5 (1981), pp. 1–110 (p. 31).

[71] John G. M'Kendrick, *Spallanzani: A Physiologist of the Last Century* (Glasgow: James Maclehose, 1891), p. 16.

[72] See René Antoine Ferchault de Réaumur, *Observations sur la Digestion des Oiseaux* (Paris: De L'Imprimerte Royale, 1752).

[73] Lazzaro Spallanzani, *Dissertations Relative to the Natural History of Animals and Vegetables*, trans. by anon., 2 vols (1780; London: John Murray, 1784), vol. 1, pp. 198–217.

[74] Ibid., p. 217.

with an emphasis on the importance of experiment over 'precarious hypotheses'. Indeed, material research not only offered new evidence on the nature of digestion, it challenged the tendency, in the 'writings of the ancient and modern physicians' to speculate—to make suppositions based on moralistic bias. Spallanzani conducted a number of experiments on himself. To get samples of his own gastric fluid, he fasted then vomited. He developed 'such a repugnance for the operation, that [he] was absolutely incapable of repeating it, notwithstanding [his] earnest desire of procuring more gastric liquor'.[75] Spallanzani had better success with swallowing various articles, and he reached the point where he was able to swallow a number of perforated wooden tubes at a time (he was afraid that tin tubes would poison him). What he claimed he could prove through such procedures was that digestion was not a kind of putrefaction, or fermentation, as had been assumed since the early-seventeenth-century research of Johan Baptista Van Helmont;[76] nor was food broken down by muscular action as it was in some species of bird (the mechanical theory popularized by Giovanni Alphonso Borelli).[77] Instead, it was a process where gastric fluid interacted with the chemicals in food and allowed solid matter to dissolve gradually.

Parallel with these material discoveries was Spallanzani's equally vital work on the use of controlled observation, experimentation, and the quest for objectivity in biological research. John Senebier observed in 1805:

When we have read nature with precision, we must interpret her with fidelity; analyse, by means of the understanding, the phenomena anatomised by the senses; attend to the species, while studying the individual; and anticipate general propositions, in considering insulated facts. In this case, prudence and circumspection are not always securities against error, did not an ardent love of truth assay observations with their consequences, and reduce to scoria everything that is not the truth.

Such was Spallanzani in all his researches.[78]

---

[75] Ibid., p. 229.

[76] Gillespie noted in 1898 that, for Van Helmont, 'the whole body was under the influence of an "archeus Influus", or vital principle, which resided in the stomach [...] During the process of digestion in the stomach the local "archeus" generate[s] a ferment whereby an acid [is] produced to dissolve the food. This "fermentum acidum" caused the necessary changes to take place in the food'; A. Lockheart Gillespie, The Natural History of Digestion (London: Walter Scott, 1898), pp. 11–12. See also Michael Foster, *Lectures on the History of Physiology* (1901; New York, NY: Dover, 1970), pp. 136–9; Karl E. Rothschuh, *Gerschichte der Physiologie*, trans. as *History of Physiology* by Guenter B. Risse (1953; New York: Robert E. Krieger, 1973), pp. 59–60; Porter, *Flesh in the Age of Reason*, pp. 53–4.

[77] The argument, according to Gillespie, was that, 'as the pressure capable of being excited by the human thumb is very considerable, and as the superficies of the stomach wall is much more extensive, so the pressure which can be exercised by the coats of that organ is correspondingly greater' (*Natural History of Digestion*, p. 12). See also Foster, *History of Physiology*, p. 166.

[78] John Senebier, introduction to Lazzaro Spallanzani, *Memoirs on Respiration*, ed. by Senebier (London: Thomas Cox, 1805), pp. 19–21.

The 'precision', 'fidelity', and 'truth' of Spallanzani's research were, according to Senebier, built upon a cognitive journey from specific examples to general principles. Contrary, for example, to those interpretations of the Irish Hunger which would process the meaning of individual cases deductively using general rules based on theories of political economy, Spallanzani mastered a process of reasoning inductively, fathoming nature's laws through the study of 'phenomena anatomised by the senses'. His experiments thus tethered the idea of scientific truth or fidelity to both material research and the rejection of 'precarious hypotheses'.

Significantly, Spallanzani came into conflict with John Hunter when the Scottish surgeon criticized him for taking the inductive method too far. Spallanzani's experiments were 'in themselves conclusive', Hunter noted, but he complained that,

> like all experiment-makers, [...] he multiplies them most unnecessarily. [...] I think we may set it down as an axiom, that experiments should not be often repeated which tend merely to establish a principle already known and admitted; but that the next step should be, the application of that principle to useful purposes. If Spallanzani had employed half his time in this way, and had considered digestion under all the various states of the body and stomach, with all the varieties of food, both natural and artificial, he had employed his time much better than in making experiments without end.[79]

Hunter's criticism reveals a problem with the multiplication of experiment only in the sense that it delayed the practical application of research. Spallanzani's response, in *Una Lettera Apologetica in Risposta alle Osservazioni del Signor Giovanni Hunter* (1788), was to pick holes in the scientific objectivity of Hunter's own methods, implying, predictably, that his English counterpart would have done better to spend more time researching his subject before testing its impact in the hospital wards. This was a difference of opinion fuelled by the fact that Hunter, unlike Spallanzani, saw and treated sick patients. Richard Owen, Professor of Anatomy and Physiology, and conservator of Hunter's collection at the Royal College of Surgeons, insisted that Hunter was a 'philosopher conscious of the extent of his powers, and of the kind of knowledge which the right exercise of those powers was adapted to acquire'. Being conscious of the need to apply research to the treatment of patients allowed Hunter to 'explain many of the phaenomena of digestion more satisfactorily than had been done by his predecessors Spallanzani and Reaumur'.[80]

---

[79] John Hunter, *Observations on Certain Parts of the Animal Œconomy* (1786; Philadephia: Haswell et al., 1840), p. 117.

[80] Richard Owen, Preface to Hunter, *Animal Œconomy*, p. 17. L. S. Jacyna has discussed the various acknowledgements of Hunter's excellence by nineteenth-century medical figures in 'Images of John Hunter in the Nineteenth Century', *History of Science*, 21 (1983), pp. 85–108.

In spite of their differences, Spallanzani and Hunter were part of the same drive to develop an accurate, materialist understanding of the digestive process. In his important *Lectures on the Principles of Surgery* (1786–7) Hunter expanded on the kind of inductive, atomizing reasoning employed by Spallanzani:

> Animals and vegetables have a power of action within themselves, are capable of increasing their own magnitude, and possess the power, as it were, of working themselves into form and a higher state of existence. This power of action and capability requires a supply of materials, as well as the increase as for the waste arising from action.[81]

There are two major ideas here. The first is that life is self-iterating: living matter is characterized by its 'power of self-formation'; it is, as François Duchesneau elegantly puts it, 'a kind of *Bildungstrieb* [...] architectonic in character'.[82] The second point, which is more important for the direction of my discussion, is that life is self-*reiterating*: living matter is distinguished by its self-determining ability to resist 'waste arising from action'. Bichat hypothesized a few years later that the materials of the body were constantly dying and regenerating; his famous definition of life was that it was 'the sum total of functions which resist death'.[83] In fact, Bichat, like Hunter, converted an old theory of 'the physical degradation of the starving', the 'bestial metamorphosis',[84] into an experimentally verifiable phenomenon. But there was a crucial difference between Bichat's and Hunter's work. The latter's definition of life as 'the principle of preservation in the animal preserving it from putrefaction' identified waste as a pathological process kept at bay by nourishment.[85] In Bichat's thought, waste and regeneration were normal and ongoing. John Abernethy, surgeon and Hunter devotee, claimed in 1814 that Hunter saw life not as an energy that was constantly extinguishing and reigniting, as Bichat did, but as one that was perpetually resisting 'the chemical decomposition, to which dead animal and vegetable matter is so prone'. A living egg, for example, 'does not putrefy under circumstances that would rapidly cause that change in a dead one'.[86] Hunter had performed a number of experiments on

---

[81] Hunter, *Lectures*, pp. 13–14.

[82] François Duchesneau, 'Vitalism in Late Eighteenth-Century Physiology: The Cases of Barthez, Blumenbach and John Hunter', in *William Hunter and the Eighteenth-Century Medical World*, ed. by W. F. Bynum and Roy Porter (1985; Cambridge: Cambridge University Press, 2002), pp. 259–95 (p. 284).

[83] Xavier Bichat, *Reserches Physiologiques sur la Vie et la Mort* (1800), quoted in J. M. D. Olmsted, *François Magendie: Pioneer in Experimental Physiology and Scientific Medicine in XIX century France* (New York, NY: Schuman's, 1944), p. 25.

[84] Camporesi, *Bread of Dreams*, p. 33.   [85] Hunter, *Lectures*, p. 23.

[86] John Abernethy, *An Enquiry into the Probability and Rationality of Mr. Hunter's Theory of Life* (London: Longman et al., 1814), p. 17. Abernethy was an avid populariser of the idea that the stomach was the centre of animal life. See Ian Miller, *A Modern History of the Stomach: Gastric Illness, Medicine and British Society, 1800–1950* (2011; London: Routledge, 2015), pp. 14–16.

chicken eggs in 1757 in which he observed that 'whenever an egg was hatched, the yolk, which is not diminished in the term of incubation, remains sweet to the last [...] But if the egg did not hatch, I observed that it became putrid nearly in the same time that other dead animal matter does'.[87] Contrary to what had been written by mechanist natural philosophers,[88] action and movement were not the basis of the living principle; rather, nutrition leading to the living principle—the resistance of waste and death—constituted the real essence of life. According to Catherine Packham, for Hunter 'it was blood' which 'gave the body, in all its parts, the power of preservation, the susceptibility to impressions, and its ability to act and to react—all actions which collectively enabled it to resist disease, restore itself to health after injury and undertake other vital acts'.[89] And yet it was the process of digestion that allowed the blood to do its vital work: 'Digestion', Hunter noted, is 'the first step towards vivification'; the stomach is 'the converter of the food by hidden powers into part of ourselves'.[90] As one early biographer notes, the stomach is the organ 'Hunter considers to be the essential part of every animal'.[91] The work on digestion, added Owen, 'convey[ed] perhaps the best idea of the extent of Hunter's researches in Comparative Anatomy, and of the soundness of his reasonings in general physiology'.[92]

In 'Some Observations of Digestion', an article he appended to 'On the Stomach itself being digested after Death' (1772) and published in *Observations on Certain Parts of the Animal Œconomy* (1786),[93] Hunter discounted the major theories of human digestion that preceded his own. The mechanical theory, which had suggested that food is ground by the internal structure of the stomach, was incorrect because, like many animals, humans chew their food before it enters the stomach, thus removing any need for internal mechanical action. Van Helmont's popular theory was also unlikely to be true because fermentation 'is that natural succession of changes by which vegetable and animal matter is reduced to earth [and] therefore must be widely different from digestion which converts both animal and vegetable substances into chyle [a milky compound of gastric fluid and food matter]'.[94] The chemical theory, the one favoured by Spallanzani, had failed to

---

[87]   Hunter, *Lectures*, p. 22.

[88]   See Joseph Priestley, *Disquisitions Relating to Matter and Spirit* (London: J. Johnson, 1777), and Sharon Ruston, *Shelley and Vitality* (2005; Basingstoke: Palgrave Macmillan, 2012), pp. 27–8. Bichat's important claim was that 'sensibility and contractility [were the] properties universally characteristic of living things'. Olmsted, *François Magendie*, p. 29.

[89]   Packham, *Eighteenth-Century Vitalism*, p. 114.

[90]   Hunter, *Lectures*, pp. 27, 42. The same idea was mentioned in both Hippocrates and Aristotle. See Rothschuh, *History of Physiology*, pp. 6–7, 10.

[91]   Drewry Ottley, *The Life of John Hunter* in *The Works of John Hunter, F.R.S.*, ed. by James F. Palmer, 5 vols (London: Longman et al., 1835), vol. 1, p. 162.

[92]   Owen, Preface, p. 18.

[93]   'On the Stomach itself being digested after Death' was originally read to the Royal Society and published in their *Philosophical Transactions* (volume 62) in 1772.

[94]   Hunter, *Animal Œconomy*, pp. 135.

STARVATION SCIENCE AND POLITICAL ECONOMY 41

account for the generative force of digestion, in which new matter is produced: 'the digestive organ is evidently constructed in a different manner in different animals',[95] Hunter pointed out, but in humans, there occurs 'a species of generation [with] two substances making a third', namely chyle.[96] The fermentation and chemical theories of digestion could not explain how the digestive tract 'transformed', in the words of Robert Mitchell, 'food into a form (or forms) that could be engaged by the body'.[97] This last process was a *living* process, one in which the body resisted the *dead* courses of waste and chemical decomposition. As Cross explains:

> The first function of the stomach is to 'animalize' common matter; its second is to confer upon the resulting newly formed animal matter specific vital properties, a process Hunter calls 'vivification'. The blood—in fact the chyle prior to that—is thus considered to be alive; it is the result of the transformation of common matter into animal matter endowed with the inherent properties of life. [...] Only when deprived of the living principle are animal [...] parts susceptible again to the 'common' (chemical) processes of degradation.[98]

Unholy Starvation

Hunter's 'vivification' theory offered scientific validation for an idea that had been around at least as far back as Galen.[99] It would be identified in the 1810s as 'assimilation' by vitalist physician and chemist William Prout. Best known for his work on metabolism and for discovering hydrochloric acid in animal gastric juice, Prout believed, in harmony with Hunter, that:

> blood begins to be formed, or developed from the food, in all its parts from the first moment of its entrance into the duodemum, or even, perhaps, from the first moment of digestion, and that it gradually becomes more perfect as it passes through the different stages to which it is subjected, till its formation be completed in the sanguiferous tubes, when it represents an aqueous solution of the principal textures and other parts of the animal body to which it belongs.[100]

---

[95] Ibid., p. 113.   [96] Ibid., p. 135.

[97] Robert Mitchell, *Experimental Life: Vitalism in Romantic Science and Literature* Baltimore, MD: Johns Hopkins University Press, 2013), p. 112.

[98] Cross, 'John Hunter', p. 41.

[99] 'Nutrition, in Galen's view, was absolutely necessary in order to replace the living substance of the body which was continuously lost': Rothschuh, *History of Physiology*, p. 20.

[100] William Prout, 'Inquiry into the Origins and Properties of Blood', *Annals of Medical Surgery*, 1 (1816), 10–26 (p. 20); W. H. Brock, *From Prolyte to Proton: William Prout and the Nature of Matter* (Bristol and Boston, MA: Adam Hilger, 1985), p. 48.

As we shall see later in this chapter and in Chapter 4, respectively, it would take the interventions of Justus von Liebig and Edward Smith to link the rate of assimilation (or 'metamorphosis of tissues', as Liebig termed it) to the loss of vitality caused by physical activity. Karl Marx seized upon this very idea to suggest that workers were drained of vital energy by the long hours they served in the factory: 'Capital is dead labour', he said, 'that, vampire-like, only lives by sucking living labour, and lives the more, the more labour it sucks':

> Children of nine or ten are dragged from their squalid beds at two, three, or four o'clock in the morning and compelled to work for a bare subsistence until ten, eleven, or twelve at night, their limbs wearing away, their frames dwindling, their faces whitening, and their humanity absolutely sinking into a stone-like torpor, utterly horrible to contemplate. [...] Food is given to the labourer as to a mere means of production, as coal is supplied to the boiler, grease and oil to the machinery.[101]

Earlier in the century, the claim that digestion generated 'a supply of materials' to restore 'the waste arising from action' had implications for the way starvation was perceived both as a desire and, in providentialist terms, as a corrective. Although there would continue to be medical figures who fully subscribed to the providentialist approach to hunger,[102] the vivification or assimilation theory suggested that the *resistance* of waste (not its creation) was the basis of a natural, healthy economy. It demonstrated, to use Cheyne's statement of the obvious, that health was about 'growing continually healthier'[103] rather than growing, as the providentialists believed, in pestilent and famished numbers.

In 1822, the Leeds surgeon Charles Thackrah, best known for his later work on occupational health,[104] delivered a series of lectures on physiology to the Philosophical and Literary Society of his home town. Feeling that the information contained in his lectures on digestion was 'urgently required' by the world, he published them in 1824. In that volume, Thackrah outlined the process of starvation in great detail. It involves, he said, 'constipation of the bowels and [the opposite experience] tenesmus, swelling of the legs, extreme weakness of the muscles, a hollow and ghastly appearance of the face, dizziness, excessive inclination for

---

[101] Karl Marx, *Das Kapital*, trans. as *Capital*, ed. by David McLellan (1867; Oxford: Oxford University Press, 2008), pp. 149, 154, 163.

[102] Dublin surgeon D. J. Corrigan argued in an important pamphlet on famine and fever that nature created famines and epidemic fevers in order to control population numbers. It was possible, however, for medical experts to predict the arrival of such 'checks' and to alleviate their worst effects. He refused to accept that such 'checks' were a positive thing in the long run. *On Famine and Fever as Cause and Effect in Ireland* (Dublin: J. Fannin, 1846).

[103] Cheyne, *English Malady*, p. 26.

[104] See Charles Turner Thackrah, *The Effects of the Arts, Trades, and Professions and of the Civic States and Habits of Living, on Health and Longevity* (London: Longman et al., 1832).

sleep, debility of sense and intellect'.[105] He cited an 1818 case which had been outlined by the German physician Christoph Wilhelm Friedrich Hufeland, where a thirty-two-year-old merchant, depressed by 'severe reverses of fortune',[106] went into the woods near his home and committed suicide by fasting. In the man's pocket was found a journal in which he had kept a record of the symptoms he experienced over the fourteen days he went without food and water. On the third day he wrote: 'I yet live; but how have I been soaked in the night, and how cold it has been! O God! when will my sufferings terminate!!' Three days later: 'How hard is this, no one knows; and my last hour must soon arrive. Doubtless, during the heavy rain, a little water has got into my throat […yet] I have none even of this for six days, since I am no longer able to move from the place.' The last entry read:

> Finally, I here protest, before the all-wise God, that, notwithstanding all the misfortunes which I have suffered from my youth, I yet die very unwillingly; although necessity has imperiously driven me to it. Nevertheless I pray for it. Father, forgive him, for he knows not what he does! More can I not write, for faintness and spasms: and this will be the last.[107]

Hufeland's case study became famous among physiologists, not because of the spiritual raptures of the young man or the pathos of his sufferings, but for what it told them about the material process of starvation. Thackrah, for instance, drew out the information on the man's physiological experiences:

> It is hence evident that consciousness and the power of writing remained till the *fourteenth day* of abstinence.—The operation of famine was aggravated by mental distress, and still more by exposure to the weather. This indeed seems to have produced his most urgent sufferings. Subsequent to the common cravings and debility of hunger, his first physical distress seems to have been the sensation of cold; then cold and thirst; lastly, faintness and spasms. In this case, we find no symptoms of inflammation. A want of nervous energy, arising from the reduction in the quantity or quality of the blood, appears to have been the principal disease. The effort of swallowing, and the oppression of food on the exhausted stomach, completed the catastrophe.[108]

The interpretation of the merchant's 'principal disease' as a 'want of nervous energy, arising from the reduction in the quantity or quality of the blood' may seem fairly unsympathetic to his mental and spiritual sufferings, yet the merchant's own account of his distress was similarly focussed, interestingly, on the physicality of

[105] Charles Turner Thackrah, *Lectures on Digestion and Diet* (London: Longman et al., 1824), p. 39.
[106] Ibid., p. 41.   [107] Ibid., pp. 42–3.   [108] Ibid., p. 43. Italics in original.

his experience: the causes of anguish are cold, faintness, spasms, cravings, debility, and physical sensation. God remains 'all-wise', and any disorder is felt to be in the flesh rather than the spirit. Indeed, the case was ideally suited to Thackrah's seeming intention to speak about starvation in a way that stressed its materiality:

> In extreme abstinence, we learn that the whole alimentary canal is contracted, and the walls close on the empty abdomen; that the gastric and pancreatic juices, the mucus of the intestines, and even the serum of the peritoneum are partially absorbed. Nay, from the ulcerated state of the villous coat, it seems, that the Conservative Power of the constitution, distressed by the want of nourishment, urges the absorbents to prey upon the live intestine. The blood is said to be depraved.[109]

This last word, 'depraved', is very suggestive. Thackrah means it to denote a form of breaking down, or corruption, in the integrity of the blood, yet, combined with his general tone, 'depraved', when applied to material phenomena, suggests that hunger is an offensive and unnatural process: when we starve, our viscera cannibalize themselves—the gut becomes a place of warfare as the intestine is predated by the 'Conservative Power' of the constitution.

In contrast to instances, mainly in the past, where hunger was used as a mortification of the flesh and a spiritualizing link with God, starvation, in scientific works, was largely stripped of its ennobling qualities and made physical, filthy, and offensive. The key result of this reformulation was the disassociation of hunger with salubrity. In the same decade in which Thackrah was insisting upon the horrors of starvation, *Kirby's Wonderful and Eccentric Museum; or Magazine of Remarkable Characters* included an account of the 1816 story of Ann Martin.[110] Ann, it is reported, 'came from Lewes some time back, with an artillery soldier'. She had left him and, 'being destitute of money, and oppressed by fatigue, she, in a fit of despair, laid herself down to die'.[111] This was in the month of September. Eleven days later, having eaten nothing, she was found alive, but

> in such a situation as excited the most shuddering sensations of horror and disgust, mixed with surprise, that a human being could retain any portion of animation under such complicated sufferings of want and wretchedness. She was almost in a state of putrefaction, large maggots were feeding on every part of her frame. Exposed to the attacks of flies, her nostrils, and even her mouth, were infested by them; behind her ears, between her fingers, and between her toes,

---

[109] Ibid., p. 38.

[110] Charles Dickens owned a copy of the volume edition from 1820. John H. Stonehouse, *Catalogue of the Library of Charles Dickens from Gadshill* (London: Piccadilly Fountain Press, 1935), p. 68.

[111] Unsigned, 'Preservation of Ann Martin', *Kirby's Wonderful and Eccentric Museum; or Magazine of Remarkable Characters*, 6 vols (London: R. S. Kirby, 1820), vol. 6, pp. 143–4.

they were crawling in sickening quantities; and her clothes were literally rotten from long exposure to the varying and humid atmosphere.[112]

Thanks to the ministrations of a surgeon in Rochester, Ann made a full recovery. The references to waste—putrefaction, rotten clothes, and maggot and fly infestations—all underscore how there is nothing 'salutary' about starving. Instead, such disgusting imagery reminds us of the medical claim that nourishment is what allows living organisms to resist degeneration and decomposition.

In *The Physiology of Digestion Considered with Relation to the Principles of Dietetics* (1836), Scottish physician Andrew Combe hoped to create a system of dietetics based on the idea that life was maintained by the correct balance of matter. Whereas Cheyne had sought to manage dietetics not as an academic discipline but as a means of restoring health, Combe aimed to make nutrition a subject of rigorous physiological research. Since the 1820s, chemists had been dividing foodstuffs into carbohydrates, fats, and proteins. In 1827, William Lambe proposed the classification of food into sugars and starches, oily bodies, and albumen. (The term *protein* was coined by Gerrit Jan Mulder in 1838, and carbohydrates would be identified by Carl Schmidt in 1844.[113]) Combe's physiological approach concentrated on a balanced diet as the thing needed to ward off somatic decay: 'Throughout every department of Nature waste is the inevitable result of action', he said. It 'goes on in living bodies not only without any intermission, but with a rapidity immeasurably beyond that which occurs in inanimate objects'; yet, '*living* bodies [...] possess the distinguishing characteristic of being able to repair their own waste and add to their own substance':

If man, whose system throws out every day five or six pounds of substance by the ordinary channels of excretion, possessed no means of repairing the loss, his organization would speedily decay and perish. This very result is frequently witnessed in cases of shipwreck and other disasters where, owing to the impossibility of obtaining food, death ensues from the body wasting away till it becomes incapable of carrying on the operations of life.[114]

Such had been the unhappy experiences of Hufeland's merchant and Ann Martin. Some years later, in *The Physiology of Common Life* (1859), George Henry Lewes argued that 'life is waste':

---

[112] Ibid., pp. 143–4.

[113] See Harmke Kamminga and Andrew Cunningham, 'Introduction: The Science and Culture of Nutrition', in Kamminga and Cunningham (eds), *The Science and Culture of Nutrition, 1840–1940* (Amsterdam: Rodopi, 1995), pp. 1–14; Catherine Price, 'Probing the Mysteries of Human Digestion', *Distillations*, 4:2 (2018), pp. 27–35.

[114] Andrew Combe, *The Physiology of Digestion Considered with Relation to the Principles of Dietetics* (1836; Boston: Marsh, Capen, Lyon and Webb, 1840), pp. 17–19, 20. Italics in original.

In every living organism there is an incessant and reciprocal activity of *waste* and *repair*. The living fabric, in the very actions which constitute its life, is momentarily yielding up its particles to destruction, like the coal, which is burned in the furnace: so much coal to so much heat, so much waste of tissue to so much vital activity. You cannot wink your eye, move your finger, or think a thought, but some minute particle of your substance must be sacrificed in doing so. Unless the coal which is burning be from time to time replaced, the fire soon smoulders, and finally goes out; unless the substance of your body, which is wasting, be from time to time furnished with fresh food, Life flickers, and at length becomes extinct.

Hunger is the instinct which teaches us to replenish the empty furnace.[115]

In Skibbereen, during the height of the Irish Hunger, the physician Daniel Donovan identified what he called 'famine cachexia [wasting], or *lingering* starvation'. According to Charlotte Boyce: 'Famine cachexia caused the starving body to become autophagous—to cannibalise itself'.[116] What Combe, Lewes, and Donovan, following Hunter, all illustrated was how the 'characteristic of being able to repair [one's] own waste' was a 'distinguishing characteristic' of the 'living body'; it was a natural and a normal process to replenish the empty furnace. The impossibility of obtaining food, as in cases of shipwreck, is decidedly abnormal because it causes one to waste, to flicker, and become extinct.

Such dedication to the decomposition theory illustrates how that idea endured just as much as Malthus's population theory did. (The latter had some help from the ideologies feeding into, and seeping out of, the New Poor Law (1834), but so too did physiological theory, as we shall see.) We remember Ebenezer Scrooge's heartless injunction that those who refuse to go into the workhouse ought to get on with dying 'and decrease the surplus population'.[117] Lord Henry Kames, Scottish advocate, judge, and philosopher, said, likewise, that 'if a few [aged and helpless] should die of want [...] it would be of no importance, *or rather it would be an advantage*; for the example of such, left to perish, would tend more to reformation than the most pathetic discourse from the pulpit'.[118] The alternative view of extreme poverty as a disorder and a violation of nature's laws can be traced back to the view of starvation that was developed through medicine and physiology. I do not claim that all philanthropic and radical thought on poverty has its roots in biological science (just as all conservative or punitive thinking did not all

[115] George Henry Lewes, *The Physiology of Common Life*, 2 vols (London: William Blackwood and Sons, 1859), vol. 1, p. 8. Italics in original.

[116] Charlotte Boyce, 'Representing the "Hungry Forties"', p. 431. Italics in original.

[117] Charles Dickens, *A Christmas Carol* (1844), in *Christmas Books*, ed. Glancy, pp. 1–90 (pp. 11–12).

[118] Quoted in William Pulteney Alison, *Reply to the Pamphlet entitled 'Proposed Alteration of the Scottish Poor Law Considered and Commented on, by David Monypenny, Esq. of Pitmilly'* (Edinburgh: William Blackwood and Sons; London: Thomas Cadell, 1840), p. 6. Italics in original.

come from Malthusian political economy), but I do suggest that physiological ideas offered both an alternative way of thinking about hunger and an exploration of the ways in which it might be interpreted.

The Social and Political Climate

In recent times, Juan Manuel Garrido has said that 'hunger means the fact of being alive', and 'to live precisely means to be constantly and structurally dying of hunger'.[119] Lesa Scholl has added that 'some form of hunger seems an inevitable part of the human condition, from the gentle prod of a healthy appetite to dire starvation'.[120] It may seem that such ideas are consummate with the waste theories explored in the previous section, yet medical specialists of the eighteenth and nineteenth centuries would have agreed neither that 'dire starvation' and 'dying from hunger' are part of the 'fact of being alive', nor that they are 'inevitable'. The gentle prod of a healthy appetite they would have seen as the cue to rectify a diminished amount of energy; what was normal was the maintenance of a nourished body, not the experience of a hungry one. The details of accounts such as Hufeland's merchant or Ann Martin were extreme examples, yet they underscored how hunger was a *pathological state*; they also underscore, for us, how vital the materialist view became to challenging entrenched opinions about hunger as something that might be left to its own devices because it was natural. If people starved to death, according to medical men, they did so not in accordance with natural laws, but in breach of them. If, therefore, social policy was to be driven by perceptions of nature's teachings, it stood to reason that, like the body, the state should be seeking to avoid starvation rather than form an unholy alliance with its fictive inevitability. In his *Address to Journeymen and Labourers* (1816), Malthus's most persistent critic, William Cobbett, explored similar ideas in his radical claim that 'labourers and their families have a *right*, they have a *just claim*, to relief from the purses of the rich'; 'poverty is not a crime', he added, 'and though it sometimes arises from faults, it is not, even in that case to be visited by punishment beyond that which it brings with itself'.[121] A year after the passing of the New Poor Law, William Wordsworth wrote in a postscript to his collection of poems *Yarrow Revisited* (1835) that 'all persons who cannot find employment, or procure wages sufficient to support the body in health and strength, are entitled to maintenance

---

[119] Juan Manuel Garrido, *On Time, Being and Hunger: Challenging the Traditional Way of Thinking Life* (New York, NY: Fordham University Press, 2012), p. 84.

[120] Lesa Scholl, *Hunger Movements in Early Victorian Literature: Want, Riots, Migration* (London: Routledge, 2016), pp. 4, 8.

[121] William Cobbett, *Address to Journeymen and Labourers* (1816) and *Advice to Young Men and (Incidentally) Young Women in the Middle and Higher Ranks of Life* (1830), quoted in James P. Huzel, *The Popularization of Malthus in Early Nineteenth Century England: Martineau, Cobbett and the Pauper Press* (Aldershot: Ashgate, 2006), p. 135.

by law'. The new law 'proceeds too much upon the presumption that it is a labour-ing man's own fault if he be not, as the phrase is, beforehand with the world'.[122] As John M. Ulrich notes, Cobbett's radical re-visioning of the Condition of England question 'may be seen as advocating a materialist version of the social body meta-phor, one that recentres the national body around individual [...] laborers and the satisfaction of their material needs'.[123] In Cobbett's view, political economists and politicians excluded the material body from their discourses and duly 'render[ed] that body vulnerable to inanition and neglect'.[124] By putting the body back into such discussions, he followed the discursive pattern we have already observed at work in biological research, where social questions were discussed through the bodies of individuals; it was an inductive form of reasoning set firmly against the abstract deductions of the most conservative political economists.

It follows that, by suggesting how it is 'normal' for bodies to resist cachexia, medical figures supported the picture of the modern industrial world, with its harsh working hours and unequal distributions of wealth, as putting too much strain upon the bodies of the labouring classes. Combe notes, for example:

> Among the operative part of the community we meet with innumerable examples of [a...] condition of the system, where, from excess of labour, a greater expend-iture of energy and substance takes place than what their deficient diet is able to repair. It is true that the disproportion is generally not sufficient to cause that immediate wasting which accompanies actual starvation, but its effects are nevertheless very palpably manifest in the depressed buoyancy, early old age, and shorter lives of the labouring classes. Few, indeed, of those who are habitually subjected to considerable and continued exertion survive their forty-fifth or fiftieth year. Exhausted at length by the constant recurrence of their daily task and imperfect nourishment, they died of premature decay long before attaining the natural limit of human existence.[125]

In this picture of industrialized Britain, working men and women do not live (or breed) beyond their means; nor do they have their own weaknesses or follies to blame for their burdens. They have instead little choice but to chafe against an impoverished bodily economy whose physical expenditure far outweighs the nourishment needed to counteract 'the waste arising from action'. Combe insists upon *palpable* effects and *actual* starvation: 'Minute acquaintance with the laws

---

[122] Quoted in Stephen Gill, *Wordsworth's Revisitings* (Oxford: Oxford University Press, 2011), p. 207. Italics in original. Hazlitt makes the same point much earlier in *A Reply to the Essay on Population*, pp. 315–19; and Gallagher argues that a similar view was held by Coleridge. See *Body Economic*, pp. 13–14.

[123] John M. Ulrich, *Signs of their Times: History, Labor, and the Body in Cobbett, Carlyle, and Disraeli* (Athens, OH: Ohio University Press, 2002), p. 36.

[124] Ibid., p. 36.   [125] Combe, *Physiology of Digestion*, pp. 41–2.

by which [the cachexia economy] is regulated', he adds, reveals a subtle but sure process of malnutrition. Concrete details—symptoms such as 'depressed buoyancy', premature ageing, and death in middle age—allow him to shift the onus of responsibility from the poor themselves. Robert Southey, another of Malthus's detractors, denied the efficacy of political economy on the basis that it sought 'political and social improvement in a manner which implicitly attributed poverty, famine and disease to "the will of God" rather than "human institutions"'.[126] What physiological language such as Combe's promised was that the focus on human institutions could be placed on a scientific footing, with the weight of material evidence and reasoned analysis behind it.

Reasoned Analysis

It would be unfair to the political economists, and a gross simplification of what they set out to achieve, to say that they were incapable of reasoned analysis, or that their labours did not seek to be every bit as rigorous as those of their medical counterparts. That such allegations were made against them in the nineteenth century is no reason for us to accept them without reflection. Yet political economy's attachment to the idea of natural providentialism did seem to offer a means of sidestepping the kind of critical self-scrutiny that became common in physiology and medicine. Political economy relied upon the idea of a higher, guiding power—Adam Smith's invisible hand, say, or Nature's law. This belief encouraged the perception of evidence (especially statistics) as plain truth; there was no need for discussion or the kind of scrutiny that comes with the acknowledgement of the fallibility of interpretation. In *Observations on the Management of the Poor in Scotland* (1840), physician William Alison argued that the 'fallacy' of such speculation was that it 'thwarted or prevented such improvements as the sense of duty and feelings of humanity would otherwise have introduced'. What was needed was 'experience', not 'speculation'.[127] 'Medical men', he wrote in a later text, were 'the most intelligent and impartial witnesses of the actual condition of the poor'.[128]

In 'Some Observations of Digestion', published as part of *Animal Œconomy*, John Hunter had been keen to criticize scientists who were 'directed by what is best suited to their fancy'; 'the connexion, arrangement, mode of action, and uses of the whole, or of particular organs, have more commonly been reserved for the consideration of those whose views have extended further, and whose powers

---

[126] Philip Connell, *Romanticism, Economic and the Question of 'Culture'* (Oxford: Oxford University Press, 2005), p. 40.

[127] William Pulteney Alison, *The Management of the Poor in Scotland and its Effects on the Health of the Great Towns* (Edinburgh: William Blackwood and Sons; London: Thomas Cadell, 1840), pp. iv, vi.

[128] William Pulteney Alison, *Reply to the Pamphlet*, p. 41. Italics in original.

of reasoning ha[ve] been enlarged by habits of observation and inquiry'.[129] According to Owen, Hunter, 'instead of dogmatising [...] endeavour[ed] to analyse the vital forces peculiar to each organic element, and to classify, as it were, the phænomena of which life consists'.[130] Despite Hunter's attachment to the idea of a 'life principle' drawn from vitalist theories, there was a marked turn in his work from abstractions, unfounded theories, and deductions, and towards materiality, quantifiable evidence, and induction. Indeed, the experimental standards of his physiology illustrate how the methods of science offered something of a challenge to the 'dogmatized' notions of Malthus's less-ruminative disciples. While John Stuart Mill, advocate of deduction, looked forward to a time when 'the well-being of mankind may almost be measured by the number and gravity of the truths which have reached the point of being uncontested',[131] positivists such as George Henry Lewes argued for a 'hermeneutics of suspicion': 'The fundamental move of all positivisms is akin to Descartes' establishment of the Great Doubt', George Levine explains; they do not believe we have 'access to the "essence" of things, and that abstract nouns create an illusion of essence that is merely the creation of human methods of perception and ordering'.[132] In his study *Comte's Philosophy of the Sciences* (1853), Lewes defined positivism as 'principally distinguished from the theologico-metaphysical philosophy by a constant and irresistible tendency to render *relative* all the notions which at first were *absolute*', and noted that 'the relative character of scientific conceptions is inseparable from the true notion of natural laws'.[133]

For Lewes, as for Comte and William Alison, the implementation of a scientific view was inseparable from the analysis and remedying of social problems: 'All the sciences—physical and social' are, according to Comte, 'branches of one Science, to be investigated on one and the same Method'.[134] Methodologically speaking, there was not much of a difference between the micro and the macro for Comte and Lewes. The tools used by men like Hunter to observe bodies were just as relevant to the large and diverse populations studied by Malthus. Political economy, however, had been subservient to 'the theological or metaphysical spirit' that typified the 'infancy of human reason', and this had led to its being more 'speculative' than 'positive':

[129]   Hunter, *Animal Œconomy*, p. 112.
[130]   Owen, Preface, p. 16.
[131]   Quoted in George Levine, 'In Defence of Positivism', in *Realism, Ethics and Secularism: Essays on Victorian Literature and Science* (Cambridge: Cambridge University Press, 2008), pp. 136–64 (p. 141).
[132]   Ibid., pp. 144, 146. In spite of his comments about doctrines which are no longer disputed, Mill appears to have approved of these ideas in Auguste Comte's writing.
[133]   George Henry Lewes, *Comte's Philosophy of the Sciences: Being an Exposition of the Principles of the Cours de Philosophie Positive of Auguste Comte* (London: Henry G. Bohn, 1853), p. 250. Italics in original.
[134]   Quoted in ibid., p. 10.

When we leave the world of entities for real speculations we perceive how the economic and industrial analysis of society cannot be positively accomplished apart from its intellectual, moral, and political analysis. The predilection which the human mind seems to manifest in our days for what is called political economy, must be considered in reality a symptom of the want felt of at least submitting social studies to really *positive* methods.[135]

What was needed, in fact, was a 'necessary and permanent subordination of the imagination to observation which specially constitutes the scientific spirit'.[136] The scientific spirit, for Lewes, consisted of observation, experimentation, and comparison.

Starvation Statistics

In her study *A History of the Modern Fact* (1998), Poovey has observed how statistical knowledge, in nineteenth-century discussions of population and economics, was an attempt to put the stamp of scientific verifiability on a range of theoretical assertions. Malthus, in particular,

> admitted that the first edition [of his *Essay*] was 'written on the spur of the occasion, and from the few materials which were then within my reach in a country situation [...]'. Immediately upon completing the first edition, Malthus determined to test what had essentially been a deduction against the kind of numbers he had wanted all along.[137]

Subsequent editions of the *Essay* featured a greater amount of statistical research, and there grew among his followers the impression that statistics could be relied upon to tell the plain truth. In *Elements of Medical Statistics* (1829), surgeon F. Bisset Hawkins wrote:

> Statistics has become the key to several sciences, opening in a manner the most convincing, simple, and summary, their gradual progress, their actual condition, their relations to each other, the success which they have attained, or the deficiencies which remain to be supplied. Its application to the objects of government has created political economy and there is reason to believe, that a careful cultivation of it, in reference to the natural history of man in health and disease, would materially assist the completion of a philosophy of medicine, by pointing out to the physicians of every part of the world the comparative merits of

---

[135] Ibid., pp. 249, 248.   [136] Ibid., pp. 249–50.
[137] Poovey, *History of the Modern Fact*, p. 290.

various modes of practice, the history of disease in different ages and countries, the increase and decrease of particular maladies, the tendency of certain situations, professions, and modes of life to protect or to expose; and by indicating, as the basis of prognosis, those extended tabular views of the duration and termination of diseases, which are furnished, at successive periods, by hospitals and civic registers.[138]

Hawkins is mindful of the need to execute statistical research carefully (and not to reduce theories to a simple row of numbers), and his sense of what statistics can achieve is seemingly difficult to find fault with. And yet, words like *convincing*, *simple*, and *summary* would no doubt have met with short shrift from the critics of the statistical method; Carlyle's *Past and Present* (1843) described statistics as an 'ever-whirling chaos of Formulas',[139] and his earlier *Chartism* (1839) dismissed them as follows:

A witty statesman said you might prove anything by figures. We have looked into various statistical works, Statistic-Society Reports, Poor-Law reports, Reports and Pamphlets not a few, with a sedulous eye to this question of the Working Classes and their general condition in England; we grieve to say, with as good as no result whatever. Assertion swallows assertion according to the old Proverb, 'as the *statist* thinks, the bell clinks!' Tables are like cobwebs, like the sieve of the Danaides; beautifully reticulated, orderly to look upon, but which will hold no conclusion. Tables are abstractions, and the object a most concrete one, so difficult to read the essence of.[140]

In one passage in *Past and Present*, Carlyle satirized how statisticians believed their work to be the flesh and blood of 'Human Life': formulas, he writes ironically,

are real as the very *skin* and *muscular tissue* of a Man's Life; and a most blessed indispensable thing, so long as they have *vitality* withal, and are a *living* skin and tissue to him! No man, or man's life, can go abroad and do business in the world without skin and tissues.[141]

In using corporeal terms, Carlyle unwittingly pinpoints the key difference between statistics and the biological sciences: the reference to *vitality* is a reference to the days of vitalist medicine, when the essence of life was abstract, intangible, and vaguely defined; offset against this are 'skin and tissues', a vocabulary

---

[138] F. Bisset Hawkins, *Elements of Medical Statistics* (London: Longman et al., 1829), pp. 2–3.

[139] Thomas Carlyle, *Past and Present* (New York: William H. Colyer, 1843), p. 102.

[140] Thomas Carlyle, *Chartism* (1839; London: James Fraser, 1840), pp. 9–10.

[141] Carlyle, *Past and Present*, p. 77.

that invokes the science of Bichat, and drives home the point, made in *Chartism*, that there is a yawning chasm between tabular abstractions and the concreteness of real life. That 'assertion swallows assertion' is a sign, for Carlyle, of how abstraction means summary, simple, and *un*convincing verification: one might, as the statesman says, prove anything with figures.

William Farr vs. Edwin Chadwick

In the 1820s and '30s, statistics became the dominant method of measuring starvation in Britain; in 1837, the Registrar General's Office (RGO) had been established, as James Vernon points out, 'to record what was confidently expected to be the increasing health of Britons (evident from the new civil registration of births, deaths, and marriages)'.[142] It was through the statistics of starvation, however, that a problem was identified with the use of numerical evidence in social reform. Starvation formed the basis of a disagreement between the medical statistician and epidemiologist William Farr and chief administrator of the Poor Law Commission, Edwin Chadwick. Farr believed, along with Bisset Hawkins, in the power of arithmetic in understanding social health and human behaviour, but he also recognized the importance of combining statistical research with accounts of individual cases, and, most importantly, of recognizing when the latter contradicts the former. According to John M. Eyler, Farr had 'a sensibility more finely tuned by human sympathy' than some of his contemporaries: like Carlyle, he appears to have 'rejected the mindless garnering of numbers and had nothing but scorn for the empiric who throws heaps of tables in our faces, and asserts that he can prove anything by figures'.[143] In a report to the office of the Registrar General, Farr demonstrated that being 'finely tuned by human sympathy' meant being familiar with specific cases:

> Medical practitioners meet with many distressing cases of starvation in this metropolis. I will mention one. In the winter of 1838 I was requested, in the middle of the night, to see a woman, who, it was said, was dying for want of help. I followed the messenger through a labyrinth of narrow passages, near Fitzroy market, and found in the corner of an attic a young woman, thinly clad, lying on a straw bedspread upon the floor. She had given birth to a child, then at her feet. Three children lay on the same bed, under a single rug. It was intensely cold. She had no fire, no candle, no food, and, if I recollect right, had not more than three

---

[142] James Vernon, *Hunger: A Modern History* (Cambridge, MS and London: Belknap Press of Harvard University Press, 2007), p. 81.

[143] John M. Eyler, *Victorian Social Medicine: The Ideals and Methods of William Farr* (Baltimore, MD: Johns Hopkins University Press, 1979), p. 29.

half-pence in money to meet the exigencies of child-birth. The lodgers in the
room below had been aroused by her groans.[144]

Christopher Hamlin has shown how such descriptions were not absent in the
later work of Chadwick; the *Sanitary Report* of 1842, for example, contained a
substantial number of detailed descriptions of individual cases.[145] Indeed, Eyler is
near the mark when he suggests that what differentiated Farr's approach from
that of Chadwick was the former's 'sophisticated understanding of statistics' and a
'greater willingness' than the latter to discuss the philosophical indications of
tabular information. Eyler is also right to put this more critical approach down to
Farr's medical training.[146] Farr had been educated as a physician in Paris during
the years when Magendie's and Bichat's physiological approaches were the dom-
inating trends in practice and research. Although, as Hamlin notes, Farr took an
interest in the 'broad set of social (and economic) determinants of health and
illness,[147] his fuller, more nuanced accounts of starvation relied, as it did for
medical experimentalists, upon evidence that could be, in the words of John
Senebier, 'anatomised by the senses'. In 1837, while in the employ of the RGO,
Farr complained to Chadwick that the Poor Law Commission was 'too much
occupied, and [had] too little acquaintance—practical acquaintance—with the
subject' of real poverty.[148] Two years later, he compiled and published a report on
the health and longevity of Britons, in which he wrote:

> It will be seen with regret that in the half-year the deaths of 63 individuals were
> ascribed (principally at inquests) to starvation; this is almost 1 annually to a
> population of 11,000. The want of food implies the want of everything else—
> except water—as firing, clothing, every convenience, every necessary of life, is
> abandoned at the imperious bidding of hunger. Hunger destroys a much higher
> proportion than is indicated by the registers in this and in every other country;
> but its effects, like the effects of excess, are generally manifested indirectly, in the
> production of diseases of various kinds. The privation is rarely absolute.[149]

Farr's report suggested that for all their arithmetical power, statistics were unable
to capture the range of complications attendant on malnutrition. Chadwick, who

[144] William Farr, letter to T. H. Lister (1840), in D. V. Glass, *Numbering the People: The Eighteenth-Century Population Controversy and the Developments of Census and Vital Statistics* (Farnborough: D. C. Heath, 1973), pp. 161–7 (p. 163).
[145] Christopher Hamlin, *Public Health and Social Justice in the Age of Chadwick: Britain, 1800–1854* (Cambridge: Cambridge University Press, 1998).
[146] Eyler, *Victorian Social Medicine*, p. 29.
[147] Christopher Hamlin, 'Could You Starve to Death in England in 1839? The Chadwick-Farr Controversy and the Loss of "Social" in Public Health', *American Journal of Public Health*, 85:6 (1995), pp. 856–66 (p. 856). See also Hamlin's *Public Health and Social Justice*, pp. 144–6.
[148] William Farr, letter to Edwin Chadwick (1837), in Glass, *Numbering the People*, p. 148.
[149] Quoted in Glass, *Numbering the People*, p. 146.

had helped Farr secure his position at the RGO, was not pleased. With the removal of outdoor relief, and the strict use of punitive diets in union workhouses, the poor, he believed, responded to hunger by taking measures to secure work, to help each other, and to be more prudent. If people starved to death, as Farr suggested they did, then it meant that the deliberate austerities of the new legislation were a failure at best, and a cruelty at worst.[150] There was certainly no shortage of commentators willing to confirm either to be the case, perhaps unfairly. As both Hamlin and Poovey have shown, Chadwick was no Malthusian. While he prided himself, like Malthus did, on his empirical research, his statistical approach was not as pessimistic as Malthus's. Hamlin notes that Chadwick 'differed from many political economists in his optimism for industrial growth. For Chadwick, there was no "surplus population", no limited fund of wages, but an economy that could always absorb workers provided they were released from the bondage of antiquated paternalism'.[151] Poovey has noted how Chadwick cherished 'Reason as the outcome of extensive inquiry; as the inductive fruit of a "mass of facts," Reason stands opposed to the deductive—and therefore "interested"—theories of Malthus and Chalmers, which consist of "general principles" deducted from erroneous assumptions'.[152]

Nonetheless, the interpretations of the Poor Law Commission were challenged by Farr's recognition of the difficulty of drawing a line between starvation and 'secondary' pathologies; he implied that the use of statistics suited pre-established commitments to consequentialist political economy and thus amounted to narrow dogmatism. Chadwick hit back in a letter to T. H. Lister, Farr's supervisor. Farr's findings, he said, were 'calculated to produce a belief that the provisions of the law, which are intended to bring relief within the reach of every one needing it, are either inadequate to their object or improperly administered'.[153] He and the other commissioners set about discrediting the young doctor's report. Not all of its sixty-three starved individuals were sourced in coroner's reports, they found; of that sixty-three, at least thirty-six were infants who had died during weaning. Farr later conceded that he was wrong to attribute all of his results to coroners' inquests, but he reminded the commissioners that if just one person had died of starvation in a country that had not had a national famine for almost a hundred years, then surely that one was a death too many. He admitted that thirty-six of the sixty-three had been infants, and wondered how far these deaths might be attributed to the harsh environments of the poverty-stricken or to the

---

[150] See John V. Pickstone, 'Dearth, Dirt and Fever Epidemics: Rewriting the History of the British "Public Health", 1780–1850', in *Epidemics and Ideas: Essays on the Historical Perception of Pestilence*, ed. by Terence Ranger and Paul Slack (1992; Cambridge: Cambridge University Press, 1995), p. 137; Huzel, *Popularization of Malthus*, pp. 139–40; Vernon, *Hunger*, pp. 18–19.

[151] Hamlin, *Public Health and Social Justice*, pp. 33, 87.

[152] Mary Poovey, *Making a Social Body: British Cultural Formation, 1830–1864* (Chicago IL and London: Chicago University Press, 1995), p. 108.

[153] Edwin Chadwick, letter to T. H. Lister (1839), in Glass, *Numbering the People*, pp. 150–1 (p. 150).

famishment of nursing mothers. And what of the rest? At least thirteen people in the table provided by the commissioners were acknowledged to have died from malnourishment: 'whether starvation occurred therefore in infants, or in the aged', Farr concluded, 'whether it was accidental, inevitable, or the result of negligence, the fact itself remained unchanged; it was still starvation'. And, 'if there should be one death the less, "for the future", I ask no other vindication'.[154]

To be clear, Farr's issue with the Poor Law Commission did not concern the use of statistics, but rather the disingenuous way in which the data had been interpreted. More vitriolic in his attack on statistics, Charles Kingsley later noted in a letter to his wife:

> *we* may choose to look at the masses in the gross, as subjects for statistics [...but] there is One above who knows every thirst and ache, and sorrow, and temptation of each slattern, and gin-drinker, and street boy. The day will come when He will require an account of these neglects of ours not in the gross.[155]

Like many of his contemporaries, including Carlyle, Kingsley saw the statistical view as falling short of the standard of truth required in discussions of the experiences and sufferings of the poor. As he noted in the *North British Review* in 1850:

> The truth is, in statistics, as in every other physical science, a little learning is a dangerous thing. An enormous number of facts must be collated before anything like a sage general law can be deduced from them. The man of genius may, indeed, hit off instinctively on a world-wide law from a single phenomenon; but he will keep it to himself for years, rack and torture it by every possible mode of verification, before he gives it to the world.[156]

Kingsley appears to be advocating for the use of experimentation as a more reliable mode of research than statistics. While he does not mention the Farr–Chadwick debate, the following observation of Kingsley's is supported by the fact that both Farr and Chadwick reached opposing conclusions from the same set of data: '"There is no romance [...] like the romance of statistics"—the art of "*combler les numeros*," of "cooking returns," by which the most utterly contradictory propositions can be proved with equal certainty'.[157] Although Farr believed 'that the phenomena of life and death were law-abiding',[158] and that they could be recorded in statistical form, he 'struggle[d] with the problem of making a classification system that was unambiguously exclusive, [...] that was exhaustive [...], and that facilitated empirical inference'.[159] In a letter to Lister he suggested that

---

[154] Farr, letter to Lister, pp. 164, 167.   [155] Kingsley, *L&M*, vol. 1, p. 180. Italics in original.
[156] [Charles Kingsley], 'The Agricultural Crisis', *North British Review*, 14 (1850), pp. 85–121 (p. 87).
[157] Ibid., p. 87.   [158] Eyler, *Victorian Social Medicine*, p. 32.
[159] Hamlin, 'The Chadwick-Farr Controversy', pp. 858–9.

some subjects were too complicated, or too concrete, as Carlyle would have put it, to be held within the boxes created by statisticians: the effects of hunger, in particular, 'manifested indirectly' and were linked to 'diseases of various kinds'. What his disagreement with Chadwick encapsulates is a determination to develop a more solid, materialist approach to poverty and to use a language of complexity, or difficulty, in approaching the subject.

Famine Fever

Richard Baron Howard was a physician at the Ardwick and Ancoats Dispensary in Manchester in the late 1830s. He had previously been the resident medical officer at the Manchester Poor House, and in 1839 published *An Inquiry into the Morbid Effects of Deficiency of Food* after noticing how 'the public in general have very inaccurate ideas of the marks by which this state [starvation] is distinguished, and the singular symptoms which often attend it'.[160] Even, he continues, 'if any suspicion is aroused that a person has died of starvation, and a *post mortem* examination instituted to ascertain its probability; [...] it is too generally assumed, as a matter of course, that death has arisen from natural causes'.[161] As Farr had suggested, starvation was a difficult condition to pin down because it was linked to a wide range of 'secondary' conditions. According to surgeon James Bower Harrison, in extreme cases of hunger 'life terminates' through a 'gradual failure of the circulation of the blood'.[162] Physician William Carpenter believed, by contrast, that 'death by starvation [is] really death by cold' due to the fact that the body loses up to 94 per cent of its body fat.[163] As Howard illustrated, an individual dying from heart failure or hypothermia was unlikely to have his or her death attributed to starvation, even after a post-mortem examination. The same applies to tuberculosis, dysentery, and paraplegia—just three of the more serious conditions that he observed in his malnourished patients. In an article that appeared in Dickens's journal *All the Year Round* in 1865, it was noted of the victims of the Irish Hunger that they

> did not all die in the same manner. With some, the symptoms were concentrated in the chest; they were choked by coughs or suffocated by water suffusions. Others were carried off by diarrhœa. A few, after several hours' lethargic sleep,

---

[160] Richard Baron Howard, *An Inquiry into the Morbid Effects of Deficiency of Food, Chiefly with Reference to their Occurrence amongst the Destitute Poor* (London: Simpkin, Marshall, et al., 1839), p. 1.

[161] Ibid., p. 40.

[162] James Bower Harrison, *The Medical Aspects of Death and the Medical Aspects of the Human Mind* (London: Longman et al., 1852), p. 45.

[163] William Carpenter, *Principles of Human Physiology*, ed. by Henry Power (1842; Philadelphia: Henry C. Lea, 1876), p. 123. This comment probably belongs to Power as it does not appear in earlier editions of the earlier editions of *Principles* overseen by Carpenter.

expired without apparent pain. Many sunk under the first attacks of an intermittent fever, which was sure to assume a pernicious character in systems so impoverished as those.[164]

There is irony in the fact that such causes of death are reported, and identified, and yet each contribute to a general impression of inconclusiveness over what exactly causes death from starvation. It is another confirmation, if we needed one, of the failure of individual cases and statistical aggregations to speak a language that applies to all. In 1856, it was written in *The Times* that:

> It is difficult to ascertain the deaths by actual starvation, because much mortality that is referred to fever, to cholera, and other maladies is primarily due to the insufficiency of food; and then, again, those deaths which are attributed to 'infirmity, debility, and old age,' and which in the years of famine are very numerous—in 1847, for example, being more than 22,000—are not easily distinguished from the cases of downright starvation. We may therefore be pretty sure that in enumerating the deaths arising from pure hunger we shall very much understate the mortality. Now, the deaths in England that result from privation of food are less than 100 annually,—a large number, no doubt; but it sinks into insignificance beside the figures of the Irish famine. Mark how the numbers rise. In 1842 the deaths were 187; in 1845 they were 516; in 1846 they amount to 2,041; in 1847 they reached the greatest height—6,058; in the two following years together they amount to 9,395, and so gradually diminished, although there is not much room, after all, for congratulation, seeing that in the first quarter of 1851—that year of grace, that *annus mirabilis*, which has been described as if it were the jubilee of the world—there were not less than 652 deaths attributed to starvation.[165]

This correspondent finds matter to be believed and doubted in statistics; the death rates, he suggests, make grim reading in themselves, but the links between hunger and pestilence indicate this to be only half of the story. Starving predisposes the body to infection by weakening it: 'In persons laboring under an impaired state of health from deficiency of food', claimed Howard, 'there is a remarkable susceptibility to the effects of contagion [...]; and it is this class which always suffers most severely, during the prevalence of endemic, epidemic, or contagious disorders.'[166] Ireland was seen to offer the clearest evidence that there was link between famine

---

[164] Unsigned, 'Poverty', *All the Year Round*, 13 (1865), pp. 512–15 (p. 514).

[165] Unsigned, 'As the Famine which brought the Israelites', *The Times*, 16 September 1856, p. 6.

[166] Howard, *Morbid Effects*, p. 38. Anne Hardy has argued that there is no primary link between instances of fever and starvation in the nineteenth century; typhus, she argues, is more likely to be connected to the aggregation of people in urban environments and poor sanitation. See 'Urban Famine or Urban Crisis? Typhus in the Victorian City', *Medical History*, 32 (1998), pp. 401–25.

and fever. D. J. Corrigan's pamphlet *On Famine and Fever*, published in Dublin in 1846, was the most significant piece of work on the links between hunger and contagion up to that point. 'As want appeared' in Ireland, it claimed, 'so certainly did Pestilence follow. The two have kept pace with one another; as the degree of want, so has been the extent of fever.' He coined the famous axiom 'if there be no famine, there will be no fever'.[167] Epidemiologist William Budd, writing in *The Lancet*, identified a specific strand of typhus unique to Ireland which he imaginatively called '*Irish typhus*'.[168] In 1847, in the less-specialized context of the family periodical *Fraser's Magazine*, typhus was identified as '*road sickness*' because of the way it attacked Irish labourers who had 'to walk some three or four miles, on an average, to their work [...] on an empty stomach', and were often found dead on the side of the road.[169]

The most common term for infections related to starvation, however, was simply 'famine fever', and for every author who was willing to argue that pestilence had an iron-bound relationship with hunger, there were plenty of others who were prepared to deny any such link. As Hamlin has illustrated, the New Poor Law Commission in England was keen to argue that disease and fever were the result of environment, not destitution. Chadwick's *Sanitary Report* subscribed to the pythogenic (miasmatic) theory of disease, where contagion is attributed to the poisonous gases caused by the putrefaction of organic matter. *The Times* alleged that 'the commissioners, carefully conceal[ed] the fact that the increase of disease among the poor is mainly attributable to *starvation*'.[170] Environmental causes could be managed; dust heaps and stagnant puddles could be cleared; if fever was caused by the lack of cleanliness, moreover, responsibility could be put upon the shoulders of the impoverished people themselves: 'a cesspool or a foul privy was a scapegoat'.[171] If, however, hunger was the cause of disease, as Corrigan and his medical colleagues suggested it was, the measures of the New Poor Law, which had used hunger as a deterrent to those relying on social support, had added to the miseries of the very people it had set out to assist.

Yet medicine itself was far from certain on the links between famine and fever. In 1846, Robert J. Graves wrote a response to Corrigan's pamphlet in *The Dublin Quarterly Journal of Medical Science*. Identifying cholera as the main problem, rather than typhus, he argued that:

Great numbers of the indigent and starving poor will be daily brought together for the purpose of being fed, and thus people in multitudes will be assembled,

[167] Corrigan, *Famine and Fever*, pp. 14, 33.
[168] William Budd, 'On Intestinal Fever', *The Lancet*, 2 (1859), pp. 131–3 (p. 133). Italics in original.
[169] Unsigned, 'Famine in the South of Ireland', *Fraser's Magazine*, 35 (1847), pp. 491–504.
[170] Unsigned report, *The Times*, 25 November 1840, quoted in Hamlin, *Public Health and Social Justice*, p. 131.
[171] Hamlin, *Public Health and Social Justice*, pp. 103–4 (p. 104).

and to a certainty the contagion of the cholera will be disseminated far and near. [...] In truth, wherever large numbers of starving persons are collected to receive food, it is a mere matter of accident what contagious disease may become prevalent amongst them.[172]

Of course, the shift in focus from hunger to foul environments was, according to some writers, no less of a condemnation of the Poor Law Commission's legislative recommendations than starvation was. In his *Observations on the Management of the Poor*, Alison argued: 'Districts without sewers will, naturally, be not only the dirtiest, but the cheapest: they will be inhabited by the poorest and most destitute of people, who will be huddled together in the greatest numbers in proportion to the space they occupy.'[173] Charles Murchison's important work *A Treatise on the Continued Fevers of Great Britain* (1862), however, featured a long chapter in which it was made clear that the incidence of famine fever confirms a link between hunger and typhus as well as cholera:

The result of famine has usually been, that the poor have flocked from the country districts to swell the pauper population of the large towns, which become more crowded the longer famine lasts. As this crowding increases, the fever, which results from crowding (typhus), is gradually substituted for that which is more immediately the result of destitution.[174]

Murchison added:

Under prolonged abstinence [...] the human body seems to become the subject of purely chemical changes, the process of vital renewal not taking place as in health; febrile symptoms are developed; while at the same time the deficient supply of new histogenetic materials appears to check the elimination of those which have become effete, for in no way can we account for that tendency to putrescence, manifested during life in the fetid exhalation and peculiar secretion from the skin, and after death in the rapidity with which putrefaction supervenes. [...] It is not unreasonable to suppose that under such circumstances a contagium should be generated capable of lighting up fever in the system, and communicable by the sick to those who are in health.[175]

Murchison's ideas of fever suddenly 'lighting up' might have been wide of the mark (*contagium vivum*—the theory that a microscopic living organism are

---

[172] Robert J. Graves, 'On the Progress of Asiatic Cholera', *The Dublin Quarterly Journal of Medical Science*, 2 (1846), pp. 289–316 (pp. 308–9).
[173] Quoted in Hamlin, *Public Health and Social Justice*, p. 127.
[174] Charles Murchison, *A Treatise on the Continued Fevers of Great Britain* (1862; London: Longman et al., 1884), p. 341.
[175] Ibid., p. 343.

responsible for the propagation of disease—had been suggested as early as 1856 by Budd,[176] although it was not until Louis Pasteur's 1878 demonstration of germ theory that the idea was widely accepted), yet it was not the pythogenic hypothesis which was the most dominant theory at the time, and which insisted that typhus was generated from within dirty environments and was not communicable from the sick to the healthy. Murchison's counter-theory was that the condition was a destructive energy caused, in many instances, by hunger—it was a result of chemical imbalances which made the empty stomach a volatile place.

If these conflicting arguments tell us anything it is that, in nineteenth-century medicine, nothing could be taken as a matter of course. In 1830, just as experimental medicine was taking hold in Britain and France, leading Scottish physician John Abercrombie stressed that health was an uncertain science: 'The scientific physician well knows the difficulty of ascertaining the true relations of those things which are the proper objects of his attention [...] Even in those cases where he has distinctly ascertained true relations, new causes intervene and disappoint his endeavors.'[177] It is imprudent to rely upon the testimonies of patients, Abercrombie believed, as well as the observations of medical practitioners: pathological conditions will not always follow the same course; it is often difficult to tell one condition apart from another; and there is a misleading tendency in professional interpretations to have a 'fondness for systems [...], a zeal for nosology [...as if] the characters of diseases are, to a certain extent, fixed and determined, like the botanical characters of a plant, or the chymical properties of a mineral'.[178] Abercrombie's *Inquiries Concerning the Intellectual Powers and the Investigation of Truth* (1830) ran to four editions and was very popular with medical writers. Featuring a long chapter on the 'Application of the Rules of Philosophical Investigation to Medical Science', it argued that, 'in a science encumbered with so many difficulties, and encompassed by so many sources of error, it is obvious what cause we have for proceeding with the utmost caution and for advancing from step to step with the greatest circumspection'.[179]

In 1853, in another contribution to the *Dublin Quarterly*, Thomas Purefoy suggested that such vigilance was particularly important in cases of famine fever because symptoms were not always obvious:

In almost every instance a period of general indisposition, or delicate state of health, precedes for some time the full establishment of the fever, indicated by indisposition for business, depression of spirits, unusual drowsiness, indisposition

---

[176] See Michael Dunnill, *William Budd: Bristol's Most Famous Physician, Pioneer of Preventative Medicine and Epidemiology* (Bristol: Redcliffe, 2006).
[177] John Abercrombie, *Inquiries Concerning the Intellectual Powers and the Investigation of Truth* (1830; New York, NY: Harper and Brothers, 1840), p. 30.
[178] Ibid., pp. 307–8.   [179] Ibid., pp. 299–300.

for society, loss of accustomed appetite [...] How many instances occur in daily practice to prove that a depressing influence, acting unexpectedly upon the mind of a patient ill of simple continued fever, may at once alter the disease to typhus! [...] It is to be remembered that I speak of the disease only in reference to my own experience and observations.[180]

The last sentence of this extract is intended to qualify Purefoy's conclusions by suggesting that his 'experience and observations' are necessarily 'peculiar to my locality',[181] but it also suits a claim made elsewhere in the essay that 'a diligent and careful attention to and observation of the general symptoms' was required to understand famine fever.[182] 'Utmost care and watchfulness on the part of the medical attendant' is needed, he adds:

I witnessed myself [...how] the want of clothes and fuel and all the complicated miseries of the poor, during even a temporary famine, formed a combination of circumstances well calculated to induce a morbid condition of the digestive organs primarily, which could not fail to mark very decidedly the symptoms, progress, and character of the fever, which so soon followed in the footsteps of famine,—a fever which, if not the direct result of famine, was yet unmistakeably and very closely connected with it.[183]

Comments like Purefoy's followed Abercrombie in stressing the need for close and detailed observation of the specific links between famine and disease: 'When we find two events placed in a state of contiguity to each other', Abercrombie advised, 'we should use the utmost caution in considering them as connected in the manner of cause and effect [...] and we should keep in view the various sources of fallacy [...] which encompass the whole subject of medical causation'.[184] Such a methodology was a way of talking about social problems in a way that counterbalanced the kind of programmatic thinking which Abercrombie identified as typical among political economists. Political economy, he said, is an 'uncertain science'. Unlike good medical thinking, the problem with the former is its bias or, as he put it, rather knottily, the 'different aspects in which the same measure is often viewed by different men distinguished for political wisdom and talent'.[185] Indeed, in the drawn-out attack on political economy sustained, in no insignificant part, by the Lake Poets in the early nineteenth century, the perceived intangibility of the calculations of economists came under fire as exactly the sort of narrow dogmatism that 'real experience', like that attained through medical practice, counterpointed. The twelfth book of William Wordsworth's *The Prelude*

---

[180] Thomas Purefoy, 'Observations on Remittent Fever in Ireland', *Dublin Quarterly Journal of Medical Science*, 16 (1853), pp. 318–31 (pp. 322, 324, 327–8).
[181] Ibid., p. 328.   [182] Ibid., p. 323.
[183] Ibid., pp. 325, 327.   [184] Abercrombie, *Inquiries*, p. 330.   [185] Ibid., p. 31.

(1805–6/1850), for instance, criticized 'Plans without thought' and 'false philoso-phy' (or 'Plans [...] built on theories / Vague and unsound' in the later version).[186] Smith's *Wealth of Nations* (1776) was highlighted as a progenitor of the problem, yet, as Philip Connell has argued, it was likely that Wordsworth had more interest in joining the chorus of protest, led by Coleridge, Southey, and Hazlitt, against Malthus.[187] Of particular dislike was political economy's figuration of man as an 'Abstraction, shadow, image'. It went forcibly against the poet's extolments of the virtues of the flesh-and-blood common man: 'the man whom we behold / With our own eyes' (p. 492). Wordsworth's solution, similar to the physiologists, was a special kind of observation. Connell observes:

> Against Malthus's 'artificial lights', Wordsworth claims to find a more profound truth in the insights he has derived from those 'observations' and 'notices' that have been his gift since early youth. It is not bookish speculation, but rather his unmediated experience of 'solid life', which allows Wordsworth to claim a super-ior insight into the 'human souls' of the rural poor.[188]

Of course, Wordsworth had very different objectives to men such as Abercrombie: the poet's observations were intended to celebrate the universality of human vir-tues, while the latter's were intended to explore the links between materialist thought and material workings—the blood, bones, and fibres—of animal and human life. Yet, like medical men and physiologists, Wordsworth suggested that 'solid life' requires solid observation, and the material approach offers a powerful antidote to sweeping abstractions.

Waste Economies: George Henry Lewes vs. Justus von Liebig

In same year that *The Prelude* was published, P. W. Banks wrote in *Fraser's Magazine* that political economy was 'less capable of exactness than the physical [sciences], and cannot be brought to the point of rendering the same degree of satisfaction to the inquiring mind'.[189] Banks was not simply offering another stick with which to beat Malthus and his followers, but was noticing, more importantly, how the inexactness of political economy was linked to physical science's seem-ingly more successful approach to the same range of topics. The satisfaction, or dissatisfaction, of the inquiring mind was all-important here. On the subject of

---

[186] Both quotations come from a parallel edition of the text: William Wordsworth, *The Prelude*, ed. by J. C. Maxwell (1805–6/1850; London: Penguin, 1982), pp. 492, 493. Subsequent references to this edition will be given in the text, in the same format of pagination where both editions are quoted.
[187] See Connell, *Question of 'Culture'*, p. 55.   [188] Ibid., p. 52.
[189] 'Morgan Rattler' [P. W. Banks], 'Touching Opinion and Evidence', *Fraser's Magazine*, 41 (1850), pp. 237–49 (p. 247).

digestion, George Henry Lewes insisted in *The Physiology of Common Life* that the matter required the liberal mental cultivation that comes only with the physiological approach. The strength of medical research was its ability to begin with the assumption that the body and its processes are too complicated for any single-minded or narrow approach to fathom. In his chapters on food and drink, he made substantial use of the work of the German chemist Justus von Liebig. At the 1842 meeting of the British Association for the Advancement of Science, professor of botany Lyon Playfair delivered an abstract of Liebig's paper on 'Organic Chemistry applied to Physiology and Pathology'. Playfair would himself play no insignificant role in the diagnosis and prognosis of Ireland potato blight in 1845. Along with John Lindley, editor of the *Gardener's Chronicle and Horticultural Gazette*, he was dispatched by the government to ascertain the nature and extent of the problem. Playfair wrote to Robert Peel, then Prime Minister, that 'the account is melancholy and it cannot be looked upon in other than a most serious light. We are confident that the accounts are under-rated rather than exaggerated [...] I am sorry to give you so desponding a letter, but we cannot conceal from ourselves that the case is much worse than the public supposes.'[190] As a former student of Liebig's, Playfair had up-to-date knowledge on the chemistry of food and nutrition. Liebig had delivered some of his early findings at the British Association's 1837 conference in Liverpool. As Kenneth J. Carpenter notes: 'The association expressed great interest in his ideas and asked him to prepare a report. This has frequently been taken as the stimulus that completely changed Liebig's interests and caused him to write *Organic Chemistry in Its Relation to Agriculture and Physiology*, which appeared in 1840.'[191] At the 1842 meeting, unable to attend himself, Liebig asked Playfair to illustrate how his research was suggesting that, in the kind of plants eaten by man and graminivorous animals, the three nitrogenized compounds (fibrin, albumen, and casein) were '*absolutely identical with the chief constituents of the blood*'.[192] How beautifully simple, Playfair pointed out, 'does nutrition appear! These vegetable constituents which are used by animals to form blood, contain the essential ingredients for blood ready formed.'[193] After a warm reception both at the British Association and in his native Germany, Liebig published a synthesis of his major ideas in *Familiar Letters on Chemistry* (1843). Written in English, and edited by the surgeon John Gardner, the work was 'written for the especial purpose of [...] promoting, by every means, the study of a science so intimately connected with the arts, pursuits and social well-being of modern civilized

---

[190] Quoted in Woodham-Smith, *Great Hunger*, pp. 44–5.

[191] Kenneth J. Carpenter, *Protein and Energy: A Study of Changing Ideas of Nutrition* (Cambridge: Cambridge University Press, 1994), p. 47.

[192] Lyon Playfair, 'Professor Liebig's Report on "Organic Chemistry applied to Physiology and Pathology", *Report of the Twelfth Meeting of the British Association for the Advancement of Science* (London: John Murray, 1843), pp. 42–54 (p. 47). Italics in original.

[193] Ibid., p. 22.

nations'.[194] Thanks to 'accurate' and 'certain' research,[195] and to an 'alliance of chemistry and physiology', Liebig said, it was now possible to have 'a clear conception of the causes of hunger, of the exact nature of death; and [not be], as formerly, obliged to content ourselves with a mere descriptions of their symptoms'.[196]

Echoing the theories of both Hunter and Bichat on waste restoration, and Prout on assimilation, Liebig suggested that all animal organisms undergo 'perpetual change':

> These changes take place in the healthy animal body during every moment of life; a waste and loss of substance proceeds continually; and if this loss is to be restored, and the original weight and substance repaired, an adequate supply of materials must be furnished from whence the blood and wasted tissues may be regenerated. This supply is obtained from the food.[197]

Liebig hypothesized that in a healthy and successful species, a balance between the nitrogenized and the non-nitrogenized elements allows 'perpetual waste' to be resisted. In instances of starvation, however, the battle has been lost:

> If we deprive an animal of food, the weight of its body diminishes during every moment of its existence. If this abstinence is continued for some time, the diminution becomes apparent to the eye; all the fat of the body disappears, the muscles decrease in firmness and bulk, and, if the animal is allowed to die starved, scarcely any thing but skin, tendon, and bones remain.[198]

Liebig intended his observations to be applied to the human world. When our species moved from hunting and gathering to farming and shepherding, we found the necessary balance between the nitrogenized and the non-nitrogenized, for assimilation and respiration, in the smallest possible space.[199]

In seeming anticipation of Spencer's Social Darwinism, Liebig concluded that an unbalanced diet was characteristic of 'savages who live by the chase alone':

> Cultivation is the economy of force. Science teaches us the simplest means of obtaining the *greatest* effect with the *smallest* expenditure of power [...] The unprofitable exertion of power, the waste of force in agriculture, in other branches of industry, in science, or in social economy, is characteristic of the savage state, or of the want of knowledge.[200]

[194] Justus von Liebig, *Familiar Letters on Chemistry, and its Relation to Commerce, Physiology, and Agriculture* (Philadelphia: James M. Campbell, 1843), p. 3.
[195] Ibid., pp. 22, 29.   [196] Ibid., p. 21.   [197] Ibid., pp. 43–4.   [198] Ibid., p. 43.
[199] Ibid., p. 34.   [200] Ibid., pp. 33, 34. Italics in original.

Liebig intended for his *Letters* to be useful among political economists,[201] yet it is clear from what he writes that he had found *their* work to be useful in the formulation of *his* ideas: nations and tribes who fail to balance the nitrogenized and the non-nitrogenized were 'utterly incapable of increasing [their] number beyond a certain point, which is soon attained'.[202]

Without undervaluing the labours of Liebig, a man he greatly admired, G. H. Lewes was troubled by the way the former had assumed that the laws of chemistry would apply to physiology:

> The researches into the nature of Food have been extensive and minute, but they have been almost exclusively confined to alimentary substances, which have been analysed, weighed, and tabulated with great labour, and in a chemical point of view with considerable results; but in a physiological point of view—the only one really implicated—with scarcely any results at all.[203]

Liebig 'derided physiologists as being in no position even to comment until they had also made chemists of themselves'.[204] Lewes responded with the suggestion that, if the subject of (mal)nutrition is to 'receive any practical solution', it 'must no longer be left in [the] hands' of chemists:

> The chemist may analyse fat for [the physiologist]; but he, on receiving this analysis, will request the chemist *not* to trouble him with hypotheses respecting the part played by fat in the organism; for although the chemist may accurately estimate the heat involved in the oxidation of so much fat, the physiologist has to do with a vital laboratory extremely unlike that in which the chemist works, and he has to ascertain how the fat comports itself there.[205]

Lewes's use of term *vital laboratory* is highly revealing in this context. Made oxymoronic, it is contrasted to the laboratories of chemists, where accurate estimates may be made. 'In the vital laboratory' there can be no separation of a single point of evidence from other variables:

> The organism has no glass vessels, no air-tight cylinders. Vital processes go on in tissues which, so far from isolating the substance introduced—so far from protecting it from interference, do invariably interfere, and are *themselves involved* in the very changes undergone by the substance.[206]

---

[201] Ibid., p. 3.   [202] Ibid., p. 33.
[203] Lewes, *Physiology of Common Life*, vol. 1, pp. 56–7.
[204] Carpenter, *Protein and Energy*, p. 52.
[205] Lewes, *Physiology of Common Life*, vol. 1, pp. 58–9.   [206] Ibid., p. 112. Italics in original.

And even when Science shall have established laws on this point, such as may accurately express the general value of each substance as food, there will always remain considerable *difficulty in applying those laws*, owing to that peculiarity of the vital organism [...]—namely, that the differences among individuals are so numerous, and often so profound, as to justify the adage, 'one man's meat is another man's poison'.[207]

Lewes saw physiology as a means, not only of classifying and understanding natural phenomena, but of bringing into prominence the notion of 'variation of phenomena under varying conditions' as well.[208] In his later work *The Problems of Life and Mind* (1877), he extended Darwin's idea of natural selection to include the laws of physiology: what is true of species, he said, is also true of the organs in the body: they develop, succeed, and fail depending on the elements they interact with.[209] And what is true of materials is also true of processes. Digestion and hunger will vary according to 'environment' (in this case, general health, the functioning of other organs, the nature of food ingested, and so on). In *The Physiology of Common Life*, Lewes said 'we all know what Hunger is [...] but Science as yet has been unable to furnish any sufficient explanation of it'. A man 'under certain conditions will not survive six days' fasting, and under other conditions, he will survive six weeks'.[210] Against the confidence of a scientist like Liebig, he presented physiology as a field full of caution: it was able to tell a great deal about the stages of hunger, but only, to return to the words of P. W. Banks, if it was able to offer 'satisfaction to the inquiring mind'. In focusing on chemistry as a point of contrast with physiology, Lewes seems to have chosen a very different science to that of political economy to critique, and yet his identification of the problems in chemistry are the same that others saw in the reasoning of men who followed the principles of providentialist philosophy uncritically. Dedication to a catch-all theory relies upon the construction of a dogmatic laboratory, where evidence is brought in, subjected to a uniform set of sanitized processes, and repackaged as predictable hypotheses. In the vital laboratory of medical and physiological research anything may happen—evidence is brought in, is allowed to infect, grow, and seep beyond the vessels created for it; it is cautiously sent into the world with a hypothesis and a methodological appendix attached. Biological research was no less positivist or materialist than chemistry; in acknowledging how complete accuracy and objectivity was beyond its abilities, however, it developed a hermeneutics that could challenge, sometimes through accident and sometimes through design, the unreflecting commitments to laissez faire which dominated nineteenth-century perceptions of poverty.

---

[207] Ibid., p. 121. Italics added.
[208] George Henry Lewes, *The Problems of Life and Mind*, 3 vols (1877; Boston, MA and New York, NY: Houghton Mifflin, 1891), vol. 2, p. 6.
[209] Ibid., vol. 2, p. 124.   [210] Lewes, *Physiology of Common Life*, vol. 1, pp. 3, 9.

2

Charles Kingsley

'The Symbolism and Dignity of Matter'

In *Alton Locke* (1850), Kingsley's fictional autobiography of a tailor, poet, and Chartist, we are informed that 'grim and real is the action and the suffering'.[1] Working in the sweatshop system and in the world of literary hack-work, the eponymous hero experiences real starvation:

> And, here let me ask you, gentle reader, who are just now considering me ungentle, virulent, and noisy, did you ever, for one day in your whole life, literary, involuntarily, and in spite of all your endeavours, longings, and hungerings, *not get enough to eat*? If you ever have, it must have taught you several things.
>
> (p. 195; italics in original)

The address has much in common with Kingsley's review of *Mary Barton* (1848), discussed in my Introduction, which assumes that a well-off readership will have little understanding of, and have much to learn from, the sensation of *actual* hunger. The author's use of italics in '*not get enough to eat*' emphatically differentiates the *idea* of hunger from the reality: going without food is not the same as the usual 'endeavours, longings, and hungerings' of everyday life. The night that the starving Alton is banished from his mother's home for having intellectual desires that offend her narrow evangelicalism, he encounters a policeman who assumes he has been drinking:

> Before I had proceeded a quarter of a mile, a deadly faintness and dizziness came over me. I staggered, and fell against [some] railings.
>
> 'And have you been a-drinking arter all?'
>
> 'I never—a drop in my life—nothing but bread-and-water this fortnight.'
>
> And it was true. I had been paying for my own food, and had stinted myself to such an extent, that between starvation, want of sleep, and over-exertion, I was word to a shadow, and the last drop had filled the cup; [...] I dropped on the pavement, bruising my face heavily.   (p. 58)

---

[1] Charles Kingsley, *Alton Locke, Tailor and Poet. An Autobiography*, ed. by Elizabeth A. Cripps (1850; Oxford: Oxford University Press, 1983), p. 19. Subsequent references to this edition will be given in the text.

The Science of Starving in Victorian Literature, Medicine, and Political Economy. Andrew Mangham, Oxford University Press (2020). © Andrew Mangham.
DOI: 10.1093/oso/9780198850038.001.0001

This episode is similar to the real case of John Cooke, which was reported in *The Morning Chronicle* in 1828. (Kingsley was a reader of the *Chronicle* by the early 1830s, when he and many others read Henry Mayhew's journalistic accounts of the London poor.) Cooke died from what was believed to be 'want of food'; his body, when viewed by the coroner's jury, was described as having 'presented a most deplorable appearance—the bones nearly protruding through the skin'. So hungry had been the man that he was mistaken for a drunk by a watchman: 'He was lying on the pavement quite insensible; the watchman dragged him along the street, and, swearing dreadful oaths at him, called him a cursed drunken old scoundrel.'[2] Fortunately for Alton Locke, he and the policeman encounter two medical students soon after they encounter each other. The first assumption of the students is that the prostrate young man is a corpse, and that he might be appropriate furniture for their anatomist's table:

'What's that? Work for us? A demp unpleasant body?'

'I'll tell you what, Bromley, this fellow's very bad. He's got no more pulse than the Pimlico sewer. [...]'

'We shall have this fellow in phrenitis, or laryngitis, or dothen-enteritis, or some other it is, before long, if he's aggravated.'   (pp. 58–60)

Bromley and his companion revive Alton in a nearby gin shop. The first-person narrator then addresses the students as follows:

I have never met you again, but I have not forgotten you. Your early life may be a coarse, too often a profligate one—but you know the people, and the people know you: and your tenderness and care, bestowed without hope of repayment, cheers daily many a poor soul in hospital wards and fever-cellars—to meet its reward some day at the people's hands. You belong to us at heart, as the Paris barricades can tell. Alas! for the society which stifles in afterlife too many of your better feelings, by making you mere flunkeys and parasites, dependent for your livelihood on the caprices and luxuries of the rich.   (pp. 61–2)

These last words clearly belong to a narrator with Chartist sensibilities, yet they also demonstrate Kingsley's admiration for medicine as a panacea for social and spiritual diseases. In 'The Physician's Calling', a sermon he delivered in the 1870s for St. George's Hospital, he said that

healing of disease was an integral part of our Lord's mission. [...] If all classes did their work half as simply, as bravely, as determinedly, as unselfishly, as our

---

[2] Unsigned. 'Dreadful Case of Starvation', *Morning Chronicle*, 25 February 1828, p. 4.

medical men of Great Britain—and, I doubt not, of other countries in Europe—this would be a far fairer place than it is likely to be for any a year to come.[3]

In another scene in *Alton Locke*, the protagonist meets two agricultural labourers:

As we came up to the fold, two little boys hailed us from the inside—two little wretches with blue noses and white cheeks, scarecrows of rags and patches, their feet peeping through bursten shoes twice too big for them, who seemed to have shared between them a ragged pair of worsted gloves, and cowered among the sheep, under the shelter of a hurdle, crying and inarticulate with cold.

'What's the matter, boys?'

'Turmits is froze, and us can't turn the handle of the cutter. Do ye gie us a turn, please?'

We scrambled over the hurdles, and gave the miserable little creatures the benefit of ten minutes' labour. They seemed too small for such exertion: their little hands were purple with chilblains, and they were so sorefooted they could scarcely limp. I was surprised to find them at least three years older than their size and looks denoted [...]

I went on, sickened with the contrast between the highly-bred, over-fed, fat, thick-woolled animals, with their troughs of turnips and malt-dust, and their racks of rich clover-hay, and their little pent-house of rock-salt, having nothing to do but to eat and sleep, and eat again, and the little half-starved shivering animals who were their slaves.   (pp. 256–7)

In accordance to what the author believed about the importance of medical work, *Alton Locke* is most forceful when it focuses on bodies. There is anger over the disparity between the comfort of the sheep and the wretchedness of the boys, and Kingsley makes his feelings on the subject most apparent in the way he focusses on the boys' blue noses, white cheeks, chilblains, and sore feet. In his philosophy, 'spiritual good' comes from 'physical evil' once it is acknowledged how 'the salvation of our souls' depends upon 'the health of our bodies'.[4] He was 'famous', according to Christopher Hamlin, 'for trying to square the physical with the spiritual', and he was devoted to questions of sanitary reform.[5]

It might seem that the idea of 'the salvation of our souls' being dependent upon 'the health of our bodies' is yet another iteration of that ancient maxim

[3] Charles Kingsley, 'The Physician's Calling' in *The Water of Life and other Sermons* (London: Macmillan, 1879), pp. 14–26 (pp. 16, 18).

[4] Ibid., p. 16.

[5] Christopher Hamlin, 'Charles Kingsley: From Being Green to Green Being', *Victorian Studies*, 54:2 (2012), pp. 255–81 (p. 259). See also Pamela K. Gilbert, *Cholera and Nation: Doctoring the Social Body in Victorian England* (New York, NY: State University of New York Press, 2008), pp. 155–85.

'cleanliness is next to godliness'; yet what the representations of hunger in Kingsley's work suggest is that the subject of health involved more than the advocacy of sanitation or the attempt to find a place for a compromise between the physical and the spiritual. Health debate, for Kingsley, included a meditative attention to the scientific way of looking. He wrote in the *North British Review* in 1850: 'In proportion to a man's real inductive genius, whether in chemistry, anatomy, or any other inductive science, will be his cautious and reverent abstinence from hasty generalization.' In words prefiguring those that would be used by G. H. Lewes in *The Physiology of Common Life* (1859), he added that science requires 'continual self-distrust, continual watchfulness lest effects be attributed to wrong causes, continual suspicion of unperceived influences at work; the energies of a whole mind, and the labour of a whole life.'[6] As Will Abberley notes in his excellent essay on Kingsley and natural theology, 'studying [nature] could form part of humankind's elevation toward godly truthfulness.'[7] But only, I add, if humankind adopted the methodological scepticism that was integral to, and appropriated from, the human sciences.

Materialist Christianity

For Kingsley it was an essential belief that all intellectual roads lead to God and scientific study was, therefore, a tribute to the all-wise creator. It followed, then, that human perception was ultimately inferior to that of a higher truth. Later, in the 1860s, truth would become the basis of the author's famous disagreement with John Henry Newman. Although both men would turn the conflict into a debate about high church versus low, and Newman would write *Apologia pro Vita Sua* (1864) as a pre-emptive strike against suggestions that he had been dishonest in preaching Anglican creeds prior to his conversion to the Roman faith, the original topic on which their argument hinged was the nature of material truth. In a *Macmillan's Magazine* review of J. A. Froude's massive *History of England from the Fall of Wolsey to the Death of Elizabeth* (1856–70), Kingsley noted that 'Truth for its own sake, had never been a virtue with the Roman clergy, Father Newman informs us that it need not, and on the whole ought not to be.'[8] Newman was notoriously thin-skinned when it came to his religious conversion, and he took the comment as an attack on the constancy of his religious beliefs. Writing to the publishers of *Macmillan's*, he complained that 'there is no reference at the foot

---

[6] Kingsley, Charles. 'The Agricultural Crisis', *North British Review*, 14 (1850), pp. 85–121 p. 87.

[7] Will Abberley, 'Animal Cunning: Deceptive Nature and Truthful Science in Charles Kingsley's Natural Theology', *Victorian Studies*, 58:1 (2015), pp. 34–56 (p. 43).

[8] [Charles Kingsley], 'Froude's History of England, vols. VII and VIII', *Macmillan's Magazine*, 9 (1863–4), pp. 211–24 (p. 217).

of the page to any words of mine, much less any quotation from my writings'.[9] Shortly afterwards, he received a letter from Kingsley stating that his (Newman's) opinions on truth had been gleaned from the sermon 'Wisdom and Innocence', which had been published in *Sermons Bearing on the Subjects of the Day* (1843). Kingsley offered a rather tepid apology in *Macmillan's Magazine*, and both men would go on to write heated pamphlets defending their theological positions. It is worth looking closely at Kingsley's original argument that truth was not important to Catholicism or, at least, to Newman. The latter believed, according to Kingsley, that 'cunning is the weapon which Heaven has given to the saints wherewith to withstand the brute male force of the wicked world which marries and is given to marriage'.[10] Newman's insistence that such a view could not be found in any of his writings is only partly true; his sermon 'Wisdom and Innocence' did suggest that 'cunning', along with 'fleetness; or [...] a certain make and colour; or certain habits of living', was given to 'inferior animals' by God as compensation for 'their want of strength',[11] but nowhere does he say that cunning was given to the saints as a defence against the brute force of the non-celibate. Kingsley was on firm ground, however, with his citation of the seemingly opposing view that 'Truth, *for its own sake*, had never been a virtue with the Roman clergy'. Newman's sermon had preached a curious sort of epistemological laissez faire, where good Christians are expected to leave larger questions to the trust of the Almighty and satisfy themselves with a serene donothingism:

> Truth has in itself the gift of spreading, without instruments; it makes it way in the world, under God's blessing, by its own persuasiveness and excellence; 'So is the kingdom of God,' says our Lord, 'as if a man should cast seed into the ground, and should sleep, and rise night and day, and the seed should spring and grow up, he *knoweth not* how' [Mark 4.27].[12]

It was this advocacy of sitting back and watching truth find its own way that appears to have nettled Kingsley most. Whatever anti-Catholic mud he decided to fling later, his original antagonism was based on Newman's conception of truth, which went directly against his own.

As we shall see, Kingsley saw a productive, almost harmonic relationship between religion and the quest for truth in material science. Although generally sympathetic towards science, Newman was critical of the idea, then gaining traction (or so he believed), that devotion to the study of the natural world could

---

[9] Quoted in Ian Ker, *John Henry Newman: A Biography* (1988; Oxford: Oxford University Press, 1990), p. 533.

[10] Kingsley, 'Froude's History', p. 217.

[11] John Henry Newman, 'Wisdom and Innocence', in *Sermons Bearing on the Subjects of the Day* (London: J. G. F. and J. Rivington, 1843), p. 333.

[12] Ibid., pp. 303–4. Italics in original.

replace religious feeling. In a series of letters written to *The Times* in February 1841, responding to Robert Peel's opening of a new library and reading room in Tamworth, he criticized the materialist belief

> that the mind is changed by a discovery, or saved by a diversion, and can thus be amused into immortality,—that grief, anger, cowardice, self-conceit, pride, or passion, can be subdued by an examination of shells or grasses, or inhaling of gases, or chipping of rocks [...] If virtue be a mastery over the mind, if its end be action, if its perfection be inward order, harmony, and peace, we must seek it in graver and holier places than in Libraries and Reading-rooms.[13]

Contrary to what Kingsley believed, Newman insisted that those who 'give their leisure and curiosity to this world, [...] will have none left for the next'.[14]

Just a few years later, Kingsley was writing in *Alton Locke* that

> all analyses [...] whether of appearances, of causes, or of elements, only lead us down to fresh appearances—we cannot see a law, let the power of our lens be ever so immense. The true causes remain just as impalpable, as unfathomable as ever, eluding equally our microscope and our induction.   (p. 368)

It was in the context of a fairy tale, *The Water-Babies* (1863), that Kingsley was best able to demonstrate how 'there are a great many things in the world' which are invisible to the empiricist enterprise.[15] Here, as Jessica Straley observes, Kingsley 'recruits the scientific method's own principle of observation on behalf of an argument for possibilities that escape that method's reach'.[16] Addressing the child reader, Kingsley says:

> You must not talk about 'ain't' and 'can't' when you speak of this great wonderful world round you, of which the wisest man knows only the very smallest corner, and is, as the great Sir Isaac Newton said, only a child picking up pebbles on the shore of a boundless ocean. [...] You must not say that this cannot be, or that that is contrary to nature. You do not know what Nature is, or what she can do; and nobody knows; not even Sir Roderick Murchison, or Professor Owen, or Professor Sedgwick, or Professor Huxley, or Mr. Darwin, or Professor Faraday, or Mr. Grove, or any other of the great men whom good boys are taught to

[13] John Henry Newman, 'The Tamworth Reading Room', in *Discussions and Arguments on Various Subjects* (London: Basil Montagu Pickering, 1872), pp. 254–305 (p. 268).

[14] Ibid., p. 280.

[15] Charles Kingsley, *The Water-Babies*, in *The Water-Babies and Glaucus* (London: Dent, 1949), p. 41. Subsequent references to this edition will be given in the text.

[16] Jessica Straley, 'Of Beasts and Boys: Kingsley, Spencer, and the Theory of Recapitulation', *Victorian Studies*, 49:4 (1997), pp. 583–609 (p. 598).

respect. They are very wise men; and you must listen respectfully to all they say: but even if they should say, which I am sure they never would, 'That cannot exist. That is contrary to nature', you must wait a little, and see; for perhaps even they may be wrong. [...] Wise men are afraid to say that there is anything contrary to nature, except what is contrary to mathematical truth; for two and two cannot make five, and two straight lines cannot join twice, and a part cannot be as great as the whole, and so on (at least, so it seems at present): but the wiser men are, the less they talk about 'cannot'.   (p. 42–3)

Certainty does not apply to the natural world. Nature, Kingsley argued in his book on marine science *Glaucus; or, the Wonders of the Shore* (1855), is full of contradictions: things regress as well as progress, they move in cycles, and they produce matter for great curiosity. Such is evidence of an 'Infinite Maker [...] drawing ever fresh forms out of the inexhaustible treasury of the primeval mind'.[17] The complexity inherent to all living forms means that science has the privilege of teaching us what we do not know. In his letters, Kingsley wrote '*complete* nothing can be on this side of the grave' and 'a man [...] cannot sit down to speak the truth without disturbing in his own soul a hornet swarm of lies'.[18] In the absence of the *complete*, we ought to become more mindful of the significance of the partial. In his first novel, *Yeast* (1848), Claude Mellot, an artist, is advised:

> Follow in the steps of your Turners, and Landseers, and Stanfields, and Creswicks, and add your contribution to the present noble school of naturalist painters. [...] These [men have a] patient, reverent faith in Nature as they see her, their knowledge that the ideal is neither to be invented nor abstracted, but found and left where God has put it, and where alone it can be represented, in actual and individual phenomena. [...] The universal symbolism and dignity of matter, when in man or nature.   (p. 162)

Typical of Kingsley's writing, this is a passage that becomes revealing through its complexity and contradictions. On the one hand, the text appears to value a realism of sorts as the 'naturalist painters' know that the 'ideal' is not 'invented, or abstracted, but found and left where God has put it'—a good definition, we might say, of realism. However, what the novel seems to value, more than holding a mirror up to nature, is artistic subjectivity; it seeks a picture of nature as Turner and others see it, rather than how it might be captured with complete accuracy. The idea of a subject being '*represented* in *actual* and individual phenomena' is clearly

---

[17] Charles Kingsley, *Glaucus, or the Wonders of the Shore (1855)* in *The Water-Babies and Glaucus* (London: Dent, 1949), p. 252.

[18] Kingsley, letter to unknown correspondent (1840) and letter to Frances Kingsley (1848), in Kingsley, *L&M*, vol. 1, pp. 29, 142. Italics in original.

contradictory: if a phenomenon is actual, then it cannot also be a representation. This leads to the conclusion that realism is a form of interpretation in which the faculties of criticism and judgement are active. The term 'symbolism and dignity of matter' captures a powerful and seemingly oxymoronic idea: as well as having a dignity, by which we might read definition or wholeness, matter is also symbolic. It did not constitute, as Newman alleged, a rejection of higher feeling.

Though this is a philosophical point that cuts widely, it can be illustrated by the starving body which, as we have seen, symbolized different things to different readers. In Christian iconography, the emaciated body symbolized religious fervour, a mortification of the cumbersome flesh. It was simultaneously a rejection of the body and an embracing of its symbolic power. Claude Mellot is the only character, along with his wife Sabine, to appear in more than one of Kingsley's novels. First appearing in *Yeast*, he re-emerges in *Two Years Ago* (1857). In the later work he has become a photographer and a critic of the Pre-Raphaelite Brotherhood. Following nature, he says, the Pre-Raphaelites create a 'wilful ugliness of form' (p. 171) and appear to confirm, in their literalism, Newman's worst fears concerning the age's swing towards materialism:

> You must paint, not what is there, but what you see there. They forget that human beings are men with two eyes, and not daguerreotype lenses with one eye [...]; the only possible method of fulfilling the pre-Raphaelite ideal would be, to set a petrified Cyclops to paint his petrified brother.   (pp. 172–3).

Seemingly dismissive of his own art, Mellot appears to have learned the lesson that was taught to him in *Yeast*: having two eyes provides humans with conflicting images which, when combined in the brain, provide the impression of depth. The Pre-Raphaelites, Mellot argues, paint literally what is present rather than what their human subjectivities, the basis of the understanding of depth, teaches them. Like Turner and the other artists he was told to emulate, the true seers are those who are willing to acknowledge the act of perception as enriched and enlightened by the filter of human intellection.

Kingsley's attack on Newman, like his implied disparagement of naïve realism and literalism, were part of his insistence upon the recognition of the dynamic characters of natural phenomena and the sciences tasked with understanding them. The protagonists of his three social novels *Yeast*, *Alton Locke*, and *Two Years Ago* must each come to realize the larger philosophical and critical interpretations of matter before they can be successful in the social missions they undertake. In *Yeast*, Lancelot Smith learns this lesson through a mysterious prophet figure based on the Christian-Socialist theologian Frederick Denison Maurice. In response to Lancelot's complaint 'I have listened long to Nature's voice' but 'I hear nothing in her but the grinding of the iron wheels of mechanical necessity' (p. 180), the prophet asks:

> But do you remember what the prophet saw in the Valley of Vision? How first that those same dry bones shook and clashed together, as if uneasy because they were disorganised; and how they then found flesh and stood upright: and yet there was no life in them, till at last the Spirit came down and entered into them? Surely there is shaking enough among the bones now! [...] And as for flesh, what new materials are springing up among you every month, spiritual and physical, for a state such as 'eye hath not seen nor ear heard?'—railroads, electric telegraphs, associate-lodging-houses, club-houses, sanitary reforms, experimental schools, chemical agriculture, a matchless school of inductive science, an equally matchless school of naturalist painters,—and all this in the very workshop of the world!   (pp. 178–9)

The world's 'chaos of noble materials' are looking, the prophet says, for the 'one inspiring Spirit to organize, and unite, and consecrate this chaos' (p. 179). In Kingsley's philosophy, this inspiring spirit is bound up, as we might expect, with the teachings of Christianity; yet it is also comprised of the very human ability to labour: telegraphs, chemical agriculture, sanitary reform, like the dry bones in an anatomist's workshop, are materials to be worked with. A parable from *The Valley of Vision*, a book of prayers and devotions, is brought up-to-date for the nineteenth century and is fastened to that familiar term 'the workshop of the world', suggesting that the materials of the age are in a perpetual state of manufacture, modification, and repair and that the 'idea which shall reform the age' (p. 180) will be the one that acknowledges the dynamic, ever-changing, and conditional nature of things.

In Kingsley's next social novel, Alton Locke must come to a similar realization in order to find a spiritual fulfilment that will cohere with his socialist values. During his attendance at the Chartist demonstration of 1848, he becomes ill and feverish; his delirium includes an extraordinary series of Lamarckian dreams, the first of which has him imagining himself in the role of Sisyphus:

> An enormous, unutterable weight seemed to lie upon me. The bedclothes grew and grew before me, and upon me, into a vast mountain, millions of miles in height. Then it seemed all glowing red, like the cone of a volcano. I heard the roaring of the fires within, the rattling of the cinders down the heaving slope. A river ran from its summit; and up that river-bed it seemed I was doomed to climb and climb for ever, millions and millions of miles upwards, against the rushing stream. The thought was intolerable, and I shrieked aloud. A raging thirst had seized me. I tried to drink the river-water: but it was boiling hot—sulphurous—reeking of putrefaction.   (pp. 334–5).

Alton later dreams himself to be 'the lowest point of created life; a madrepore', plus various other creatures that might be arranged, depending on one's criterion, in a scale of ascending sophistication culminating with 'a baby-ape in Borneon forests'. After this stage of transmutation, Alton's 'self', in the dream, begins to degenerate. It is an extraordinary, if racially prejudiced, episode that will reward our detailed consideration:

> I saw my face reflected in the pool—a melancholy, thoughtful countenance, with large projecting brow—it might have been a negro child's. And I felt stirring in me, germs of a new and higher consciousness—yearnings of love towards the mother ape, who fed me and carried me from tree to tree. But I grew and grew; and then the weight of my destiny fell upon me. I saw year by year my brow recede, my neck enlarge, my jaw protrude; my teeth became tusks; skinny wattles grew from my cheeks—the animal faculties in me were swallowing up the intellectual. I watched in myself, with stupid self-disgust, the fearful degradation which goes on from youth to age in all the monkey race, especially in those which approach nearest to the human form. Long melancholy mopings, fruitless stragglings to think, were periodically succeeded by wild frenzies, agonies of lust and aimless ferocity. I flew upon my brother apes, and was driven off with wounds. I rushed howling down into the village gardens, destroying everything I met. I caught the birds and insects, and tore them to pieces with savage glee. [...] Then my cousin came—a hunter missionary; and I heard him talk to [his wife, Alton's unrequited love Lillian] with pride of the new world of civilization and Christianity which he was organizing in that tropic wilderness. I listened with a dim jealous understanding—not of the words, but of the facts. I saw them instinctively, as in a dream. She pointed up to me in terror and disgust, as I sat gnashing and gibbering overhead. He threw up the muzzle of his rifle carelessly, and fired—I fell dead, but conscious still. I knew that my carcase was carried to the settlement; and I watched while a smirking, chuckling surgeon dissected me, bone by bone, and nerve by nerve. And as he was fingering at my heart, and discoursing sneeringly about Van Helmont's dreams of the Archæus, and the animal spirit which dwells within the solar plexus, Eleanor glided by again, like an angel, and drew my soul out of the knot of nerves, with one velvet finger-tip.
>
> (pp. 340–1)

Eleanor Lynedale acts as Alton's social conscience throughout the novel, challenging the hero, for instance, when he seems ready to sacrifice his radical principles for the sake of commercial and critical success as a poet. In the closing stages of the novel she becomes a moral-force Chartist and convinces Alton that true social labour begins with spiritual work. The image of her plucking out Alton's soul from a 'knot of nerves' suggests that it is she who best understands the communion between body and soul. According to Rosemarie Bodenheimer, 'Alton's journey to "whole manhood" requires that he leave his lustful, violent, envious body behind';[19] Josephine Guy adds that the dream sequence 'clearly relates to Kingsley's emphasis on social reform through spiritual transformation' and 'jars so oddly with the verisimilitude of other parts of the novel'.[20] That the narrative fantasizes about a form of holy ascension is clear enough, but this is not a vision where the material is left behind. More specifically, corporeality and objects refuse to be shaken off: bed clothes become stifling, drinking water runs into reeking putrefaction, and the only ascension that happens with any success is the Sisyphean climbing of a volcano, or the perceived rise up an evolutionary scale. Moving forward, or upward, seems to involve accepting (and doing battle, as may be) with one's physical state. The image of the degenerating ape is one that advocates a sense of moral value as inseparable from a physiological or animal condition. The surgeon refers to Jan Baptist Van Helmont's *archæus* sneeringly because this was the term the seventeenth-century chemist gave to the vital principle or the 'spirit that he supposed existed in the body, for the purpose of regulating and keeping in order the innumerable glands, ducts and vessels'.[21] *Alton Locke*'s surgeon, we can assume, is a materialist, and his suggestive 'fingering' of Alton's heart is juxtaposed with Eleanor's 'velvet finger-tip', which is able to recognize Alton's spirit among his complex nerve tissues. This is not an allegory of matter being taken leave of, then, but of salvation being found among the intricate strands of the physical body. What is advocated is neither the materialism of the surgeon nor the vitalism of Van Helmont, but the critically sophisticated understanding of the material typified in the subjectivity of Eleanor Lynedale.

Finally, Kingsley's 'cholera novel' *Two Years Ago* is, in many senses, a gospel to Muscular Christianity. Although Kingsley himself rejected the term,[22] 'muscular Christian' is the perfect description for Tom Thurnall, the hero of the novel. He is a well-travelled physician, veteran of the Crimean War, and a lover of seaside studies. On a number of occasions, he is compared to his former schoolfellow, the poet Elsley Vavasour, a man whose poetry is dismissed by the narrative as impotent claptrap. 'Thank Heaven!' the poet says to Thurnall, 'that it was not my lot to become a medical man':

> Tom looked at him with the quaintest smile: a flush of mingled anger and contempt had been rising in him as he heard the ex-bottle boy talking sentiment: but he only went on quietly—

---

[19] Rosemarie Bodenheimer, *The Politics of Story in Victorian Social Fiction* (1988; Ithaca, NY and London: Cornell University Press, 1991), p. 148.

[20] Josephine M. Guy, *The Victorian Social-Problem Novel* (Basingstoke: Macmillan, 1996), p. 176.

[21] Unsigned. Review of *Culina Famulatrix Medicinæ* by Ignatius, *Edinburgh Review*, 6 (1805), pp. 350–7 (p. 356).

[22] In a letter to a fellow clergyman, Kingsley called the term 'painful' to him and 'offensive'. See Kingsley, *L&M*, vol. 2, p. 74.

'No, sir; with your more delicate sensibilities you may thank Heaven that you did not become a medical man; your life would have been one of torture, disgust, and agonising sense of responsibility.' (p. 192)

Kingsley, an excellent poet himself, was not likely to be dismissive of verse as a whole. As we shall see, he saw poetry as having important work to do, but only if it was rooted, like physical science, in the material world. As Thurnall says to Vavasour:

I often wonder why you poets don't take to the microscope, and tell us a little more about the wonderful things which are here already, and not about those which are not, and which, perhaps, never will be. [...] I always like to read old Darwin's 'Loves of the Plants'; bosh as it is in a scientific point of view, it amuses one's fancy without making one lose one's temper, as one must when one begins to analyse that microscopic ape called self and friends. (p. 190)

Thurnall is able to see, in line with Kingsley's own thinking, a world in which poetry is a form of science, and science a form of poetry, exactly as it had been for Erasmus Darwin.

Yet the hero of *Two Years Ago* also has his journey towards enlightenment to make. He boasts that he is 'F.R.C.S. London, Paris, and Glasgow' and that he has

been medical officer to a poor-law union, and to a Brazilian man-of-war. Have seen three choleras, two army fevers, and yellow-jack [yellow fever] without end. Have doctored gunshot wounds in the two Texan wars, in one Paris revolution, and in the Schleswig-Holstein row; beside accident practice in every country from California to China, and the round the world and back again. (p. 89)

Notwithstanding these impressive attainments, the narrative becomes critical of Thurnall's hyper-materialist approach to more 'moral' questions:

To whomsoever he met he must needs apply the moral stethoscope; sound him, lungs, heart, and liver; put his tissues under the microscope, and try conclusions on him to the uttermost. They might be useful hereafter; for knowledge was power: or they might not. What matter? Every fresh specimen of humanity which he examined was so much gained in general knowledge. Very true, Thomas Thurnall; provided the method of examination be the sound and the deep one, which will lead you down in each case to the real living heart of humanity: but what if your method be altogether a shallow and a cynical one, savouring much more of Gil Blas than of St. Paul, grounded not on faith and love for human beings, but on something very like suspicion and contempt? You will be but too likely, Doctor, to make the coarsest mistakes, when you fancy yourself most penetrating; to mistake the mere scurf and disease of the character for its healthy organic tissue, and to find out at last, somewhat to your confusion, that there are more things, not only in heaven, but in the earthiest of the earth, than are dreamt of in your philosophy.   (p. 112)

We are reminded of the passage in *The Water-Babies* instructing the reader to 'not talk about "ain't" and "can't" when you speak of this great wonderful world round you'. Thurnall's main infraction against Kingsley's 'pond-trawling, insect-watching Christianity'[23] is his confidence in his method of examination which, it is implied, is neither sound nor deep. Nor will it lead 'to the real living heart of humanity' which, typically of Kingsley, is presented as an idea, and an objective, that may be found in the 'earthiest of the earth' as long as one's methodology involves careful thought. In offering the pious character Grace Harvey his hand in marriage, Thurnall is given a chance at redemption. He realizes through her that 'our knowledge [does] not belong to us, but to Him who made us, and the universe' (p. 581) which is not a total abandonment of materialism or, as Straley suggests, an illustration of how 'scientific explanations are inadequate unless supplemented by aesthetic ideas',[24] but rather an acknowledgement, in tune with the teachings of physical scientists, that the material approach is always provisional and in need of humble self-examination.

1848

The year 1848 was one of considerable political activity for the young Kingsley. In April he travelled to London with the lawyer John Ludlow to witness the Chartist demonstration first hand. He was so overcome with what he saw that he wrote a notice addressed to the 'Workmen of England' in which he argued that, while the workers had been served badly by their government, the assembly of a vast number of disgruntled artisans was unlikely to meet with any happy result. As Larry Uffelman records, Kingsley's placard

proclaimed that true freedom cannot exist without virtue, nor 'true science without religion', nor true 'industry without the fear of God, and love to [one's] fellow citizens'. He declared that freedom comes with wisdom, because when the workmen are wise, they '*must* be free, for [they] will be *fit* to be free'.[25]

[23] Valentine Cunningham, 'Soiled Fairy: *The Water-Babies* in its Time', *Essays in Criticism*, 35:2 (1985), pp. 121–48 (p. 123).
[24] Straley, 'Beasts and Boys', p. 599.
[25] Larry K. Uffelman, *Charles Kingsley* (Boston, MS: Twayne, 1979), p. 19. Italics in original.

When the Charter failed, Kingsley liaised with Ludlow and Maurice on how to form a response to the problems of the working poor in a way that was based upon Christian, rather than revolutionary, principles. The result was the Christian Socialist movement. Maurice, the group's main voice, believed, in the words of Edward Norman, that 'the evil conditions of living and labour into which competitive economic practice had allowed the large majority of [his] brothers to fall was not only in itself disgraceful: it was a blasphemy, a denial of the intentions of God for his creatures'.[26] Christian Socialism was 'actively concerned with life, liberating and freeing men by causing them to acknowledge the reality of God and the society revealed by God through the Bible'.[27] The 'emphasis upon the spiritual condition of men [...] made [some] secular Socialists sceptical of its political seriousness',[28] yet Maurice insisted that 'the spiritual is also the practical' and that 'it was as needful to prove that the ladder had its foot upon the earth, as that it had come down from heaven'.[29] For Kingsley, more importantly, much of the good, practical work to be undertaken was supported by the methodological powers of physical science. In a short poem entitled 'A Parable from Liebig', written in 1848 and comprised of two stanzas, a picture of social and spiritual crisis is leavened by the ideas of the German chemist:

> The church bells were ringing, the devil sat singing
> On the stump of a rotting old tree;
> 'Oh faith it grows cold, and the creeds they grow old,
> And the world is nigh ready for me'.
> The bells went on ringing, a spirit came singing,
> And smiled as he crumbled the tree;
> 'Yon wood does but perish new seedlings to cherish,
> And the world is too live yet for thee.'[30]

Thematically, the poem anticipates the spiritual crisis of Matthew Arnold's more famous 'Dover Beach' (1867); yet, in terms of the intellectual response it makes to science, Kingsley's verse could not have been more different. Where the latter's 'naked shingles' symbolize the rawness of the age's crisis of faith, similar cycles of nature in Kingsley's poem (the rotting tree, the perishing wood) offer comfort against a bleak social backdrop. Specifically, Kingsley's poem was based on ideas from Liebig's *Chemistry: Its Application to Agriculture and Physiology* (1840).

[26] Edward Norman, *The Victorian Christian Socialists* (Cambridge: Cambridge University Press, 1987), p. 8.
[27] Uffelman, *Charles Kingsley*, p. 41.   [28] Norman, *Victorian Christian Socialists*, p. 6.
[29] Quoted in Norman, *Victorian Christian Socialists*, p. 8.
[30] Charles Kingsley, 'A Parable from Liebig' (1848), *Poems by Charles Kingsley* (New York, NY: J. F. Taylor, 1908), p. 257.

This work provided 'the first convincing explanation of the role of soil nutrients [...] in the growth of plants'.[31] As one of Liebig's earliest biographers, William Ashwell Shenstone, explains:

> Liebig pointed out that [...] all organised bodies after death suffer a change in consequence of which their remains gradually vanish. From the smallest twig to the largest tree all vegetables disappear after a few years, whilst animal matters once deprived of life and if exposed to the air are dissipated in a much shorter time, leaving only their mineral matter behind them. [...] They are then in the forms in which they can serve as food for new generations of plants and animals. [...] The death followed by the dissolution of one generation is the source of life for a succeeding generation.[32]

Liebig's research gave scientific weight to theories of natural circulation that had been the subject of literature for years. Alexander Pope wrote in his *An Essay on Man* (1734):

> See dying vegetables life sustain,
> See life dissolving vegetate again:
> All forms that perish other forms supply
> (By turns we catch the vital breath, and die,)
> Like bubbles on the sea of Matter born,
> They rise, they break, and to that sea return.[33]

Erasmus Darwin similarly wrote in *The Temple of Nature* (1803) that 'organic matter, unreclaim'd by Life, / Reverts to elements by chemic strife'.[34] And, in an 1850 article for *Household Words*, Percival Leigh updated *Hamlet*'s gravedigger scene to suit the age of Liebig. Narrated by a disgruntled undertaker, the article argues: 'science [...] is hammering into people's heads truths which they have been accustomed merely to gabble with their mouths—that all flesh is indeed grass, or convertible into it; and not only that the human frame does positively turn to dust, but into a great many things besides'.[35] The speaker is not happy with this turn of events as his trade relies upon the more Pagan view 'that what is buried, is the actual individual, the man himself'.[36] What Liebig's theories

---

[31] John Bellamy Foster and Fred Magdoff, 'Liebig, Marx, and the Depletion of Soil Fertility: Relevance for Today's Agriculture', *Monthly Review*, 50:3 (1998), pp. 43–60 (p. 44).

[32] William Ashwell Shenstone, *Justus von Liebig: His Life and Work (1803–1873)* (1895; London: Cassell, 1901), p. 66.

[33] *The Works of Alexander Pope*, 8 vols. (London: Longman et al., 1847), vol. 4, pp. 1–160 (p. 88).

[34] Erasmus Darwin, *The Temple of Nature; or, the Origin of Society* (London: J. Johnson, 1803), p. 44.

[35] [Percival Leigh], 'Address from an Undertaker to the Trade', *Household Words*, 1 (1850), pp. 301–4 (p. 302).

[36] Ibid., p. 303.

confirmed was that that which is buried is merely material: 'fluids and tissues' which 'decompose rapidly, and are dissipated, so that what is now part of the body of a Caesar or a Venus, may literally within a week become a turnip or a potato'.[37]

While Liebig's theory may seem to encourage the pessimistic outlook, to paraphrase Tennyson, that life fails beyond the grave, Kingsley's 'A Parable from Liebig' saw in the chemist's materialism something vital and hopeful. The theory offered the promise of regeneration and, as such, could be converted into a parable of the good work that remains to be done in the world, as long as one adopts the right way of interpreting its materials. The devil sitting on the stump of a tree sees only rotting matter, but the singing spirit, a symbol of scientific empiricism, sees life. Indeed, the line 'the world is too live yet for thee' embodies the findings of science, which, literally in Liebig's theories of decomposition, suggested 'life' continues after death.

Theories of decomposition shared with physiology the ability to blend subject and method. Chemists saw decay as a dynamic event in the 'life' of an organism, and this justified the claim of science that matter 'sings': it is alive with information to be gathered. As we saw in Chapter 1, physiologists similarly saw in cachexia, the living waste of starvation, a process that justified empirical interpretation; George Henry Lewes suggested, in response to Liebig, that human science was uniquely capable of understanding the larger meanings and ramifications of these ideas. 'A Parable from Liebig' is indicative of how Kingsley appropriated similarly complex epistemological questions: written in the turbulent year of 1848, the poem is a parable from Christian Socialism: the materialist interpretation of the world's complexities, as promoted through the physical sciences, is a way of tackling questions that interweave matters of faith and knowledge. 'A Parable from Liebig' is a tale from the self-reflexive hermeneutics of observational science: as the subject is alive, and protean in meaning, so the methodological approach must be active and alert, aware of when and how to interpret.

Tailor Hunting

In June 1849, Kingsley went to London to meet William A. Guy, Dean of the Medical Faculty of King's College. The author is likely to have met Guy through Maurice who, at that time, held a chair in History and Literature and Divinity at King's. On 12 June, Kingsley wrote to his wife: 'This morning I breakfasted with Dr. Guy, and went with him Tailor hunting, very satisfactory as yet.'[38] Kingsley

---

[37] James Finlay Weir Johnston, 'The Circulation of Matter' (1853), quoted in Christopher Hamlin, 'Providence and Putrefaction: Victorian Sanitarians and the Natural Theology of Health and Disease', *Victorian Studies*, 28:3 (1985), pp. 381–411 (p. 401).
[38] Kingsley, *L&M*, vol. 1, p. 167.

was by that time an avid amateur naturalist, and he had spent many an afternoon investigating the Devonshire coast, peering under rocks and seashells for rare zoophytes and plants. The natural—or, rather, unnatural—curiosity he was in search of in London was the starving tailor, the subject of both his tract *Cheap Clothes and Nasty* (1849), which had drawn heavily on Mayhew's *Morning Chronicle* articles, and the novel *Alton Locke*. In contrast to the 'honourable tailors' in the West End of the London, the East End workers were known to be employed by the 'dishonourable' sweating system. 'The greater part of the work, if not the whole', Kingsley's explains in his tract,

> is let out to contractors, or middle men—'*sweaters*', as their victims significantly call them—who, in their turn, let it out again, sometimes to the workmen, sometimes to fresh middlemen; so that out of the price paid for labour on each article, not only the workmen, but the sweater, and perhaps the sweater's sweater, and a third, and a fourth, and a fifth, have to draw their profit. And when the labour price has been already beaten down to the lowest possible, how much remains for the workmen after all these deductions, let the poor fellows themselves say![39]

The system gave rise to the worst sort of working environment: a place where tailors were effectively imprisoned while waiting for work to be allocated. As one of the tailors encountered by Kingsley reports:

> 'A man must not leave the premises when [not required to work],—if he does, he loses his chance of work coming in. I have been there four days together, and had not a stitch of work to do.' [...] It's generally remarked, that however strong and healthy a man may be when he goes to work at that shop, in a month's time he'll be a complete shadow, and have almost all his clothes in pawn. By Sunday morning, he has no money at all left, and he has to subsist till the following Saturday upon about a pint of weak tea, and four slices of bread and butter per day!!![40]

Another tailor recounts:

> *I worked for one sweater who almost starved the men; the smallest eater there would not have had enough if he had got three times as much. They had only three thin slices of bread and butter, not sufficient for a child, and the tea was both weak and bad. The whole meal could not have stood him in 2d. a head, and what made*

[39] Parson Lot [Charles Kingsley], *Cheap Clothes and Nasty* (1849; London: William Pickering, 1850), p. 5. For Mayhew's account, see 'London and the Poor', *The Morning Chronicle*, 14 December 1849, p. 5.
[40] Ibid., p. 7.

it worse was, that the men who worked there couldn't afford to have dinners, so that they were starved to the bone.[41]

Kingsley could not have selected a better guide for seeking out these unfortunates, for getting a good measure of their medical conditions, and for asking them the right kind of questions. William Guy was honorary secretary of the Statistical Society, an association that had, at one time or another, counted Nassau Senior, William Farr, and Thomas Malthus among its members. However much Farr's and Guy's medical expertise put them at odds with men like Malthus and Senior, the Society dedicated the majority of its time and energy to 'determining the state of English society. Studies of the living conditions of the urban poor were especially common' in the 1830s and '40s.[42] Guy later described the 1840s as a time when 'by lectures, by speeches, by printed appeals, and by all the legitimate machinery of a wholesome and successful agitation, I bore my part in that labour of love.'[43] He also held a chair in the relatively new science of forensic medicine and had written the pioneering *Principles of Forensic Medicine* in 1845. The book featured a chapter entitled 'Death from Starvation', in which Guy's main concern is with the use of hunger in criminal offences. For example, he outlines the 1753 case of Elizabeth Canning, an eighteen-year old who had been imprisoned then starved by the procuress 'Mother Wells'. According to Guy, Wells

> thrust [Elizabeth] into a back-room, or hay-loft, where she was confined for twenty-eight days, without fire, and with no food but some pieces of bread, amounting altogether to about a quarter of a loaf, about a gallon of water in a pitcher, and a small minced pie which she happened to have in her pocket. Canning further stated, that no human being had visited her during this time, and that, when her provision of bread and water was exhausted, she broke down a window-shutter which was fastened with nails, got out of the window onto a sort of pent-house, and thence jumped to the ground, nine of ten feet below. She reached home by walking as fast as her little remaining strength allowed.[44]

Imprisoned, starved, and exploited, Elizabeth experiences a similar ordeal to the sweatshop workers. Her case 'excited the sympathy and indignation of the public' and, in line with the zero-tolerance nature of the eighteenth century's penal code, Madam Wells was sentenced to death.[45] The Lord Mayor, Sir Crisp Gascoyne,

[41] Ibid. Italics in original.
[42] John M. Eyler, *Victorian Social Medicine: The Ideas and Methods of William Farr* (Baltimore, MD and London: The Johns Hopkins University Press), 1979, p. 16.
[43] William A. Guy, *Public Health: A Popular Introduction to Sanitary Science* (London: Henry Renshaw, 1870), p. 3.
[44] William A. Guy, *Principles of Forensic Medicine* (London: Henry Renshaw, 1845), p. 390.
[45] Guy, *Forensic Medicine*, p. 390.

commuted the sentence on the basis that Elizabeth's own account of her starvation was physiologically implausible:

> It was now Canning's turn to be put on her trial, for it was clear, that if the old woman was innocent, Canning must be guilty. She was accordingly indicted for perjury.
>
> A physician and an apothecary were examined as to her state of health at the time of her alleged escape from Mother Wells's loft. They stated that she appeared like one who had suffered extreme hunger, thirst, cold, but they acknowledged that a person might be as she was from other causes. After mature consideration of all the circumstances of the case, the jury brought a verdict of 'wilful and corrupt perjury', and the prisoner was sentenced to transportation for seven years.[46]

Guy concurred that the medical evidence was, on the whole, rather thin: 'there were many circumstances on which medical science might have thrown much light', yet, based on what proof there was, he saw the outcome as the correct one: 'life might have been prolonged for twenty-eight days, or even more, on this scanty supply of nourishment; but it is extremely improbable that, at the end of this time, she would have had strength enough left to effect her escape'.[47] As I have written elsewhere, one of the main tasks facing forensic medicine in the nineteenth century was making seemingly detached scientific methods work within a legal system that traditionally relied upon 'common-sense' ideas of right and wrong.[48] In contrast to ideas of 'obvious truth', forensic specialists such as Guy believed that, in cases where forensic evidence was important, expert interpretation of the clues left by bodies and circumstantial proof was vital to a successful prosecution. Hence, following Guy's account of Elizabeth Canning's story, there is, in his textbook, a list of the things to be looked for in cases of extreme hunger:

> *The Symptoms produced by protracted Abstinence* are pain in the epigastrium, relieved by pressure; emaciation, the eyes and cheeks sunken, the bones projecting, the face pale and ghastly, the eyes wild and glistening, the breath hot, the mouth dry and parched, intolerable thirst, delirium, extreme prostration of strength.
>
> After a longer interval the body exhales a foetid odour, the mucous membranes of the outlets become red and inflamed, and death takes place in a fit of maniacal delirium, or in horrible convulsions.[49]

In accordance with the medical idea of hunger as a form of corporeal wasting, Guy's description makes starvation look like decomposition: emaciation, sunken

---

[46] Ibid., p. 390.   [47] Ibid., p. 391.

[48] Andrew Mangham, *Dickens's Forensic Realism: Truth, Bodies, Evidence* (Columbus, OH: Ohio State University Press, 2016).

[49] Guy, *Forensic Medicine*, p. 389. Italics in original.

cheeks, a pale and ghastly face, a fœtid odour. As a man dedicated to forensic science and reform enterprises, Guy had an understanding of such evidence, ghastly though it was, as part of a moral crusade. In *Forensic Medicine*, the understanding of facts associated with malnourished bodies allows justice to be done in the courts of law; in more general terms, the focus on corporeal matter fits with Kingsley's notion, explored in his Liebigian parable, of knowledge of physical processes as being consummate with spiritual good.

Like many of his contemporaries, Kingsley had been moved by Mayhew's accounts of the labouring poor in *The Morning Chronicle*. After visiting the cholera districts of Bermondsey, which had been the focus of one of the *Chronicle*'s most alarming articles, Kingsley wrote to his wife, 'London is perfectly *horrible*':

> Oh God! What I saw! people having no water to drink—hundreds of them—but the water of the common sewer which stagnated full of [Mrs. Kingsley censors the description here], dead fish, cats and dogs, under their windows. At the time the cholera was raging, [we] saw them throwing untold horrors into the ditch, and then dipping out the water and drinking it!! [...] And mind, these are not dirty, debauched Irish, but honest hard working artizans. It is most pathetic [...] to see the poor souls' struggle for cleanliness, to see how they scrub and polish their little scrap of pavement, and then go through the house and see '*society*', leaving at the back poisons and filth—such as would drive a lady mad, I think, with disgust in twenty-four hours.[50]

There is hysterical energy in Kingsley's oscillations between the moral and the material in this letter. On the one hand, he uses a high language of disgust and prejudice, yet on the other, he employs a coarser language, tactfully expurgated by Mrs. Kingsley, describing what the filth actually consists of. Kingsley appears to be in search of some form of continuity between the materiality of the rotting bodies, the effluvia, the 'flesh and blood', and his moral indignation.[51] In an account of an Irish tailor's dwelling in *Alton Locke*, Kingsley writes:

> The stench was frightful—the air heavy with pestilence. The first breath I drew made my heart sink, and my stomach turn. But I forgot everything in the object which lay before me, as Downes tore a half-finished coat off three corpses laid side by side on the bare floor.
>
> There was his little Irish wife:—dead—and naked; the wasted white limbs gleamed in the lurid light; the unclosed eyes stared, as if reproachfully, at the husband whose drunkenness had brought her there to kill her with the pestilence; and on each side of her a little, shrivelled, impish, child-corpse,—the wretched man had laid their arms round the dead mother's neck—and there

---

[50] Kingsley, *L&M*, vol. 1, pp. 166, 177. Italics in original.   [51] Ibid., p. 177.

they slept, their hungering and wailing over at last for ever; the rats had been busy already with them—but what matter to them now?

'Look!' he cried; 'I watched 'em dying! Day after day I saw the devils come up through the cracks, like little maggots and beetles, and all manner of ugly things, creeping down their throats; and I asked 'em, and they said they were the fever devils.'

It was too true; the poisonous exhalations had killed them. The wretched man's delirium tremens had given that horrible substantiality to the poisonous fever gases.   (pp. 331–2)

The focus of this scene is tangible matter: air has a physiological effect on the narrator as he notices, in turn, the limbs, eyes, and postures of Downes's dead family. The rats have similarly looked upon the bodies as matters of mere flesh and used them as a means of assuaging their own hunger. There is, nonetheless, and in keeping with the teachings of Maurice and Guy, some attempt to turn away from matter and to link the sad and horrible spectacle to higher and more spiritual thoughts, as when the rhetorical question 'but what matter to them now?' asserts the belief that the body is but a shell and the spirit has departed. Downes attempts to convert chemical processes into 'fever devils', but corporeality refuses to be shaken off even here: the devils turn into 'maggots and beetles', and Alton confirms they are nothing more remarkable than the poisonous miasmas produced in squalid waters.

With seemingly nothing left to live for, Downes leaps into the squalid ditch at the back of his home:

We rushed out on the balcony. The light of the policeman's lantern glared over the ghastly scene—[...] with phosphorescent scraps of rotten fish gleaming and twinkling out of the dark hollows, like devilish grave-lights—over bubbles of poisonous gas, and bloated carcases of dogs, and lumps of offal, floating on the stagnant olive-green hell-broth—over the slow sullen rows of oily ripple which were dying away into the darkness far beyond, sending up, as they stirred, hot breaths of miasma—the only sign that a spark of humanity, after years of foul life, had quenched itself at last in that foul death. I almost fancied that I could see the haggard face staring up at me through the slimy water; but no, it was as opaque as stone.   (p. 333)

An attempt to overlay the scene with a dark language of poetry is stunted by the persistence of organic materials. For instance, the haggard face staring upward is, for all its forceful corporeality, a product of fancy; yet the way in which the ditch's slimy murk swallows up Downes's story is an indication of how the material is all-powerful, even in investigations, like those in *Alton Locke*, which seek emotional and moral explication. In the novel's descriptive accounts of the most poverty-stricken, humanitarianism is met with objects and environments which confirm the author's faith in the realist approach while simultaneously portraying the material world's refusal to be made simple and parabolic.

Like many of his contemporaries, Kingsley was sympathetic to the theoretical and political forces of Chartism yet deeply ambivalent about most forms of political and industrial action. After Alton Locke becomes involved in a rural uprising, he sickens and dies while on a voyage to America. Chastened during his illness, he repents of his radical fervour and spends his remaining days seeking spiritual redemption. Alton's most serious error of judgement, according to the novel, is his failure to seek a thoughtful balance between the material world and the immaterial one. Kingsley recognizes that, in Chartist rhetoric, there is a frequent lack of distinction between reality (starving, coldness, lack of wages) and belief or emotion (resentment, perception of workers' wrongs, pride). In the chaos of the socialist gathering in *Alton Locke*, the idea, reality, and symbol of starvation becomes the subject of a tug-of-war between rhetoric and reality. Alton narrates:

> I told them that I had come to entreat their assistance towards obtaining such a parliamentary representation as would secure them their rights. I explained the idea of the Charter, and begged for their help in carrying it out.
>
> To which they answered surlily, that they did not know anything about politics— that what they wanted was bread.
>
> [Alton tries to reason with them.]
>
> To all which they answered, that their stomachs were empty, and they wanted bread. 'And bread we will have!' [...] The murmur swelled into a roar, for 'Bread! Bread!' [...] And, amid yells and execrations, the whole mass poured down the hill, sweeping me away with them. I was shocked and terrified at their threats. [...] Trembling, I went on, prepared to see the worst; following, as a flag of distress, a mouldy crust, brandished on the point of a pitchfork.   (pp. 267–9)

What may be perceived here is a reversal of what we saw in the novel's description of Downes's hovel. Whereas in the latter the material is overwhelmingly present in the novel's moral and spiritual reflections, the riot scene converts what is real into something purely emblematic. Impervious to reason (importantly), the mob allows the feeling of hunger and the absence of bread to turn unto anger: the most apposite illustration of this translation is the crust of bread, stuck on the end a pitchfork and used as a battle standard to lead the oppressed into war. Like Joseph Rayner Stephens's famous definition of Chartism as 'a knife and fork, a bread and cheese question', it underscores the symbolic power of hunger in political conflict.[52]

[52] See Peter J. Gurney, '"Rejoicing in Potatoes": The Politics of Consumption in England During the "Hungry Forties"', *Past and Present*, 203 (2009), 99–136 (p. 100).

Alton's fatal mistake is feeling the 'maddening desire of influence' (p. 268) while on the podium. Instead of inciting the mob to remain peaceful, he articulates the view that the powerful 'rob you, crush you; even now they deny you bread' (p. 268); the magic word 'bread' does its dark work and rouses the crowd to violence. According to the teachings of Kingsley's faith, bread is both an object and a symbol—physically eaten during communion, it symbolizes the body of Christ. For Kingsley, communion was a solemn ritual,[53] one in which more unruly thoughts were disciplined by a measured understanding of the push and pull that comes, respectively, from the material and spiritual significances of the Eucharist. Writing about his anger over the treatment of East End tailors, Kingsley writes in 1849: 'If I had not had the communion at church today, I should have blasphemed in my heart, I think, and said the Devil is King!'[54] In the Condition of England debates, *Alton Locke* suggests, there needs to be a similar, solemn negotiation of the intersections between the material and the symbolic; in keeping with the principles of Christian Socialism, moreover, such negotiations learned as much from the book of matter as they did the book of God.

For all the faith Kingsley had in his ability to synthesize scientific and theological thought, however, his work often reveals the conflicts he felt he needed to square between these epistemological positions. Five or so years before he wrote *Alton Locke*, and three before he met Ludlow and Maurice, Kingsley was more concerned with rural poverty than with urban sweatshops. As 1845 faced up to the prospect of a winter famine in the south of England and news spread of the worsening condition of the potato crop in Ireland, Kingsley started up 'a small agricultural project called "our little industrial field of two acres", which created employment in the parish [of Eversley, northeast Hampshire, west of London] for four men for a month'.[55] It was about this time that he wrote a poem which I quote here in full:

THE POETRY OF A ROOT CROP
Underneath their eider-robe
Russet swede and golden globe,
Feathered carrot, burrowing deep,
Steadfast wait in charmèd sleep;
Treasure-houses wherein lie,
Locked by angels' alchemy,
Milk and hair, and blood, and bone,
Children of the barren stone.

---

[53] See Kingsley, *L&M*, vol. 1, p. 96.   [54] Kingsley, *L&M*, vol. 1, p. 180.
[55] J. M. I. Klaver, *The Apostle of the Flesh: A Critical Life of Charles Kingsley* (Leiden and Boston, MS: Brill, 2006), p. 105.

Children of the flaming Air,
With his blue eye keen and bare,
Spirit-peopled smiling down
On frozen field and toiling town—
Toiling town that will not heed
God His voice for rage and greed;
Frozen fields that surpliced lie,
Gazing patient at the sky;
Like some marble carven nun,
With folded hands when work is done,
Who mute upon her tomb doth pray,
Till the resurrection day.[56]

The conflicts in this verse crystallize Kingsley's search for some sort of balance between traditional, evangelical ideas about hunger and newer physiological and chemical approaches. In references to God's voice, angels' alchemy, surpliced fields, and a marble nun, Kingsley appears to veer into providentialist territory by speaking of heavenly judgement: famine is punishment, it seems, for 'rage and greed'. Against religious symbols, however, he juxtaposes corporeal materials: milk, hair, blood, and bone. Scientists, as we saw in Chapter 1, explored how food was 'transmuted by vital processes into [...] flesh and blood'.[57] Liebig saw in root crops the same nitrogenized compounds that formed '*the chief constituents of the blood*'.[58] What literally resides beneath the soil, then, are the seeds, or the germs, of bodily matter. But there is a symbolic interpretation even here. The way milk, hair, blood, and bone are locked into the ground signifies burial after death and reminds us of the idea of hunger as pathological. If this is a picture of God's judgement, it is not a judgement that leads, as the Bible would have it, to spiritual redemption or condemnation; things are weighed down either by their own materiality or something else's, echoing the medical view that starvation means real death and suffering, not a moral education or an abstract theory. 'The Poetry of a Root Crop' indicates how, in Kingsley's work, a battle of interpretation is fought over starvation, where old providential ideas meet new materialist ones. It would be foolish to claim that Kingsley resolved this tension in his own thinking: 'I am the strangest jumble of superstition and of a reverence for scientific induction', he wrote to one correspondent in 1857, 'a mystic in theory, and an

---

[56] Charles Kingsley, 'The Poetry of a Root Crop' (1845), *Poems*, p. 232.
[57] George Henry Lewes, *The Physiology of Common Life*, (London: William Blackwood and Sons, 1859), vol. 1, p. 52.
[58] Lyon Playfair, 'Professor Liebig's Report on "Organic Chemistry applied to Physiology and Pathology', *Report of the Twelfth Meeting of the British Association for the Advancement of Science* (London: John Murray, 1843), pp. 42–54 (p. 47). Italics in original.

ultra-materialist in practice'.[59] Yet his writings became a field in which this important tension was sown, harvested, and examined.

Yeast and Yeast

The 1848 novel *Yeast* saw Kingsley at his most radical and his most reliant on the physical sciences. The work was originally serialized in *Fraser's Magazine*, though its run was cut short because, according to the journal's editor John Parker, its radicalism upset some readers and caused a drop in sales.[60] In one chapter, Kingsley explains why he chose the title: 'these papers have been, from beginning to end, as in name, so in nature, Yeast—an honest sample of the questions, which, good or bad, are fermenting in the minds of the young of this day, and are rapidly leavening the minds of the rising generation'.[61] As J. M. I. Klaver has pointed out, the closure after just two months of *Politics for the People*, the periodical Kingsley set up with Ludlow following the failure of the Charter, was 'by no means the end of Kingsley's diatribe against the wrongs of the times. He steadily pumped everything he still wanted to say into *Yeast*, but this time without the censorship of Maurice or Ludlow'.[62] Kingsley intended his first major work to be a rousing comment on the volatile politics of the time.

His use of the yeast metaphor certainly appears to support such an interpretation. In the works on chemistry that Kingsley had read, Liebig had demonstrated that yeast (a single-cell micro-organism classified as a member of the fungus family) was an agent that was central to fermentation; it was also a volatile component which had a catalytic effect in a number of compounds. In the novel *Yeast*, Colonel Bracebridge says to the protagonist Lancelot Smith, about the possibility of the latter engaging in social debates: 'say to yourself boldly, as the false prophet in India said to the missionary, "I have fire enough in my stomach to burn up" a dozen stucco and filigree reformers and "assimilate their ashes" into the bargain, like one of Liebig's cabbages' (p. 55). Liebig's work on fermentation, decay, and assimilation suggested that yeast was a successful reagent because it was a substance 'already in a state of decomposition'.[63] His big idea, later discredited by Louis Pasteur, was that the living cells of yeast are 'always accompanied [...] by

[59] Kingsley, letter to John Bullar (1857), in Kingsley, *L&M*, vol. 2, p. 50. Italics in original.

[60] Susan Chitty, *The Beast and the Monk: A Life of Charles Kingsley* (London: Hodder and Stoughton, 1974), pp. 111–12.

[61] Charles Kingsley, *Yeast: a Problem* (1848; Dover, NH: Alan Sutton, 1994), pp. 140–41. Subsequent references to this edition will be given in the text. Hamlin notes that the title of *Yeast* suggests a 'pre-occupation with chemical transformation, and indeed the novel describes the spiritual and social transformations of its hero' ('Providence and Putrefaction', p. 402).

[62] Klaver, *Apostle of the Flesh*, p. 153.

[63] Liebig, Justus von. 'Lectures on Organic Chemistry, number 10', *Lancet*, 22 June 1844, pp. 395–8 (p. 395).

dead cells, and that it was the molecular motions of the decaying matter of [the] dead cells which was communicated to the sugar and brought about its decomposition and fermentation.[64] In the science of Liebig, yeast was paradigmatic of the emergence of new life out of old. In 'Old and New' (1848), the companion verse to 'A Parable from Liebig', Kingsley wrote:

> See how the autumn leaves float by decaying,
> Down the wild swirls of the rain-swollen stream.
> So fleet the works of men, back to their earth again;
> Ancient and holy things fade like a dream.
> Nay! See the spring-blossoms steal forth a-maying,
> Clothing with tender hues orchard and glen;
> So, though old forms pass by, ne'er shall their spirit die,
> Look! England's bare boughs show green leaf again.[65]

Reminiscent of early-modern poetry, which used an analogy with nature's cycles as a promise of individual rejuvenation, Kingsley's stanzas portray life and hope emerging from the material remains of the past. Read alongside Liebigian ideas of how microorganisms operate in fermentation, Kingsley's poem presents less of a picture of the old giving way to the new than it does of hope springing from the radical materiality of waste. In *Yeast*, social and physical corruption is the source of both disillusionment and a radical polemic:

Of all the species of lovely scenery which England holds, none, perhaps, is more exquisite than the banks of the chalk-rivers—the perfect limpidity of the water, the gay and luxuriant vegetation of the banks and ditches, the masses of noble wood embosoming the villages, the unique beauty of the water-meadows, living sheets of emerald and silver, tinkling and sparkling, cool under the fiercest sun, brilliant under the blackest clouds.—There, if anywhere, one would have expected to find Arcadia among fertility, loveliness, industry, and wealth. But, alas for the sad reality! the cool breath of those glittering water-meadows too often floats laden with poisonous miasma. Those picturesque villages are generally the perennial hotbeds of fever and ague, of squalid penury, sottish profligacy, dull discontent too stale for words.   (pp. 22–3)

In a seeming inversion of the shift that takes place in 'Old and New', glorious images of Romantic Arcadia give way to a grim reality comprised of bodily ailments and moral weaknesses. The references to 'sottish profligacy' and 'dull discontent' appear to broach the Malthusian idea that the people have only

---

[64] Shenstone, *Justus von Liebig*, pp. 72–3.   [65] Kingsley, 'Old and New' (1848), *Poems*, p. 258.

themselves to blame for their harsh living conditions, yet the narrative adds: 'There is luxury in the park, wealth in the huge farm-steadings, knowledge in the parsonage: but the poor? Those by whose dull labour all that luxury and wealth, ay, even that knowledge, it made possible, what are they?' (p. 23). Indeed, *Yeast's* radicalism uses a scientific language of materiality to challenge providentialist thinking. Of one poor man, the novel says, ironically,

> no doubt the fellow has committed an unpardonable sin in daring to come into the world when there was no call for him; one used to think, certainly, that children's opinions were not consulted on such points before they were born, and that therefore it might be hard to visit the sins of the fathers on the children, even though the labour market were a little overstocked.   (p. 76)

Out of its focus on the material and its appropriation of Liebig's chemical theories, *Yeast* ferments the more radical suggestion that extreme poverty is a socially created phenomenon linked to the 'luxury in the park' and the 'wealth in the huge farm-steadings'.

In fact, Kingsley would launch a virulent attack on Malthusian consequentialism both in a series of articles he wrote for *The Christian Socialist*, 'The Church versus Malthus' (1850), and an article he wrote for *Fraser's Magazine* in 1858, 'A Mad World My Masters'. In the former, Kingsley wrote: 'we will anathematize all doctrines whatsoever which "forbid men to marry"', adding that, as a Christian and a man who had devoted 'nine years of much thought, and somewhat extensive reading, on this very subject', he could not accept the major tenets of Malthusianism.[66] In 'A Mad World My Masters', he linked his ambivalence to his interest in science:

> [One] school of political economy, which has now reached its full development, has taken all along a view of man's relation to Nature diametrically opposite to that taken by the Sanitary Reformer, or indeed by any other men of science. The Sanitary Reformer holds, in common with the chemist or the engineer, that Nature is to be obeyed only in order to conquer her; that man is to discover the laws of her existing phenomena, in order that he may employ them to create new phenomena himself; to turn the laws which he discovers to his own use; if need be, to counteract one by another. [...]
>
> By political economy alone has this faculty been denied to man. In it alone he is not to conquer nature, but simply to obey her. Let her starve him, make him a slave, a bankrupt, or what not, he must submit, as the savage does to the hail and

---

[66] Parson Lot [Charles Kingsley], 'The Church *versus* Malthus', *The Christian Socialist*, 15 February 1851, p. 121 and 29 March 1851, p. 170.

the lightning. 'Laissez-faire', says the 'Science du neant', the 'Science de la misere', as it has truly and bitterly been called; 'Laissez- faire'. Analyse economic questions if you will: but beyond analysis you shall not step. Any attempt to raise political economy to its synthetic stage is to break the laws of nature, to fight against facts—as if facts were not made to be fought against and conquered, and put out of the way, whensoever they interfere in the least with the welfare of any human being. The drowning man is not to strike out for his life lest by keeping his head above water he interfere with the laws of gravitation.[67]

The comparison of political economy with sanitary reform, chemistry, and engineering suggests that Kingsley had a preference for hands-on activity over number-compiling. The reference to nature as an all-powerful energy that might be fought against is indicative of how he saw scientific activity: it was, he suggests, a method of challenging 'fact' as well as ascertaining it; that something was an alleged truth was no reason, in his philosophy, to accept it. In accordance with what medical experts such as William Guy were writing about the body, Kingsley saw science as giving us the tools for pulling truth apart, anatomizing its influence, and questioning its workings.

What Kingsley appears to have disliked most about political economy was its tendency to encourage donothingism. In a letter to John Bullar written the year before he wrote 'A Mad World My Masters', he argued:

It says, There are laws of nature concerning economy, therefore you must leave them alone to do what they like with you and society! Just as if I were to say, You got the cholera by laws of nature, therefore you must submit to cholera; you walk on the ground by laws of nature, therefore you must never go up stairs.[68]

Kingsley believed that the laws of nature could be managed through physical science: 'Nature must', he insisted, 'be counteracted, lest she prove a curse and a destroyer, not a blessing and a mother'.[69] In a later collection of writings, *Health and Education* (1874), he illustrated how the laws of political economy were a call to action, rather than a justification of inaction:

What physical science may do hereafter I know not; but as yet she has done this:

She has enormously increased the wealth of the human race; and has therefore given employment, food, existence, to millions who, without science, would either have starved or have never been born. She has known that the dictum of the early political economists, that population has a tendency to increase faster

---

[67] Charles Kingsley, 'A Mad World My Masters', Fraser's Magazine, 57 (1858), pp. 133–42 (p. 135).
[68] Charles Kingsley, letter to John Bullar (1857), in Kingsley, *L&M*, vol. 2, pp. 64–5.
[69] Kingsley, *L&M*, vol. 2, p. 67.

than the means of subsistence, is no law of humanity, but merely a tendency of the barbaric and ignorant man, which can be counteracted by increasing mani-fold by scientific means his powers of producing food.[70]

Kingsley was writing as a disciple of Liebig. The chemist, as we have discussed, demonstrated the importance of decomposing minerals on the development of new life. His research, significantly, was linked to the reason Malthus's prognosti-cations were not realized: the invention of artificial fertilizer allowed production, in the West at least, to keep pace with growing populations.[71] As one of Liebig's most successful students, August Wilhelm von Hofmann, said in a lecture to the Chemical Society some years later: 'Science, meantime, speaking with Liebig's voice, overruled [Malthus's] gloomy forebodings, and showed the collective organism of mankind to be a self-supporting institution.'[72] There is both a mater-ial and a philosophical point to all of this. In *Alton Locke* the protagonist asks his fellow tailor and Chartist John Crossthwaite whether he believes in 'Malthusian doctrines?' He replies, 'I believe them to be an infernal lie [...] There's room on English soil for twice the number there is now' (p. 112). Liebig's science provided evidence that discredited Malthus's prognostications, but also, through its dynamic understanding of the fluid and changeful nature of matter, it provided a paradigm for taking evidence, and not theory, as read. Kingsley later writes in *Alton Locke*:

> The frightful scenes of hopeless misery which we witnessed—the ever widening pit of pauperism and slavery, gaping for fresh victims day by day, [...] the know-ledge that there was no remedy, no salvation for us in man, that political econo-mists had declared such to be the law and constitution of society, and that our rulers had believed that message, and were determined to act upon it;—if all these things did not go far towards maddening us, we must have been made of sterner stuff than any one who reads this book. (pp. 195–6)

What is at fault here is not the hypothesis itself, but the way in which it has roamed, as truth, across social and political planes.

The Chadwickiad

The well-to-do Lancelot Smith becomes a prophet of positivism in *Yeast*, and, as Klaver rightly suggests, the hero's own lack of balanced thinking is, largely speak-ing, rather naïve: 'It takes time before [he] realizes that the mere study of nature

---

[70] Charles Kingsley, *Health and Education* (1874; New York, NY: D. Appleton, 1893), p. 290.
[71] See Robert H. Kargon, *Science in Victorian Manchester: Enterprise and Expertise* (Manchester: Manchester University Press, 1977), pp. 102–3.
[72] Quoted in Kargon, *Science in Victorian Manchester*, p. 104.

makes him "hear nothing in her but the grinding of the iron wheels of mechanical society".[73] After encountering the conditions of the labouring classes and forming a friendship with the left-leaning Tregarva, a gamekeeper, the protagonist rashly decides to dedicate his life to social reform: 'He took up, with a new interest, [Carlyle's] "Chartism"' and recontemplated 'the terrible warnings of the modern seer, and his dark vistas of starvation, crime, neglect, and discontent' (p. 53). Speaking of the impact of health science on the Condition of England question with Bracebridge, he says:

> 'What a yet unspoken poetry there is in that very sanitary reform! It is the great fact of the age. We shall have men arise and write epics on it, when they have learnt that "to the pure all things are pure", and that science and usefulness contain a divine element, even in their lowest appliances'.
> 'Write one yourself, and call it the *Chadwickiad*.'   (p. 54)

For all its irony, this passage reminds us of Kingsley's ability to see poetry in just about anything; just as he saw a curious sort of dignity in root crops, he now finds epic poetry in sanitary science—the discipline concerned with dirt and sewage, 'those real devils and "natural enemies" of Englishmen, carbonic acid and sulphuretted hydrogen' (p. 54). The lowest applications of science, it seems, contain a 'divine element', yet Lancelot's positivist confidence is, like Chadwick's comments on starvation in the 1830s, ill judged. In a conversation about religion he has with his main love interest, Argemone, he is asked:

> 'What do you believe in?' [...]
> 'In this!' he said, stamping his foot on the ground. 'In the earth I stand on, and the things I see walking and growing on it. There may be something beside it— what you call a spiritual world. But if He who made me intended me to think of spirit first, He would have let me see it first. But as He has given me material senses, and put me in a material world, I take it as a fair hint that I am meant to use those senses first, whatever may come after. I may be intended to understand the unseen world, but if so, it must be, as I suspect, by understanding the visible one: and there are enough wonders there to occupy me for some time to come.'
> 'But the Bible?' (Argemone had given up long ago wasting words about the 'Church.')
> 'My only Bible as yet is Bacon. I know that he is right, whoever is wrong. If that Hebrew Bible is to be believed by me, it must agree with what I know already from science.'
> What was to be done with so intractable a heretic? Call him an infidel and a Materialist, of course, and cast him off with horror.   (p. 90)

---

[73] Klaver, *Apostle of the Flesh*, p. 160.

This is an extraordinary dialogue, full of conflict and telling clues as to how materialism is perceived in Kingsley's work. Firstly, there is an elision between what one believes in and the strategies used to interpret the world. Living a material existence was not, as Kingsley himself admitted, tantamount to being a materialist, and yet such is what Lancelot believes when he stamps his foot on the ground and asserts that his solid foundations and his 'material senses' are reasons for him to *believe in* materialism as though it were a religion. As a young Karl Marx said, writing to his father in 1837, 'If the Gods had before dwelt above the earth they had now become its centre.'[74] Lancelot contradicts himself by suggesting that, as God 'has given me material senses, and put me in a material world, I take it as a fair hint that I am meant to use those senses *first, whatever may come after*'. There is the idea here that material is the starting point of a spiritual or epistemological (the text does not differentiate between the two) journey. Kingsley wrote in a letter to the physician and zoologist George Rolleston that 'the soul of each living being down to the lowest, secretes the body thereof, as a snail secretes its shell.'[75] The same argument gets repeated on a couple of occasions in *The Water-Babies*: 'your soul makes your body, just as a snail makes his shell'; 'you must know and believe that people's souls make their bodies, just as a snail makes its shell' (pp. 54, 135). The material, for Kingsley, was 'the expression in terms of matter' of a longer process of development which included spiritual and philosophical elements.[76] As already noted, he made no distinction between the practices of faith and abstract thinking; he adapted, in his Lamarckian episode in *Alton Locke*, the example of phylogenesis into a parable of material interpretation forming the first, crucial part of a larger enterprise which includes faith in a higher power. Where Lancelot goes wrong is in his belief that 'there are enough wonders' in the material world 'to occupy [him] for some time to come'; his materiality is not like a snail's shell, to be cast off in favour of sublime thought, but an immovable part of him: 'I am under the strange hallucination that my body is part of me, and [...] look with horror at a disembodied immortality' (p. 21). In rejecting the Bible in favour of Francis Bacon, he further offends Argemone by bringing his materialism within sight of atheism.

Herbert Spencer

During his later years, Kingsley became a devotee of Herbert Spencer, the theorist who saw 'adversity [as], in many cases, the only efficient school for the

[74] Karl Marx. Letter to Heinrich Marx, November 1837, in *Writings of the Young Marx on Philosophy and Society*, trans. and ed. by Loyd D. Easton and Kurt H. Guddat (1967; Indianapolis, IN: Hackett, 1997), pp. 39–50, p. 39.
[75] Charles Kingsley, letter to George Rolleston (1862), in Kingsley, *L&M*, vol. 2, p. 133.
[76] Kingsley, letter to Rolleston, p. 133. In *The Water-Babies*, Tom is said to swim away from his 'sooty old shell' as a 'cassid does when its case of stones and silk is bored through' (p. 47).

transgressor. [...] Nature provides nothing in vain.'[77] We can, of course, trace a direct line from Malthus to Spencer; both men saw nature as self-correcting and, when applied to human experience, famine and disease—though terrible—were not unnatural. In *Health and Education*, Kingsley noted that 'those terrible laws of natural selection, which issue in "the survival of the fittest", cleared off the less fit, in every generation, principally by infantile disease, often by wholesale famine and pestilence; and [left] on the whole, only those of the strongest constitutions to perpetuate a hardy, valiant, and enterprising race.'[78] Such views were not always a direct response to Spencer. As early as 1849 Kingsley gave three sermons on the cholera epidemic which had occurred in the same year, arguing that the pestilence was 'God's judgement, God's opinion, God's handwriting on the wall against us for our sins of filth and laziness, foul air, foul food, foul drains, foul bedrooms.'[79] On the subject of famine, then at its most destructive in Ireland, he adds:

> Famines come by a nation's own fault—they are God's plainly spoken opinion of what *He* thinks of breaking His laws of industry and thrift, by improvidence and bad farming. So when a nation becomes poor and bankrupt, it is its own fault; that nation has broken the laws of political economy which God has appointed for nations, and its ruin is God's judgement, God's plain-spoken opinion again of the sins of extravagance, idleness, and reckless speculation.[80]

Kingsley's Christian belief that the soul transcends the body after a lifetime of earthly lessons allows him to preach, in spite of his dismissals of Malthus's view of nature, the message that hunger and pestilence were two of the means through which species, populations, and individuals learn hard but salutary lessons: 'we may believe that this very cholera is meant to be a blessing; that if we will take the lesson it brings, it will be a blessing to England.'[81] In a later homily on cholera, delivered in 1866, he notes:

> God uses the powers of nature to do his work; of Him it is written, 'He maketh the winds His angels, and flames of fire His ministers.' And so this minute and invisible cholera-seed is the minister of God, by which he is visiting from house to house, searching out and punishing certain persons who have been guilty, knowingly or not, of the offence of dirt; of filthy and careless habits of living [...] This outbreak of cholera in London, considering what we now know about it,

---

[77] Herbert Spencer, *The Proper Sphere of Government* (London: W. Brittain, 1843), pp. 13, 35. See Michael W. Taylor, *The Philosophy of Herbert Spencer* (London: Continuum, 2007), pp. 56, 107. On Kingsley's love of Spencer, see Susan Chitty, *The Beast and the Monk: A Life of Charles Kingsley* (London: Hodder and Stoughton, 1974), p. 272.
[78] Kingsley, *Health and Education*, p. 2.
[79] Charles Kingsley, 'First Sermon on the Cholera', *Sermons on National Subjects* (London: Macmillan, 1880), pp. 134–43 (p. 141).
[80] Ibid., p. 140.   [81] Ibid., pp. 141–42.

and have known for twenty years past, is a national shame, scandal and sin, which, if man cannot and will not punish, God can and will.[82]

Kingsley anticipates an objection that others might have had to this rather Old Testament view: 'this cholera has not slain merely families, who were more or less responsible for the bad state of their dwellings; but little children, aged widows, and many other persons who cannot be blamed in the least'. His answer uses a quote from the Bible (John 10:50), but which, in this context, reads exactly like Spencer: 'we must believe that this cholera is an instance of the great law, which fulfils itself again and again, and will to the end of the world—"it is expedient that one die for the people, and that the whole nation perish not"'.[83]

As a general rule, the more religious Kingsley is, and the least concerned, therefore, with tangible matter, the more reactionary is his message. When drawing on scientific ideas, with the exception of Spencer's loosely scientific conclusions, he is more inclined to challenge the kind of thinking employed by providentialist political economists and biological determinists. In 'Human Soot' (1870), for instance, a sermon he delivered at the Kirkdale Ragged School in Liverpool, he returned to Liebig in order to suggest that, rather than being God's will, poverty was the refuse and responsibility of industry:

> It is no-one's fault, just because it is every one's fault—the fault of the system. But it is not the will of God; and therefore the existence of such an evil is proof patent and sufficient that we have not yet discovered the whole will of God about this matter [...] Our processes are hasty, imperfect, barbaric—and their result is vast and rapid production: but also waste, refuse, in the shape of a dangerous class. We know well how, in some manufactures, a certain amount of waste is profitable—that it pays better to let certain substances run to refuse, than to use every product of the manufacture [...] So it is in our present social system. It pays better, capital is accumulated more rapidly, by wasting a certain amount of human life, human health, human intellect, human morals, by producing and throwing away a regular percentage of human soot—of that thinking acting dirt, which lies about, and, alas! breeds and perpetuates itself in foul alleys and low public houses, and all dens and dark places of the earth.[84]

In Malthusian and Spencerian theory, waste (the production of that 'dangerous class', the poverty-stricken) is an ordinary part of nature; it is salutary in its long-term workings. Employing Liebigian ideas on dynamic decomposition allows 'Human Soot' to return to the idea, also explored in *Yeast*, that poverty constitutes

---

[82] Charles Kingsley, 'Cholera, 1866', *Water of Life*, pp. 189–202 (pp. 190–1).

[83] Ibid., pp. 191–2.

[84] Charles Kingsley, 'Human Soot' (1870), *All Saints' Day and other Sermons*, ed. by W. Harrison (London: Macmillan, 1909), pp. 302–11 (pp. 305–6).

unnatural waste. What is more, the seemingly paradoxical view that material evidence shows what is *not* known ('the existence of this evil is proof patent and sufficient that we have not yet discovered the whole will of God about this matter') derives, I argue, from the methodological scepticism of medicine. In one his most scientific sermons, 'The Physician's Calling', Kingsley argued that the medical profession was ordained from on high, the evidence being that Christ was himself a healer: 'The Gospels never speak of disease or death as necessities; never as the will of God'.[85] Directly contradicting what he says in his cholera sermons, he adds:

> The Gospels, and indeed the Scripture, very seldom palliate the misery of disease, by drawing from it those moral lessons which we ourselves do. [...] It would be a miserable world, if all that the clergyman or the friend might say by the sick-bed were, 'This is an inevitable evil, like hail and thunder. You must bear it if you can: and if not, then not'.[86]

Kingsley was never more ambivalent about disease and disorder as heavenly decrees than when he was talking about medicine and physiology. On the subject of hospitals, Kingsley writes:

> But this I have a right to say,—that whatever objections, suspicions, prejudices there may be concerning any other form of charity, concerning hospitals there can be none. Every farthing bestowed on them must go toward the direct doing of good. There is no fear in them of waste, of misapplication of funds, of private jobbery, of ulterior and unavowed objects. Palpable and unmistakable good is all they do and all they can do. And he who gives to a hospital has the comfort of knowing that he is bestowing a direct blessing on the bodies of his fellow-men; and it may be on their souls likewise.[87]

The belief in the moral spotlessness of all hospital operatives is naïve, to be sure, yet Kingsley's use of adjectives such as 'direct', 'palpable', and 'unmistakable' highlights how he saw medicine to be doing good because it was doing material, tangible work. Including high praise for doctors—'excellent men', as he calls them[88]—his sermon challenges the view that disease, filth, starvation, and paucity are all a part of God's plan by presenting social problems as physical challenges to be overcome. In *Health and Education*, he says that though Nature's 'teeth [...] are very strong', it is possible for science to 'tame her and break her in to his use'.[89] 'Only as far as we understand Nature', he says, 'are we safe from it'. Addressing Nature directly, he says: 'I find something in me which I do not find in you; which

---

[85] Kingsley, 'The Physician's Calling', p. 14.   [86] Ibid., p. 15.   [87] Ibid., pp. 22–3.
[88] Ibid., p. 17.   [89] Kingsley, *Health and Education*, p. 261.

gives me the hope that I can grow to understand you, though you may not understand me; that I may become your master, and not as you now, you mine'.[90] It was
only when he was away from his pulpit, and sitting in his library of scientific trea-
tises, that Kingsley could be so optimistic. In a letter to one correspondent he
wrote: 'A crisis, political and social, seems approaching, and religion, like a root-
less plant, may be brushed away in the struggle.' If anything, 'it is the scientific
go-ahead-ism of the day which must save us'.[91] At no point, however, does he
suggest that science, man, or reason will have an easy time of it in the years to
come. References to nature's sharp teeth and to struggle, as well as the perceived
need to tame, break, master, and be safe from nature, all suggest that the materialist approach is beset with difficulties. In spite of his frequent recourse to heroic
language, Kingsley's conflicts between science and religion indicate how the strategies of pragmatism and materialism are made useful through difficult reasoning.

Flesh and Blood Poetry

In *Politics for the People*, Kingsley stated that if the socialist project was to be
taken seriously, it would need to dissociate its writings from cheap fiction:

> The other day, being in London, I said to myself, 'I will see what the Chartists are
> doing and saying just now'; and I set off to find a Chartist newspaper—and
> found one in a shop [...] Now, as a book, as well as a man, may be known by his
> companions, I looked round the shop to see what was the general sort of stock
> there—and, behold, there was hardly anything but 'Flash Songsters', and the
> 'Swell's Guide', and 'Tales of Horror', and dirty milk-sop French novels.[92]

Although the kind of popular literature described here was the subject of many a
critical attack for its salacious content, *Alton Locke* suggests that Kingsley's objection has more to do with a perceived lack of realism. In *Alton Locke*, we are taken
into the bookshop of Sandy MacKay, where the protagonist encounters 'books
books books!' (p. 34)—the nourishment he has been yearning for. Among such
treasures he encounters more wholesome companions than the trash fictions
mentioned in *Politics for the People*: 'Carlyle's works' (p. 65), naturally, and,

> in the midst of all this chaos grinned from the chimney-piece, among pipes and
> pens, pinches of salt and scraps of butter, a tall cast of Michael Angelo's well-
> known skinless model—his pristine white defaced by a cap of soot upon the top

---

[90] Ibid., pp. 262–3.
[91] Charles Kingsley, letter to Richard Powles (1846), quoted in Klaver, *Apostle of the Flesh*, p. 109.
[92] Charles Kingsley, 'Letters to the Chartists I', *Politics for the People*, 6 May 1848, pp. 28–30 (p. 28).

of his scalpless skull, and every muscle and tendon thrown into horrible relief by the dirt which had lodged among the cracks. There it stood, pointing with its ghastly arm towards the door, and holding on its wrist a label with the following inscription:—

Here stand I, the working man,

Get more off me if you can.   (p. 64)

The anatomical model's muscles and tendons, covered in dirt, look back or forward to the pauper atomies encountered in Kingsley's Bermondsey expedition, Downes's hovel, and the agricultural slums of *Yeast*. The couplet on the model's wrist reminds us that anatomical models are metonyms: MacKay intends this replica to signal the hunger of the working man, but, as a model, its function is to *signify*—to indicate something that it is not. This represents MacKay's philosophy concerning literature; prefiguring what would be written on the subject by G. H. Lewes and Emile Zola later in the century,[93] the Scotsman believes that literature ought to be a mode of representation that is mindful of its artifice yet, like an anatomical model, faithful to the original. When the young Alton Locke produces his first poem he writes fifty fantastic stanzas set on a South Sea Island. After having had it read to him, MacKay says:

What the deevil! is there no harlotry and idolatry here in England, that ye maun gang speering after it in the Cannibal Islands? Are ye gaun to be like they puir aristocrat bodies, that wad suner hear an Italian dog howl, than an English nightingale sing, and winna harken to Mr. John Thomas till he calls himself Giovanni Thomasino; or do ye tak yourself for a singing-bird, to go all your days tweedle-dumdeeing out into the lift [sky], just for the lust o' hearing your ain clan clatter? Will ye be a man or a lintic? Coral Islands? Pacific? What do ye ken about Pacifics? Are ye a Cockney or a Cannibal Islander?   (p. 86)

MacKay then takes Alton to St. Giles's, a district as well-known as Jacob's Island for its poverty and filth. What the hero finds there are bodies, smells, offal, sewage, and waste:

From the butchers' and greengrocers' shops the gas lights flared and flickered, wild and ghastly, over haggard groups of slip-shod dirty women, bargaining for

[93] I have in mind Lewes's 'Realism in Art: Recent German Fiction', in *Westminster Review*, 70 (1858), pp. 488–518, and Zola's 'Le Roman Experimental' (1880) and 'Les Roman Naturalistes (1881), both in *The Experimental Novel and Other Essays*, trans. by Belle M. Sharman (New York, NY: Cassell, 1893). For an excellent discussion of these texts in relation to the rise of realism and naturalism, see Charlotte Sleigh, 'The Novel as Observation and Experiment', in *The Routledge Companion to Nineteenth-Century British Literature and Science*, ed. by John Holmes and Sharon Ruston (London: Routledge, 2017), pp. 71–86.

scraps of stale meat and frost-bitten vegetables, wrangling about short weight and bad quality. Fish-stalls and fruit-stalls lined the edge of the greasy pavement, sending up odours as foul as the language of sellers and buyers. Blood and sewer-water crawled from under doors and out of spouts, and reeked down the gutters among offal, animal and vegetable, in every stage of putrefaction. Foul vapours rose from cowsheds and slaughter houses, and the doorways of undrained alleys, where the inhabitants carried the filth out on their shoes from the back-yard into the court, and from the court up into the main street; while above, hanging like cliffs over the streets—those narrow, brawling torrents of filth, and poverty, and sin,—the houses with their teeming load of life were piled up into the dingy, choking night. A ghastly, deafening sickening sight it was.   (p. 87)

For the most part, this is a passage that would not be out of place in Mayhew's journalism, so dedicated is it to the grim realities of the metropolis. MacKay tells Alton to study these very realities. 'Keep your eyes open' he says:

Look! there's not a soul down that yard but's either beggar, drunkard, thief, or warse. Write anent that! Say how you saw the mouth o' hell, and the twa pillars thereof at the entry—the pawnbroker's shop o' one side, and the gin palace at the other—twa monstrous deevils, eating up men, and women, and bairns, body and soul. [...] Which is maist to your business?—thae bare-backed hizzies that play the harlot o' the other side o' the warld, or these—these thousands o' bare-backed hizzies that play the harlot o' your ain side—made out o' your ain flesh and blude? You a poet! True poetry, like true charity, my laddie, begins at hame. If ye'll be a poet at a', ye maun be a cockney poet [...] Canna ye see it there?   (pp. 88, 87–9)

Poetry begins at home, but it also begins, according to MacKay, with 'flesh and blude'—material realities understood poetically. No advice could have been more Carlylean. In 1833, the 'modern seer' had written in the *Foreign Quarterly Review* that authors and poets

must, in a new generation, gradually do one of two things: either retire into nurseries, and work for children, minors and semifatuous persons of both sexes; or else, what were far better, sweep their Novel-fabric into the dust-cart, and betake them with such faculty as they have to understand and record what is *true* [...]! Poetry, it will more and more come to be understood, is nothing but higher Knowledge; and the only genuine Romance (for grown persons), Reality.[94]

---

[94] Quoted in Kathleen Tillotson, *Novels of the Eighteen-Forties* (1954; Oxford: Oxford University Press, 1961), p. 155. Italics in original.

In his 1832 review of the work of working-class poet Ebenezer Elliot (an inspiration for Alton Locke), Carlyle noted: 'The great excellence of our Rhymer [...] we take to consist even in this, often hinted at already, that he *is genuine*. Here is an earnest truth-seeking man; no theoriser, sentimentalizer, but a practical man of work and endeavour, man of sufferance and endurance'.[95] In the opening paragraphs of *Alton Locke*, the protagonist explains how he did manage to become a 'poet of the people' (p. 6). His literary efforts have been concerned with 'reeking garrets', 'workrooms', 'disease', 'brick and iron', and 'poisonous smoke'. It has been an insight, he says, 'worth buying with asthma, and rickets, and consumption, and weakness' (p. 6). In 'Signs of the Times' (1829) Carlyle famously made it clear that he was no champion of Lancelot Smith's brand of materialism: the new 'Age of Machinery', he warned, was in danger of losing sight of its rich spiritual and intellectual heritage.[96] Practical truth-seeking was Elliot's key strength, and what edified Carlyle was the poet's ability to find authenticity among the spiritual, as well as material, needs of the people; his power was in balancing the material and the spiritual without dismissing either.

In Kingsley's later novel, *Two Years Ago*, the abstract-wordsmith Elsley Vavasour is compared unfavourably with Tom Thurnall, a man who understands the poetry of nature, but is determined to deal with its worst aspects head on. Another man who measures up badly to the hero is old Dr. Heale, a physician whose practice is based mainly on fee husbandry. Heale believes, along with many of his contemporaries, that disease and death, famine and filth, are all divine judgements: 'my opinion always was with the Bible, that 'tis jidgment, sir, a jidgment from God, and we can't escape His holy will, and that's the plain truth of it' (p. 258). Having a scientific mindset, Thurnall has a different idea of 'plain truth'; 'He had heard that "'tis jidgment" from every mouth during the last few days' (p. 258). Exasperated by the fact that so many characters, including Heale, perceive the novel's cholera epidemic to be God's will, and that there was little, therefore, that might be done to control it, Thurnall tells the young priest, Frank Headley, that:

Well, I hate disease. Moral evil is your devil, and physical evil is mine. I hate it, little or big; I hate to see a fellow sick; I hate to see a child rickety and pale; I hate to see a speck of dirt in the street; [...] I hate to see anything wasted, anything awry, anything going wrong; I hate to see water-power wasted, manure wasted, land wasted, muscle wasted, pluck wasted, brains wasted; I hate neglect, incapacity, idleness, ignorance, and all the disease and misery which spring out of that. There's my devil; and I can't help it for the life of me, going right at his throat, wheresoever I meet him!   (p. 268)

---

[95] Thomas Carlyle, 'Corn-Law Rhymes', *Edinburgh Review*, 55 (1832), pp. 338–61 (p. 345). Italics in original.

[96] See Thomas Carlyle, 'Signs of the Times', *Edinburgh Review*, 49 (1829), pp. 439–59 (p. 442).

In mentioning of the waste of muscle, pluck, and brains alongside the squandering of non-human resources such as water, manure, and land, Thurnall brings together Liebig's idea on waste with the physiological concept of the wast*ing* of the corporeal. As the latter's discussion made plain that cachexia was a pathological state for all organisms, so Kingsley's association of the waste of resource and the waste of muscle, pluck, and brains, makes it clear that extreme poverty is nothing that can be termed salutary. The mention of 'disease and misery' springing out of 'neglect, incapacity, idleness, [and] ignorance' could also be read as a return to the providentialist argument put forward in the cholera sermons. However, in the novel, Thurnall is critical of the impotent verses of Elsley Vavasour, whose transports of ecstasy over abstractions and fantasies form an unfavourable comparison with the hero's desire to roll up his sleeves and get on with the work in hand. In this context, 'neglect, incapacity, idleness, [and] ignorance' are more likely to refer to the donothingism of the solvent classes than to the alleged aberrant behaviours of the poor. Material problems need material solutions, it seems, and it is in the dosomethingism of science that Kingsley finds his most consistent and philosophical vocabulary of reform.

3

Elizabeth Gaskell

'Clemming'

Mrs. Gaskell told Mr. Travers Madge that the one strong impulse to write 'Mary Barton' came to her one evening in a labourer's cottage. She was trying hard to speak comfort, and to allay those bitter feelings against the rich which were so common with the poor, when the head of the family took hold of her arm, and grasping it tightly said, with tears in his eyes: 'Ay, ma'am, but have ye ever seen a child clemmed to death?'[1]

Although there is no evidence to suggest that this anecdote, originating in an 1895 issue of *The Gentleman's Magazine*, is anything other than apocryphal, a number of scholars have argued that we have every reason to take it seriously as an insight into the social and epistemological preoccupations of Gaskell's fiction. Jenny Uglow argues that *Mary Barton* (1848) has 'all the urgency of such a confrontation; the father's voice literally gripped [the author]. [...] The book was born of her own shock and guilt.'[2] Jane Spencer, meanwhile, believes that Gaskell 'turn[ed] this potent expression of the difference between rich and poor into the starting-point for an exploration of their common humanity'.[3] That Gaskell would develop a form of social-problem fiction that took the perceived differences between the rich and poor, and the possibly of reconciliation between them, as two of its central themes is well established. Without disagreeing with the idea that the anecdote captures something very pertinent to Gaskell's work, I wish to suggest that if the labourer's question does represent a 'confrontation' and a 'shock', it does so because it introduces a form of thinking about poverty that accords more with the terms and ideas of medical experts than with the conservative assumptions of some political economists. Words of comfort, reasoning, and moral instruction are all well and good, the labouring man appears to suggest, but *actually seeing* what happens when a child starves to death is an experience that presents a different—more maddening—set of facts to interpret. Commenting at

---

[1] Unsigned, 'Mrs. Gaskell', *Gentleman's Magazine*, 279 (1895), pp. 124–38 (pp. 130–1).
[2] Jenny Uglow, *Elizabeth Gaskell: A Habit of Stories* (London: Faber and Faber, 1993), p. 193.
[3] Jane Spencer, *Elizabeth Gaskell* (London: Macmillan, 1993), p. 33. See also John Geoffrey Sharps, *Mrs. Gaskell's Observation and Invention: A Study of her Non-Biographic Works* (Sussex: Linden Press, 1970), p. 56.

The Science of Starving in Victorian Literature, Medicine, and Political Economy. Andrew Mangham,
Oxford University Press (2020). © Andrew Mangham.
DOI: 10.1093/oso/9780198850038.001.0001

either end of Gaskell's career, John Elliotson and George Henry Lewes wrote of the physiology of starvation that it was a 'frightful spectacle' and 'terrible' to witness, respectively.[4] Such 'terrible' and 'frightful' realities are not included in *The Gentleman's Magazine*'s account of Gaskell's encounter with the poor labourer, yet such details are no less powerful in their absence. In *Mary Barton*, the novel purportedly inspired by the labouring man's question, the symptoms of hunger are drawn in intense and persistent detail. Along with accounts of poor sanitation and fever, literary critics have usually considered the story's descriptive passages as a means of confronting readers with a true account of the distresses caused by the industrial way of life. Angus Easson claims, for instance, that Gaskell is 'concerned to establish a physical reality, unknown to her readers'. She 'guides readers she feels to be venturing on unfamiliar ground'.[5] Sheila M. Smith suggests that 'the ordinary middle-class and upper-class Victorian simply did not see the poor'; Gaskell thus aimed 'to make her reader see what she describes', to tell the 'truth about' poverty.[6] On the specific subject of starvation, Lesa Scholl believes that Gaskell was one of a number of authors who, 'through their fictional narratives, were able to give faces, names, and, most crucially, voices, to [...] starving figures'.[7] However, the problem that Gaskell encounters in the impoverished districts of Manchester, and which her alleged meeting with the poor labourer illustrates rather well, is that starvation already had a face and a voice for general readers; there was no need to establish a view of poverty, to make it familiar, or to lead the reader into *terra incognita* because these things were already known well—perhaps too well—through endless pages of governmental blue books, social reports, committee minutes, and journalistic accounts. What the labourer's insistence upon starving children does highlight, and which is important, is how material knowledge has the potential to destabilize a way of talking about poverty that had become too familiar and which had little to do with reality. The *Gentleman's Magazine* does not record what Gaskell's words of comfort and peace-making were; yet the fact that she aimed to allay bitter feelings against the rich is a good hint that her words may have followed the common line, inspired by political economy, that sought to move the onus of responsibility onto the poverty-stricken

---

[4] John Elliotson, *Human Physiology* (London: Longman et al., 1835), pp. 53–4; George Henry Lewes, *The Physiology of Common Life* (London: William Blackwood and Sons, 1859), p. 21. This was the year that Gaskell wrote in a letter to Charles Norton (25 and 30 October 1859) that she considered 'Mr Lewes' character & opinions [...] (formerly *at least*) so bad'; Gaskell Letters, pp. 579–82 (p. 582. Italics in original). In 1849 Gaskell attended one of Lewes's lectures at the Manchester Athenaeum. 'I did not like [him] at first', she writes in a letter to Edward Chapman, but I have liked him better every time I have seen him' (9 March 1849); Gaskell Letters, pp. 72–3 (p. 72). The lecture was not a success, she claims, due to the volume of other events taking place in Manchester the same evening.

[5] Angus Easson, *Elizabeth Gaskell* (London: Routledge and Kegan Paul, 1979), p. 75.

[6] Sheila M. Smith, *The Other Nation: The Poor in English Novels of the 1840s and 1850s* (Oxford: Clarendon Press, 1980), pp. 33, 39, 91.

[7] Lesa Scholl, *Hunger Movements in Early Victorian Literature: Wants, Riots, Migration* (London: Routledge, 2016), p. 2.

themselves—suggesting that things would be improved if the labourer was better at saving money, or if he kept a better home, or had fewer children, and so on. The labourer's response is an indication of the power that starvation, as reality, had in the 1840s: it was a protest, a confrontation, a mode of countering the laissez-faire principles that had come to dominate social discourses. As Mary Poovey notes, Gaskell approaches the Condition of England question 'as a problem of epistemology'.[8] If she did have such an encounter with a labourer, it shows in her industrial novels, all of which, I argue, demonstrate some antipathy towards proselytizing on the basis of various kinds of social, statistical, and economic theory, not because, as she disingenuously suggested, she knew 'nothing of Political Economy, or the theories of trade',[9] but because she believed the ready-made, popular rhetoric to be guilty of both obfuscating reality and discouraging the kind of critical reflection that the social problems of the age required.

Modes of Thinking

In *Mary Barton*, at the point in the narrative where Job Legh speaks to Mr. Carson about the enmity between masters and workers, the former says:

> I'm not given to Political Economy, I know that much. I'm wanting in learning, I'm aware; but I can use my eyes. I never see the masters getting thin and haggard for want of food; I hardly ever see them making much change in their way of living, though I don't doubt they've got to do it in bad times. [...] For sure, sir, you'll own it's come to a hard pass when a man would give aught in the world for work to keep his children from starving, and can't get a bit, if he's ever so willing to labour.   (p. 453)

---

[8] Mary Poovey 'Disraeli, Gaskell, and the Condition of England', in *The Columbia History of the British Novel*, ed. by John J. Richetti, John Bender, Deirdre David, and Michael Seidel (New York, NY: Columbia University Press, 1994), pp. 508–32 (p. 521). Contrary to what I argue here, Poovey sees the epistemological problem as a gendered one, where the stories of individual case histories and domestic experience offer a more valuable, and literary, insight into the problems of industrialization.

[9] Elizabeth Gaskell, *Mary Barton*, ed. by Edgar Wright (1848; Oxford: Oxford University Press, 1998), p. xxxvi. Subsequent references to this edition will appear in the text. Hilary M. Schor writes that Gaskell's 'self-denigration is what Sandra Gilbert and Susan Gubar have called a "cover story"'; in her 'disavowal of authorial aggression, we can see her carving out for herself other territory (that of earnestness and truth)'. *Scheherazade in the Marketplace: Elizabeth Gaskell and the Victorian Novel* (Oxford: Oxford University Press, 1992), pp. 21–2. See also Elizabeth D. McCausland, 'Dirty Little Secrets: Realism and the Real in Victorian Industrial Novels', *American Journal of Semiotics*, 92:2/3 (1992), pp. 149–65 (p. 150); Josephine M. Guy, *The Victorian Social-Problem Novel* (London and Basingstoke: Macmillan, 1996), pp. 140–4; Gordon Bigelow, *Fiction, Famine, and the Rise of Economics in Victorian Britain and Ireland* (Cambridge: Cambridge University Press, 2003), p. 75; Carolyn Lesjak, *Working Fictions: A Genealogy of the Victorian Novel* (Durham, NC and London: Duke University Press, 2006), p. 32.

As in Gaskell's preface to the novel, the mention of political economy here is not intended to excuse ignorance, but to suggest that the subject which is immediately apparent—starving children and other physical signifiers of distress—is more important to the discussion than abstract principles. Similarly, in *North and South* (1854–5), Margaret Hale is initially sickened by Thornton's inflexible Malthusianism, which appears (to her) to rely upon biased assumptions about what an individual may or may not achieve: 'Oh, papa', she says,

> when he spoke of the mechanical powers, he evidently looked upon them only as new ways of extending trade and making money. And the poor men around him—they were poor because they were vicious—out of the pale of his sympathies because they had not his iron nature, and the capabilities that it gives him for being rich.[10]

Not only does the little amount of sympathy Thornton feels for the workers bother Margaret, but also the way in which his belief in poverty and hardship as 'the natural punishment of dishonestly-enjoyed pleasure' (p. 85) forbids his seeing the real, complex state of affairs. A similar implication of dogmatic thinking is urged against Thornton's main opponent in the novel, Nicholas Higgins, who judges, like Lancelot Smith in *Yeast* (1848), on material evidence alone. Rejecting, for instance, Mr. Hale's insistence upon an afterlife, he says:

> Now, yo' say these are true things, and true sayings, and a true life. I just say, where's the proof? There's many and many a one wiser, and scores better learned than I am around me,—folk who've had time to think on these things,—while my time has had to be gi'en up to getting my bread. [...] The purse and the gold and the notes is real things; things as can be felt and touched; them's realities.

Higgins's naïve empiricism is exposed as problematic in the contradictions underpinning what he says next:

> If salvation, and life to come, and what not, was true—not in men's words, but in men's hearts core—dun yo' not think they'd din us wi' it as they do wi' political 'conomy? They're mighty anxious to come round us wi' that piece o' wisdom; but t'other would be a greater conversion, if it were true.   (p. 226)

On the face of it, Higgins's comments represent a rejection of political economy in favour of spiritual conversion; what ought to be preached, he says, is that which is true, vaguely, because it exists 'in men's hearts core'. But such an assumption

---

[10] Elizabeth Gaskell, *North and South*, ed. by Angus Easson (1854–5; Oxford: Oxford University Press, 1998), pp. 87–8. Subsequent references to this edition will appear in the text.

must challenge Higgins's own insistence upon 'proof' and 'real things'. The evidence in support of the life to come's not being true is to be found, Higgins suggests, in the fact that it is not advocated by those who preach political economy; his ironic comment on the latter being a 'piece o' wisdom' is intended to indicate just how mistaken he is: there is no correlation, the text implies, between the popularity of a theory and its truth or value. Also, if something is a truth embedded in 'men's hearts core', we might ask why there is a need to preach it, as some did political economy. Indeed, Higgins seems to contradict his own love of material proof in asserting that a feeling can be a truth. Overall, his speech is a cautionary example of how the commitment to preaching a subject runs the risk of convincing the speaker that his belief is a truth. Gaskell is significantly less sympathetic to both Thornton's and Higgins's way of thinking than she is of Job Legh's. The latter's empiricism comes from a healthy interest in natural history which, his granddaughter suggests, keeps him away from proselytizing; it keeps him 'silent', 'deep and eager in solving a problem' (p. 45). These preoccupations are what lead to Legh's intelligent comments on what he sees: masters never getting thin, men doing 'aught in the world to keep [their] children from starving', and so on. He is not given to political economy, nor to Higgins's brand of naïve empiricism; he prefers instead to solve the problems based on what he sees—to think sensitively about material evidence.

What Legh represents is neither the dogmatism of the political economists, nor the knee-jerk reactions of 'common-sense' socialists such as Lancelot Smith. He represents the kind of intelligent response to material evidence that natural science at that time advocated. As a characterization of a way of thinking, Legh's empiricism is explored further, and more to the point, in the inquisitive and self-scrutinizing subjectivity of Margaret Hale. The heroine's interest in the industrial culture of Milton appears to furnish the novel with an examination of its own powers of realist description. As Hilary M. Schor observes: 'the explicit "use" of the heroine as textual transmitter—as a kind of interpreter among and between the many discourses of industrialization—suggests a self-consciousness about the text and authorship'.[11] Catherine Gallagher argues, similarly, that 'the point of view of the novel is only slightly distinct from Margaret's consciousness. [...] social and familial issues [...] are first related associatively through their simultaneous presence in Margaret's mind'.[12] Eleanor Courtemanche has added that 'the ultimate belief' of social problem novels like *North and South* is that 'industrial culture can be reformed by incorporating more sensitivity to the individual point of view'.[13] When Margaret's dying mother is visited by Dr. Donaldson, we

---

[11] Schor, *Scheherazade*, p. 121.

[12] Catherine Gallagher, *The Industrial Reformation of English Fiction, 1832–1867* (Chicago, IL and London: University of Chicago Press, 1985), p. 171.

[13] Eleanor Courtemanche, '"Naked Truth is the Best Eloquence": Martineau, Dickens, and the Moral Science of Realism', *ELH*, 73:2 (2006), pp. 383–407 (p. 383). A similar argument is made by Carolyn

are told that the physician is 'a quick observer of human nature' (p. 169); the trip that Margaret makes to the Thorntons' house soon afterwards, during which she becomes involved in the threating action prompted by the strike, reveals how the heroine is similarly skilled:

> She was struck with an unusual heaving among the mass of people in the crowded road on which she was entering. They did not appear to be moving on, so much as talking, and listening, and buzzing with excitement, without much stirring from the spot where they might happen to be. [...] From every narrow lane opening out on Marlborough Street came up a low distant roar, as of myriads of fierce indignant voices. The inhabitants of each poor squalid dwelling were gathered round the doors and windows, if indeed they were not actually standing in the middle of the narrow ways—all with looks intent towards one point. Marlborough Street itself was the focus of all those human eyes, that betrayed intensest interest of various kinds; some fierce with anger, some lowering with relentless threats, some dilated with fear, or imploring entreaty; and, as Margaret reached the small side-entrance by the folding doors, in the great dead wall of Marlborough mill-yard and waited the porter's answer to the bell, she looked round and heard the first long far-off roll of the tempest;—saw the first slow-surging wave of the dark crowd come, with its threatening crest, tumble over, and retreat, at the far end of the street, which a moment ago, seemed so full of repressed noise, but which now was ominously still.   (p. 172)

> Their reckless passion had carried them too far to stop—at least had carried some of them too far; for it is always the savage lads, with their love of cruel excitement, who head the riot—reckless to what bloodshed it may lead. A clog whizzed through the air. Margaret's fascinated eyes watched its progress.   (p. 179)

The only pair of 'human eyes' not focussed on Marlborough Street in the first of these passages is Margaret's: turned in the opposite direction, they observe the observers. In the second passage, she watches the clog which has been thrown and notices how it is the 'savage lads' who resort to violence, not the calm and orderly workers. The scene is typical of Gaskell's approach throughout *North and South*: the heroine's involvement with the realities of Milton's strife allows the text to advocate a more complex, accurate engagement with the realities at the heart of social conflict. Although Gaskell, as we have seen, was ambivalent about the kinds of positivism she portrayed in Higgins, she was nevertheless drawn to a style of writing that privileged direct observation, and the detailing of material realities, over any theoretical approach.

Betensky in *Feeling for the Poor: Bourgeois Compassion, Social Action, and the Victorian novel* (Charlottesville, VA and London: University of Virginia Press, 2010), p. 14.

In two 1850 letters written by Dickens, in which he invited Gaskell to write for *Household Words*, he astutely insisted that the latter's 'reflection or observation in respect of the life around you, would attract attention and do good'; and 'the tendency to detail, where detail is an indispensable part of the art and the reality of what is written (as it decidedly is, in your case) cannot be an objection or impediment to any kind of fiction'.[14] Indeed, in Gaskell's circle of influence, there was a sense that the true, complex state of things had been obscured by the way in which pet theories had been allowed to dominate a range of social discussions. In a review of *Mary Barton*, written in 1849, one commentator said that 'the questions involved [...] have for too many years been almost shelved in order to make way for selfish and time-serving contests of political factions'. Gaskell herself is guilty of such narrow dogmatism; while 'the work is based upon the results of actual observation', it must have been of 'a somewhat limited experience'.[15] The remedy to 'intemperate partisanship', wrote Gaskell's friends William and Mary Howitt, was education 'bound to no class', but dedicated to 'the cause of Peace, of Temperance, of Sanitary reform, of School for every class—to all the efforts of Free Trade, free opinion'.[16] 'Between the employer and the employed', they claimed, 'there lies one common ground of truth and sacred right'; 'look around', they advised; 'be at once firm and patient'.[17] These comments were written in the editorial of the short-lived weekly *Howitt's Journal*, the home of Gaskell's first prose compositions,[18] and the vehicle for articles on physiology and sanitary health by William Benjamin Carpenter and Thomas Southwood Smith respectively. The *Howitts'* readers were envisaged to be middle class, or 'ambitious artisans', and the first editorial address made it clear that a more careful attention to social issues, as guide and example, was a key objective;[19] while the editors spoke about 'truth and sacred right', they also signalled education, the act of looking around, and the practising of patience as vital activities in social reform. This was not a Gradgrindian insistence upon facts, or a dogged resolution to believe only in that which is directly experienced, but rather a promotion of more considered and analytical approaches, as exemplified in medical, physiological, and sanitary science.

[14] Charles Dickens, letter to Elizabeth Gaskell, 31 January 1850 and 5 February 1820, Dickens Letters 6, pp. 21–2, 29 (pp. 22, 29).
[15] Unsigned, Review of *Mary Barton*, *British Quarterly Review*, 9 (1849), pp. 117–36, (p. 117, 121).
[16] William and Mary Howitt, 'William and Mary Howitt's Address to their Friends and Readers', *Howitt's Journal*, 1 (1847), pp. 1–2 (p. 1).
[17] Ibid., p. 2.
[18] 'Libbie Marsh's Three Eras' (1847). As stories of a labouring woman's friendship with a sickly child, and the account of a rare holiday for Manchester's mechanics, the stories are, in many ways, a forerunner of *Mary Barton*, and they were ideally suited to the Howitts' interest in social conditions and 'real life'. See also Christine L. Krueger, *The Reader's Repentance: Women Preachers, Women Writers, and Nineteenth-Century Social Discourse* (Chicago, IL and London: Chicago University Press, 1992), pp. 161–9.
[19] Laurel Brake and Marysa Demoor (eds), *Dictionary of Nineteenth-Century Journalism in Great Britain and Ireland* (Gent: Academia Press, 2009), p. 293.

Howitt's Journal and Science

Southwood Smith wrote the first article to appear in *Howitt's*, and his friend and landlady, Mary Gillies, contributed the first short story, a sad tale of a labourer's family who succumb to the insanitary conditions they are forced to live under in London: 'Let no one think there is exaggeration in this tale of misery', Gillies warned; 'such wretched homes, and such harrowing scenes, exist by hundreds and by thousands in all our large towns'.[20] Southwood Smith was, like Gaskell, a friend of the Howitts. In 1847, the year he wrote for their magazine, he was pushing the legislative bill that would eventually become the Public Health Act of 1848.[21] The purpose of his article appearing alongside Gillies's story in the same issue was to urge a more serious interest in 'the present state of the sanitary question'.[22] Southwood Smith revealed his commitment to the School of Edwin Chadwick when he argued:

> From accurate calculations based on the observation of carefully recorded facts, it is rendered certain that the annual slaughter in England alone, by causes that are preventable, by causes that produce only one disease, namely, typhus fever, is more than double the loss sustained by the allied armies in the battle of Waterloo; that 136 persons perish every day in England alone, whose lives might be saved; that in one single city, namely, Manchester, thirteen thousand three hundred and sixty-two children have perished in seven years over and above the morality natural to mankind.[23]

The conclusion Southwood Smith comes to, addressed to working classes themselves, would have sat less well, one imagines, with Chadwick:

> You should rouse yourselves and show that you will submit to this dreadful state of things no longer. Let a voice come from your streets, lanes, alleys, courts, workshops and houses, that shall startle the ear of the public and command the attention of the legislature. [...] The Government is disposed to espouse your cause; but narrow, selfish, short-sighted interests will be banded against you.[24]

These were potent words in 1847 but not, it seems, potent enough to satisfy Gillies. Her more radical conclusion to the accompanying short story, spoken by a physician, is:

---

[20] Mary Gillies, 'A Labourer's Home', *Howitt's Journal*, 1 (1847), pp. 61–4.
[21] See Gertrude Hill Lewes, *Dr Southwood Smith: A Retrospect* (Edinburgh and London: William Blackwood and Sons, 1898), pp. 48, 122.
[22] Thomas Southwood Smith, 'An Address to the Working Classes of the United Kingdom, on their Duty in the Present State of the Sanitary Question', *Howitt's Journal*, 1 (1847), pp. 3–4.
[23] Ibid., p. 3.   [24] Ibid., p. 4.

These miseries will continue [...] till the government will pass measures which shall remove the sources of poison and disease from these places. All this suffering might be averted. These poor people are victims that are sacrificed. The effect is the same as if twenty or thirty thousand of them were annually taken out of their wretched homes and put to death; the only difference being that they are left in them to die.[25]

Gillies has a similar notion of pauper conditions to Engels's *Condition of the Working Class in England* (1845), which famously referred to urban poverty as 'social murder'.[26] Like Engels, Gillies developed her radical view from a detailed account of individual experiences of poverty. The wife and mother of the careworn family in her short story is forced to use dirty water to clean her house:

The water she had so longed for was discoloured and offensive when she drew it, and a nasty black scum appeared on the top. A little which had been left in the bottom had tainted it all; and, besides, the butt was old and rotten, and enough to spoil the water had there been nothing else. Such as it was, however, it must be used; and first she set about washing up all the clothes that had been worn, meaning to finish and clear up before her husband came in. But what with the black stream, and the poor restless children, she got on very slowly; and the wet clothes were still at the door. The bad water caused the steam and the clothes to smell very badly; the baby had cried for a long time, and was still evidently too much suffering to be quieted; the supper was not laid; the passage was wet up to the door of the room, for the attempt to cleanse it had been given up in despair. Peter was nursing little Mary, who leaned her sick head on his shoulder, and Bill and Dick were complaining, in turn, of hunger, and fretting for their supper.[27]

While Southwood Smith identified government blindspots as the main problem to be solved in social reform, he also classified 'personal uncleanliness' and the 'habits of the people' as factors in the abjection of the poor.[28] In Gillies's story, however, the habits of the poor are shown to be sanitary; the children are hungry not because they are too many, but because of how they are forced to live. *Howitt's Journal* provides a picture of medicine and literature working together in social reform: Southwood Smith's specialist injunctions are fleshed out, fittingly, by Gillies's story, while the latter is given a vocabulary and a means of explication by the science which contextualizes and radicalizes its polemics.

---

[25] Gillies, 'A Labourer's Home', p. 64.
[26] Friedrich Engels, *The Condition of the Working Class in England*, ed. by Victor Kiernan (1845; London: Penguin, 1987), p. 70.
[27] Gillies, 'A Labourer's Home', p. 63.   [28] Southwood Smith, 'An Address', p. 4.

William Carpenter and Henry Holland

Carpenter's 'Physiology for the People'—fourteen essays also appearing in *Howitt's* and based upon his *Principles of Human Physiology* (1842)—made it clear that the material details of destitution were important to the social-reform aims of the journal. As Louise Henson has discussed, the Gaskells knew Carpenter through their involvement in Unitarian circles. He stayed with them while lecturing at the Manchester Mechanics Institute in 1851, and Elizabeth attended one lecture on Microscopic Research.[29] He was the son of the Dissenting preacher Dr. Lant Carpenter, brother to the social reformer Mary Carpenter, and a major figure in the rise of physiology in Britain in the early parts of the nineteenth century. In his contributions to *Howitt's Journal*, he set about explaining physiology in a language which he believed the periodical's audience would understand by using industrial metaphors for the workings of the body. Tamara Ketabgian has noted that 'in the first half of the nineteenth century the steam engine served as the dominant practical model for scientific theories of heat'.[30] In *his* section on heat, Carpenter compares the energies of the body to those of a 'factory, whose moving power is supplied by the Steam-engine' and whose 'myriads of whirling spindles, [...] noisy power-looms, [...] flying lathes, [...] thundering hammers, [...and] steadily traversing planing-tables' all become 'motionless and inert' without steam[31]—as, he said, do the pulsations, beatings, and circulations of the human body without warmth.

More literally, steam power was Carpenter's example of the extraordinary strides that had been made in the practical applications of science to industry. Physiology, by contrast, had not been taken advantage of as a means of improving knowledge of the experiences of the poverty-stricken worker. What is worth noting in the following passage is the way Carpenter sidesteps the idea that the 'masses' are to blame for their own ignorance:

> If we look around, with the advantage of but a very small amount of knowledge as to the conditions on which the preservation of health and the prolongation of life are dependent, we are at once struck with the utter neglect of those

---

[29] See Louise Henson, 'The "Condition-of-England" Debate and the "Natural History of Man": An Important Scientific Context for the Social-Problem Fiction of Elizabeth Gaskell', *Gaskell Society Journal*, 16 (2002), pp. 30–47 (p. 30). See Elizabeth Gaskell, letter to Marianne Gaskell, c. 28 March 1851, Gaskell Letters, pp. 146–7 (p. 146). T. H. Huxley said of Carpenter's microscopic research that it 'opened wide the gates of science to many people who might otherwise never have been tempted to enter therein'. Quoted in William Benjamin Carpenter, *Nature and Man: Essays Scientific and Philosophical*, ed. by J. Estlin Carpenter (New York, NY: D. Appleton, 1889), p. 67.

[30] Tamara Ketabgian, '"Melancholy Mad Elephants": Affect and the Animal Machine in *Hard Times*', *Victorian Studies*, 45:4 (2003), pp. 649–76 (p. 652).

[31] William Benjamin Carpenter, 'Physiology for the People II', *Howitt's Journal*, 1 (1847), pp. 132–4 (p. 132).

conditions which is prevalent among the masses of the people, and the continual disregard to them which is manifested by many whose example ought to be the means of directing general attention to their importance.[32]

This is a very different picture of the ignorance of the masses to that we see in Malthus and his followers. Carpenter places social responsibility on those few who ought to be setting a good example to the many. He continues: 'the ignorance and the perverseness of Man has caused him to run counter to the arrangements of Providence, and to violate in every particular the conditions which have been assigned, for good and wise purposes, as the law of his physical being'.[33] These are clearly the words of a follower of physiology rather than political economy. According to the former, pathology ran *counter* to the arrangements of providence; for the latter, it could be, as a 'check', a confirmation of its ruthless efficiency. The laws of physical being, in Carpenter's opinion, were designed to make humans healthy:

> The Creator has given to the body a certain constitution; [...] he has made it to consist of numerous parts, each having its appropriate office; [...] the mutual working-together of these parts is essential to the well-being of the whole, and [...] any disturbance in the actions of any one must necessarily influence the rest. The physiologist has [...] to show that the first development and the continued maintenance of the body are entirely dependent upon the influence which it derives from certain external agents, such as heat, light, and electricity; upon the materials which it draws from the various articles of food; and upon the constant removal of the products of its waste or decay, which should be carried off by the atmosphere, or discharged by the water, of which a free and copious supply are alike requisite for the maintenance of health.[34]

Carpenter's vision of the healthy body is, like John Hunter's concept of the animal economy, a picture of balance achieved between the fuel provided by external elements and waste. Like Xavier Bichat, he also saw vital connections between tissues and processes, meaning that occurrences such as starvation and disease were disturbances of what was natural rather than a recalibration of the same. Carpenter's reference to 'The Creator' was not, however, an example of the kind of natural theology developed by William Paley, in which God was the all-wise instigator of natural systems which ran independently of his will. In a lecture delivered in 1866, he asked: 'what but good can come from the freest search into scientific truth? What part does science play that is not in fullest harmony with the highest

---

[32] William Benjamin Carpenter, 'Physiology for the People I', *Howitt's Journal*, 1 (1847), pp. 100–2 (p. 100).
[33] Ibid., p. 100.   [34] Ibid., p. 102.

truths of religion?'[35] Like Kingsley, Carpenter believed that the act of looking at material truths was consummate with, not independent of, the search for moral and religious answers. While science, he concludes,

> is every day contributing to the *material* welfare of man, it is even more certainly benefiting him by the enlargement of his intellect, the elevation of his morale, and the strengthening of his power of spiritual discernment—all of which contribute their respective shares to the development of his religious nature.[36]

Prioritizing material objects of study over abstract ones does not amount to abandoning spiritual considerations, but rather encourages a form of perception that is better suited to engage with questions that link the moral to the material; in the context of 'Physiology for the People', the same message implies that knowledge of the body and its workings makes us better equipped to deal with the social problems that emerged as a result of industrialization and the resulting imbalance of wealth. In Gaskellian terms, Carpenter was more Job Legh than Nicholas Higgins.

As Carpenter's essays in *Howitt's Journal* are on physiology, as opposed to pathology, his interest is on the functions and structures of the *healthy* body. There is, however, one exception: the fourth essay focusses on starvation. With characteristic self-focus, he acknowledges that, in looking at something as self-evident as hunger, he might be judged as 'gratifying an idle curiosity'; yet, 'the practical applications of these principles to the welfare of Men, especially in times like the present, are very numerous and important'.[37] He believed that

> on the average of a large number of persons, from *eight to ten ounces of solid carbon* are daily set free from the lungs in the form of carbonic gas and this quantity must be supplied by the food, or else the body will gradually diminish in weight, and will waste away.[38]

According to Gaskell's cousin, the physician Henry Holland, nobody understood the 'abstruse subject' of the 'mutual relations of the physical and vital forces' better than Carpenter.[39] Writing in 1859, he said:

[35] William B. Carpenter, 'Antiquity of Man' (1866), in *Nature and Man*, p. 87.

[36] Ibid., p. 88. Italics in original.

[37] William B. Carpenter, 'Physiology for the People IV', *Howitt's Journal*, 1 (1847), pp. 198–201 (pp. 200, 201).

[38] Ibid., pp. 200–1 (p. 200). Italics in original.

[39] Henry Holland, 'The Progress and Spirit of Physical Science' (1858), in *Essays on Scientific and Other Subjects contributed to the Edinburgh and Quarterly Reviews* (London: Longman et al., 1862), pp. 1–49 (p. 15). On the family connection to Gaskell, see Henson, 'Condition-of-England', p. 31. Uglow sees Holland as a 'terrible snob' and complains that in his *Medical Notes and Recollections* (1839) he 'drops names like confetti'; Uglow, *Elizabeth Gaskell*, p. 17.

No period has been so prolific of [physiological] achievements as that in which we are now living. [...] Whoever takes up the massive volume of Dr. Carpenter [*Principles of Human Physiology*]—a work of great excellence, and the most complete we possess—will see how much is comprised in this wide domain, how profound the subjects offered to human thought, how large the voids yet left for future inquiry.[40]

Holland goes on to state that great advances had been made in understanding 'the functions of nutrition and assimilation' in particular, because these 'have been the objects of refined experiment and sedulous observation by the physiologists and physicians of our day'.[41] Holland himself was, according to Rick Rylance, 'one of a number of eminent medics [...] who formed an informal grouping with W. B. Carpenter at their head [...] Carpenter dedicated his major work *Principles of Mental Physiology* to Holland in 1874, in tribute to "the wonderful suggestiveness" of his work'.[42] Holland sat on the Council of the Royal Society and was a Fellow of the Royal College of Physicians; 'Among his patients were Queen Victoria, Prince Albert, six Prime Ministers, George Eliot and G. H. Lewes.'[43] Rylance also suggests that Holland 'was not interested in theoretical speculation',[44] which may hold true of his psychological speculations, which is Rylance's main interest, but is certainly not true of his writings on physiology. In 'Life and Organisation' (1859), an essay which he wrote for the *Edinburgh Review* (a journal the Gaskells borrowed regularly from the Portico Library in Manchester[45]), he considered the impact of recent studies into natural history, among them studies by Richard Owen and Lewes,[46] on an old debate: 'What is the principle or property', he asks, 'superadded to the known properties of matter, giving it those new conditions which create and constitute vitality? It is an enquiry which, in one form or another, has exercised every age and school of philosophy'.[47] The 'ultra-Lockean', hard-empiricist approach he has little time for, much in the same way that Gaskell unsympathetically portrays Nicholas Higgins's positivism: 'The materialist fancies himself on firm ground', he opines, 'because his argument has Matter for its foundation. [Yet] matter itself is known only by and through that mind which he assumes to create out of it'.[48] Similarly, the old vitalist approach

---

[40] Holland, 'Life and Organisation' (1859), in *Essays*, pp. 50–101 (pp. 51, 54).

[41] Ibid., p. 94.

[42] Rick Rylance, *Victorian Psychology and British Culture, 1850–1880* (Oxford: Oxford University Press, 2000), p. 128.

[43] Ibid., p. 127.   [44] Ibid., p. 129.

[45] See Barbara Brill and Alan Shelston, 'Manchester: "A Behindhand Place for Books": The Gaskells and the Portico Library', *Gaskell Society Journal*, 5 (1991), pp. 27–36 (p. 29). On the Gaskells' use of the Portico Library, see Shirley Foster, ' "We sit and read our time away": Elizabeth Gaskell and the Portico Library', *The Gaskell Society Journal*, 14 (2000), pp. 14–23.

[46] Holland reviews Owen's *On Parthenogenesis* (1849) and Lewes's *Sea-side Studies* (1858), along with other works on natural history.

[47] Holland, 'Life and Organisation', p. 55.   [48] Ibid., p. 55.

'admits of little argument or advance. [It] quit[s...] the region of the senses and of material experiment, and affirm[s] a power unknown, except in what we presume to be its effects. It is negative evidence; and, as far as we can see, never to be rendered other than such.'[49] Holland advocated a compromise between vitalist and materialist approaches, suggesting that advances in the organic sciences offered a framework for understanding the nature of thought:

> While the astronomer is soberly dealing with the great elements of space and time, which make the material of his science, the modern naturalist is rioting in rapturous language about the beauty of his zoophytes and the microscopic marvels of infusorial life. [...] That which human calculation cannot reach, has in itself a certain element of the sublime, be the subject what it may. But connected with this study, we have also the many mysterious questions which regard the manner of generation and existence of these simpler forms for animal life, and their relation to other beings of higher order;—topics well fitted to take strong hold on the mind of every thoughtful man. [...] We must repeat that the doctrine of a separate vital principle rests on negative grounds only, and little admits either of amplification or detail. The bold and active science of our day has for the most part ranged itself on the opposite side; and is ever occupied in fixing new relations and equivalents of power—the materials, it may be, of more general laws than have yet been reached by human intelligence.[50]

While Holland is cautious about the extent to which the materialist view can be extended, he nevertheless favours that approach's focus on matter over abstract philosophy. The driving force of recent science has been mystery: zoophytes might hold the key to the enigmas of creation, and natural history may uncover general laws of a higher understanding than human intelligence. More agnostic than Carpenter's thinking, it is a view that insists upon a critical approach to the truth: the facts of life are not evidences given directly to us, nor are they a sort of 'dark matter' which exists (to our understanding) in relation to its effects only. They are instead a source of further and higher thought rooted in the material. In 'Materialism as a Question of Science and Philosophy' (1875), he quotes Spinoza: 'body is not terminated by thinking, nor thinking by body'.[51]

Manchester Realism

Manchester, the great seat of material production, was central to ways of thinking about the links between approaches to social problems and physiology. As

---

[49] Ibid., p. 57.   [50] Ibid., pp. 53, 61.
[51] Henry Holland, 'Materialism as a Question of Science and Philosophy', in *Fragmentary Papers on Science and Other Subjects* (London: Longman et al., 1875), pp. 206–13 (p. 212).

Gaskell's acquaintance, James Phillips Kay-Shuttleworth, noted in 1873: 'the North of England is a great laboratory, in which research is in progress for the solution of social problems; and the wisest explorers are those who watch the processes of natural development, and make themselves interpreters of phenomena.'[52] Prior to marrying the wealthy Janet Shuttleworth, medical man James Kay had researched the links between industry, bodies, and ethics in his *Moral and Physical Condition of the Working Classes Employed in the Cotton Manufacture in Manchester* (1832). Responsible for inspiring the establishment of Manchester's Statistical Society,[53] Kay's analysis saw the moral and physical not as separate aspects of the working-class experience, but as linked through physiology:

> These artizans are frequently subject to a disease in which the sensibility of the stomach and bowels are morbidly excited; the alvine secretions are deranged, and the appetite impaired. Whilst this state continues, the patient loses flesh, his features are sharpened, the skin becomes pale, leaden coloured, or of the yellow hue [...] The strength fails, all the capacities of physical enjoyment are destroyed, and the paroxysms of corporeal suffering are aggravated by the horrors of a disordered imagination, till they lead to gloomy apprehension, to the deepest depression, and almost to despair.[54]

The reference to a 'disease' in which there is a 'sensibility of the stomach and bowels' is rather vague, yet the list of symptoms that follows is more explicit. Kay aims to show how a disturbance of the physical (a likely contingency in the harsh environments of Manchester) leads to a disturbance of the 'moral', especially a disordered imagination and depression. In the face of 'the horrors of hunger and disease', he adds, 'no modern Rousseau' is needed to rhapsodize on the happiness of the state of nature.[55] We need to focus on the physical signs because, as he puts it,

> the sensorium of the animal structure, to which converge the sensibilities of each organ, is endowed with a consciousness of every change in the sensations to which each member is liable; and few diseases are so subtle as to escape its delicate perceptive power. Pain thus reveals to us the existence of evils, which, unless arrested in their progress, might insidiously invade the sources of vital action.[56]

---

[52] James Kay Shuttleworth, *Thoughts and Suggestions on Certain Social Problems* (London: Longman et al., 1873), p. vi. On Kay Shuttleworth's connection to Gaskell See Uglow, *Elizabeth Gaskell*, pp. 22, 247. It was Kay Shuttleworth who introduced Gaskell to Charlotte Brontë in 1850.

[53] Frank Smith, *The Life and Work of Sir James Kay-Shuttleworth* (1926; Bath: Cedric Chivers, 1974), pp. 25–6.

[54] James Kay Shuttleworth, *The Moral and Physical Condition of the Working Classes Employed in the Cotton Manufacture in Manchester* (London: James Ridgeway, 1832), pp. 9, 11–12.

[55] Ibid., p. 48.   [56] Ibid., p. 3.

At this point Kay uses pain as a social metaphor: the envisaging of civic ills as bodily complaints makes 'every order immediately conscious of the evils affecting any portion of the general mass, and thus rendering their removal equally necessary for the immediate ease, as it is for the ultimate welfare, of the whole social system'.[57] The reference to pain also makes it clear that recognizing problems *as* physical, or understanding the ways in which they *become* so, is a vital part of how we think about the broader 'moral' and social aspects of the issue.

Like Holland and Kay, and to a lesser extent Carpenter, Gaskell drew upon the period's physiology to suggest that matter provokes further and higher thinking and to explore whether 'higher thinking' is incomplete, or even harmful, without some foundation in matter. I disagree with Scholl's view that Gaskell's fiction links the 'rational' and the 'theoretical' with a 'dismissal of very real human suffering'.[58] Conservative reinterpretations of political economy were based, as we have seen, not on the rational and the theoretical, but on assumptions driven by prejudices and personal interests. Gaskell saw rational and theoretical thought, as embodied in science, as one of the key solutions to social problems. It is clear from her letters and various other writings that she was wedded to the idea of what she perceived to be the 'plain truth'. In the preface to *Mary Barton* she famously asserted, 'I have tried to write truthfully' (p. xxxvi). It is a point she maintained in letters to numerous correspondents:

> I told the story according to a fancy of my own; to really SEE the scenes I tried to describe, (and they WERE as real as my own life at the time) and then to tell them as nearly as I could, as if I were speaking to a friend over the fire on a winter's night and describing real occurrences.[59]

> I was sure a great deal of [*Mary Barton*] was truth, and I knew that I had realized all my people to myself so vividly that parting with them was like parting with friends.[60]

> I believe that what I have said in Mary Barton to be perfectly true, but by no means the whole truth; and I have always felt deeply annoyed at anyone, or any set of people who chose to consider that I had manifested the whole truth; I do not think it is possible to do this in any *one* work of fiction.[61]

Gaskell's sense of realism is as cautious as Holland's materialism. She seeks what is 'real' and 'perfectly true' and she aims to 'realize' her characters, yet she is also annoyed by those who expect her work to offer the 'whole truth'. She was fully aware of her limitations as an observer tasked with describing the 'real': '*I tried to*

---

[57] Ibid., p. 4.   [58] Scholl, *Hunger Movements*, p. 53.

[59] Elizabeth Gaskell, letter to Eliza Fox, 29 May 1849, Gaskell Letters, pp. 80–2 (p. 82).

[60] Elizabeth Gaskell, letter to John Seely Hart, 28 April 1850, Gaskell Letters, pp. 114–15 (p. 115).

[61] Elizabeth Gaskell, letter to Lady Kay-Shuttleworth, 16 July ?1850, Gaskell Letters, pp. 118–21 (p. 119).

tell', she qualifies, 'as nearly as I could'. It has been acknowledged that, 'because of their implausible resolutions of problematic social situations', social-problem novels such as *Mary Barton* 'subject the novelist to charges of failing to be totally "realistic"'.[62] Yet, as Joseph W. Childers notes:

> Gaskell never purports to be representing the reality of the situation she observes; she knows this is a claim she cannot make. She writes of *Mary Barton* in an undated letter of 1848, '[...] not that I dare say it is the abstract absolute truth'. She is always aware of the limits on what she can see, and thus the limits on what she can (or should) say.[63]

Josie Billington comments on the moment, in *Mary Barton*, where the narrator says, with reference to the workers' anger: 'I know that this is not really the case; and I know what is the truth in such matters: but what I wish to impress is what the workman feels and thinks' (p. 24). According to Billington, 'Ideas are rendered first of all as perceptions before they are accounted feelings, or become truths or prejudices.'[64] Gaskell does not seek to account for 'abstract absolute truth', but is aware instead that that which is seen or felt as real has a direct bearing on what is perceived to be the larger moral and emotional truth. Like Kingsley, Carpenter, and Holland, she has a sense of the correct emotional response as dependent on a rational interpretation of the material.

Unitarianism

It could be objected that, rather than coming from medicine and physiology, Gaskell's interest in the material aspects of starvation was more likely to have stemmed from her Unitarian beliefs, which, according to Angus Easson, were 'direct, scriptural and practical'.[65] Yet, especially in the context of 1840s Manchester, the boundaries between Unitarian philosophy and the interlinking subjects of medicine and social reform were not altogether distinct. Although Gaskell was a close friend of James Martineau, the Unitarian philosopher who sought to revive a new 'emotional strain'[66] within the faith, her own approach to Unitarianism was informed by more established appeals to reason and material truth. As Henson notes, Unitarianism believed that 'education was the means by

---

[62] Deirdre David, *Fictions of Resolution in Three Victorian Novels: North and South, Our Mutual Friend, Daniel Deronda* (London: Macmillan, 1981), p. 6.

[63] Joseph W. Childers, *Novel Possibilities: Fiction and the Formation of Early Victorian Culture* (Philadelphia PA: University of Pennsylvania Press, 1995), p. 166.

[64] Josie Billington, *Faithful Realism: Elizabeth Gaskell and Leo Tolstoy: A Comparative Study* (London: Associated University Presses, 2002), p. 77.

[65] Easson, *Elizabeth Gaskell*, p. 12.   [66] Ibid., p. 8.

which mental energies could be channelled and controlled'.[67] Hence, when Gaskell writes in an undated letter to John Bright 'you know I am not (*Unitarianly*) orthodox!',[68] she was referring to a lack of sympathy with the new wave of Unitarianism, preached by Martineau, where feeling, beauty, and symbolism were prioritized over logic and reason. Gallagher notes that 'Elizabeth Gaskell and her husband, William, stayed within the old school of Unitarianism on most issues and made no decided moves towards transcendentalism'. [69] As Easson has demonstrated in what is the best account of Gaskell's religious principles, eighteenth-century Unitarianism, the creed popularized by Joseph Priestly, argued that 'since religion and reason proceed from the same God, they cannot be contrary to one another'.[70] Priestly himself 'was suspicious of mere feeling: since we are to form out life in following righteousness, mercy and truth'.[71] Uglow adds that 'the influence of the new school of thought, which gave priority to feeling, is equally strong, if not stronger' than Gaskell's emphasis on 'education, truth and lies, atonement and regeneration'.[72] Unitarianism gave the author

the feeling that humanity is engaged in a continuous process of learning, of unravelling the puzzle of life (an idea at the heart of the liberal tradition of the novel); the emphasis on enlightenment through feeling and personal relationships; the idea of Christ as nearer in nature to man than to God, which hallowed the artistic 'incarnation' of spiritual truths in the daily life of fallible mortals.[73]

As we shall see, the 'incarnations' in Gaskell's novels are more complex than 'daily life' events, and they were inspired by other, more scientific sources than the Unitarian belief in a flesh-and-blood Christ. While I agree with the claim that Gaskell was interested in life and humanity as processes of learning and puzzles to be solved, I would argue that it was not feeling and personal relationships that prompted an incarnation of spiritual truth, but a focus on the physical as a means of understanding the practical and moral puzzles of industrial life, similar to the methods employed by Carpenter, Kay, and Holland.

In *The Story of Protestant Dissent and English Unitarianism* (1899), Walter Lloyd noted:

Unitarianism is synonymous with intellectual freedom. [...] Whilst Unitarians, notwithstanding their differences of opinion upon many topics, maintain the spirit of unity and natural affection, they may avoid contracting careless indifference to truth. Indeed, their constitution furnishes them with singular advantages in pursuing it, because a change of sentiment founded upon inquiry, is not

[67] Henson, 'Condition-of-England', p. 40.
[68] Elizabeth Gaskell, letter to ?John Bright, undated, Gaskell Letters, pp. 784–5 (pp. 784–5).
[69] Gallagher, *Industrial Reformation*, p. 64.   [70] Easson, *Elizabeth Gaskell*, p. 5.
[71] Ibid., p. 7.   [72] Uglow, *Elizabeth Gaskell*, p. 131.   [73] Ibid., p. 134.

attended with a painful separation from former religious connections; and while by uniting as *Worshippers of the Father only*, they are free from those impediments to further investigation which would arise from a sub-division into parties, they have every opportunity for assisting one another by friendly discussion, and the mutual communication of their sentiments.[74]

This 'undogmatic Unitarianism' is what allowed the dissenting movement to find a common ground with science; both were interested in the prospect of vision that was as free as was possible from 'impediments to further investigation'. 'The influence of natural science upon the trend of Unitarian opinion', notes one historian, 'has hardly been second to that of Biblical criticism'.[75] According to Robert H. Kargon, the dissenting chapels of central Manchester were the driving force of much of the scientific activity that took place in the city.[76] And we can see why. Unitarianism did not deify human vision, as Uglow suggests, but rather encouraged a superior criticalness of understanding—a greater interpretive engagement with reality. As William Gaskell said, in an 1862 sermon to the Supporters of the British and Foreign Unitarian Association:

In our day and generation let us seek to be as true; never paltering with principle, never listening to any selfish time-serving pleas, never taking for a proof of liberality that loose grasp of opinions which is only a proof of indifference, never yielding to that charity for all forms of faith which is fidelity to none, never giving way to that weak tolerance of wrong which is sheer treason to right, but ready, through cloud and sunshine, through honour and dishonour, through evil report and good report, everywhere and at all times, to follow the truth, and in the spirit of our holy Master to 'bear witness to it'![77]

As summarized by Carol Lansbury, 'Truth to a Unitarian was the torch that would eventually illuminate the whole of mankind. [...] It was not difficult for a Unitarian scientist like Charles Lyell or an industrialist like John Fielden to find a harmony between their work and their religion.'[78] As we saw in Kingsley's work, and in William Carpenter's contributions to *Howitt's Journal*, science appeared to offer a set of tools for substantiating theological notions of truth. As George Sydney Smythe, MP, said in a speech to the Manchester Athenaeum in the 1840s,

---

[74] Walter Lloyd, *The Story of Protestant Dissent and English Unitarianism* (London: Philip Green, 1899), pp. 221–2. Italics in original.

[75] W. G. Tarrant, *Unitarianism* (Texas: Grindl Press, 2015), p. 67.

[76] Robert H. Kargon, *Science in Victorian Manchester: Enterprise and Expertise* (Manchester: Manchester University Press, 1977), p. 27.

[77] William Gaskell, 'Unitarian Christians Called to Bear Witness to the Truth: A Sermon Preached Before the Supporters of the British and Foreign Unitarian Association at their Annual Meeting, in Essex-Street Chapel, London, June 11, 1862' (London: Edward T. Whitfield, 1862), p. 23.

[78] Carol Lansbury, *Elizabeth Gaskell: The Novel of Social Crisis* (London: Paul Elek, 1975), p. 14.

here, at this very hour, we are proclaiming the banns of a marriage which represents the primeval alliance between the spirit and the matter [...] It is a marriage between an industry which has conquered the world, and overspread it [...] and an intellect which is young, which is of the people, and which, by God's help, shall continue pure.[79]

Manchester, with its obsessive love for raw materials and the manufacture of saleable things, plus its perennial need for social reform, was the perfect environment for the 'marriage' between matter and spirit to flourish. This congress appealed to material science as much as applied to material production.

Unitarian materialism perceived hunger to be a topic that begins with individual bodies and then, as a subject, broadens to suggest vital things about the state of the nation. (This was very different to Malthus's demography, which performed the opposite manoeuvre of applying broad population theories to individual case histories.) *Howitt's Journal*, for instance, went into print during the Irish Hunger's most destructive period. In one of his own contributions, 'The Fast and the Famine' (1847), William Howitt rejected the claims, made often at the time, that Irish families earned their distress by committing various crimes of improvidence against the laws of nature. The Howitts identified as Quaker during this time and had, as part of a sister dissenting group, a number of beliefs in common with Unitarians. Among these was the belief in the importance of habits of observation, especially of nature, as having an influence on the health of the spirit of the observer. In 'The Fast and the Famine', Howitt saw starvation not as representing any will of God, or nature, but as a national disgrace caused by governmental incompetence. The English, he alleged, ought to be 'heartily ashamed of our criminal neglect' of Ireland.[80] 'There is famine in Manchester and the manufacturing districts', he adds, and 'we must resolve, if we will put an end to the recurrence of the famine, which is now stalking not alone through Ireland, but through the manufacturing districts of England, to look Truth and God in the face'.[81] Howitt's writing brings three major topics together: materiality, spirituality, and selfhood. The reform project, for him, involves not only looking to the streets of Manchester as potential breeding grounds of famine fever, but also of looking 'Truth and God' in the face as a form of self-analysis: seeing reality involves being ashamed of ourselves for what we have failed to see in the past ('our criminal neglect'). In the minds of Victorian dissenters such as Howitt, spiritual links with God were achieved through a self-reflexive or self-aware engagement with a perception of material realness: what I suggest is that, in Gaskell's work, physiology

[79] George Sydney Smythe, 'Speech to the Manchester Athenaeum', in *Athenaeum Addresses 1843–1848* (Manchester: Manchester City News, 1875), pp. 31–7 (p. 37).
[80] William Howitt, 'The Fast and the Famine', *Howitt's Journal*, 1 (1847), pp. 181–2 (p. 182).
[81] Ibid., pp. 181, 182.

became a central part of this search for 'Truth and God'. That she intended for her works to have a moral and emotional weight is well established, and obvious from the most cursory of glances at her plots; what has been acknowledged less, and yet is just as important, is the way medicine and physiology coalesced with Unitarian principles in Gaskell's fiction and suggested that poverty, understood in all its grim reality, requires a greater degree of critical engagement than that typified in the dogmatic or deductive strategies used in consequentialist political economy.

Gaskell's Realism

In *Mary Barton*, after the failure of the Chartist march to London in which John Barton participates, we are informed:

> In times of sorrowful or fierce endurance, we are often soothed by the mere repetition of old proverbs which tell the experience of our forefathers; but now, 'it's a long lane that has no turning', 'the weariest day draws to an end', &c., seemed false and vain sayings, so long and so weary was the pressure of the terrible times. Deeper and deeper still sank the poor; it showed how much lingering suffering it takes to kill men, that so few (in comparison) died during those times. But remember! we only miss those who do men's work in their humble sphere; the aged, the feeble, the children, when they die, are hardly noted by the world; and yet to many hearts, their deaths make a blank which long years will never fill up. Remember, too, that though it may take much suffering to kill the able-bodied and effective members of society, it does *not* take much to reduce them to worn, listless, diseased creatures, who thenceforward crawl through life with moody hearts and pain-stricken bodies.   (p. 130)

Old maxims appear to have lost their relevance in the modern settings Gaskell describes.[82] Proverbs, in this context, have a lot in common with the laziest interpretations of political economy in that they offer blank prognostications based on a limited understanding of the true state of affairs. *Mary Barton*, by contrast, seems eager to draw attention to what is *not* seen as much as what is: the suggestion that we seldom remember the aged, the feeble, and the infantile in times of sorrow reminds us of the Chadwick-Farr debate of the 1830s, wherein statistics had managed to be highly selective in what they revealed about starvation. It would be easy to assume that Gaskell makes a point about the limitations of such

---

[82] For an excellent discussion of folklore and natural science in *Mary Barton*, see Amy Mae King, 'Taxonomical Cures: The Politics of Natural History and Herbalist Medicine in Elizabeth Gaskell's Mary Barton', in *Romantic Science: The Literary Forms of Natural History*, ed. by Noah Heringman (New York, NY: State University of New York Press, 2003), pp. 255–70.

observations as a preface to the hidden realities her work will uncover, but I think the passage aims to caution us against taking the evidence of our own eyes for granted. As in the argument between Chadwick and Farr, starvation is the focal point of a reminder that appearances cannot always be trusted, that the meanings and interpretations of poverty are unstable, and that the realist approach, for all its power, should have no easy time of it.

The first picture of actual famishment we encounter in *Mary Barton* is the famous outline of the Davenports' cellar, where a critical, realistic approach is called for. Gaskell's rich, descriptive prose relies, as others have noted, upon the language of sanitary science,[83] but its incarnation of hunger, as both a physiological and a moral concern, invokes questions about perception and knowledge:

> In that dim light, which was darkness to strangers, [the children] clustered round Barton, and tore from him the food he had brought with him. It was a large hunch of bread, but it vanished in an instant. [...] The children clamoured again for bread; but this time Barton took a piece first to the poor, helpless, hopeless woman, who still sat by the side of her husband, listening to his anxious miserable mutterings. She took the bread, when it was put into her hand, and broke a bit, but could not eat. She was past hunger. She fell down on the floor with a heavy unresisting bang. The men looked puzzled. 'She's well-nigh clemmed,' said Barton. 'Folk do say one mustn't give clemmed people much to eat; but, bless us, she'll eat nought.'   (pp. 67-8)

In the dim light, where perception is no simple enterprise, the men manage to see one of starvation's major paradoxes: that one may be starving, yet also unable to eat. Barton appeals to what 'folk do say' and, in this case, common knowledge is backed up with medical opinion: John Elliotson explained the failure to eat in cases of starvation by saying 'the pain of hunger ceases' and 'relaxation of the stomach [causes] debility'.[84] Davenport's condition is identified as 'a low, putrid, typhoid kind' (p. 68), which corresponds with medical ideas of famine fever, where 'pestilential diseases must certainly follow in the wake of a famine, and carry off a far greater number than perish from actual starvation'.[85] These aspects of hunger, its contradictions and its close relationship with secondary conditions, make it a paradigm of unstable knowledge. After visiting Mr. Carson to ask for a hospital order, Wilson returns to the foetid cellar to find Davenport a 'skeleton of a body' (p. 69): 'Wilson looked. The flesh was sunk, the features prominent, bony, and rigid. The fearful clay-colour of death was over all. But the eyes were open and sensible, though the films of the grave were settling upon them' (p. 80). The picture of the starving man is painted in such a way that it is difficult to have a

---

[83] See Childers, *Novel Possibilities*, pp. 163, 167.
[84] Elliotson, *Human Physiology*, pp. 53-4.   [85] Ibid., pp. 53-4.

reaction that is not analytical: the light is dim and the men are 'puzzled' by some of the physiological effects they perceive; Davenport is both dead and alive: he is skeletal, yet his eyes are 'open and sensible', and these have the film of death over them. What appears to be discouraged—made impossible, in fact—is any kind of unreflecting interpretation of the scene: we cannot apply proverbs like 'it's a long lane that has no turning' or 'the weariest day draws to an end', the novel concludes, because the witnessing of starvation requires a self-questioning attention to facts that mislead as much as they guide: Wilson and Barton frequently appeal to each other's knowledge, both of the process of starvation and of the immediate case in hand: 'There's a change comed over him', says Barton, 'is there not?' (p. 79).

There is little wonder, then, that the root of the social problems in *Mary Barton* are found to be in the lack of a reasoned response to poverty from both the working and the middle classes. During their demonstration in London, 'the starving multitudes' discover 'that the very existence of their distress had been denied in Parliament' (p. 97), a lack of sympathy that is played out in the scene where the young Harry Carson sketches the workers in a satirical cartoon. In spite of its instrumentality in the major arc of the narrative, the scene acts as a parable of the problems of perception that take place across the classes. Young Carson's diagram is described as 'an admirable caricature of them—lank, ragged, dispirited, and famine-stricken', illustrating how hunger is both seen *and* seen with an 'admirable' accuracy by Carson's class. He passes the drawing around the mill owners who have gathered to hear the workers ask for better wages, then he tears 'the back of the letter on which it was drawn in two, twisted them up, and flung them into the fireplace; but, careless whether they reached their aim or not, he did not look to see they fell just short of any consuming cinders' (p. 216). This carelessness proves to be Harry's undoing, and it also signifies how lightly the famishment of the workers is taken by the propertied class. With their 'heads clustered together' in ominous signification of their dangerous plotting, the workers 'gaze at and detect the likenesses' in the recovered sketch:

> 'Well' said John Slater, after having acknowledged his nose and his likeness; 'I could laugh at a jest as well as e'er the best on 'em, though it did tell again myself, if I were not clemming' (his eyes filled with tears; he was a poor, pinched, sharp-featured man, with a gentle and melancholy expression of countenance), 'and if I could keep from thinking of them at home, as is clemming; but with the cries for food ringing in my eyes, and making me afeared of going home, and wonder if I should hear 'em wailing out, if I lay cold and drowned at the th' bottom of the canal, there,—why, man, I cannot laugh at aught.'   (pp. 219–20)

Carson's sketch and Slater's reaction make a complex point about the meaning and the perception of starvation. Having misjudged the severity of the facts standing plainly in front of him, Carson produces a representation whose sole purpose is comedy. Slater's experience and knowledge of his own and his family's hunger prevents *him* from having the intended response; he feels, instead, the emotions that Carson ought to have experienced in the first place. Gaskell thus highlights the broken links between reality, representation, and feeling, suggesting a relationship between physical knowledge of hunger and the correct emotional response to the same. On the other side of the coin, she draws a line between bad feeling and misjudgements of reality. Harry's sketch, like Parliament's rejection of the Charter, signifies a way of looking at poverty that reads its clues too lightly, too casually, and in a way that, according to Gallagher, 'obscures the tragedy'.[86] We know from the older Carson's issue of Davenport's hospital order that he is not entirely ignorant of or unsympathetic to the plights of the most distressed; yet, his son's sketch is an illustration of the dangers of reading material indications of poverty without both exploring their meaning and dissecting the processes that are used to see, know, and interpret them.

Hunger and Anger

Of course, if Carson's sketch is indicative of a response to social problems that is too cool, Barton's anger is suggestive of a response that is too warm. We have already seen that, for all its melodrama, John Slater's response to the experience and witnessing of hunger is the correct one. Barton says, portentously, 'it makes me more than sad, it makes my heart burn within me, to see that folk can make a jest of striving men' (p. 220). In Gaskell's novels, hunger is one of the key incitements to socialist anger, and Barton's storyline clearly shows that the author had some ambivalence towards the use of 'reality' or the 'common sense' approach as a militant position. Barton's rage is tied to the experience of real starvation and to the understanding of that horrible event as a reality. He explains how his son died 'for want of better food that I could give him' (p. 8). Later, he says 'we're thinking we'n been clemmed long enough' (p. 99); there is 'many a little one clemming at home in Lancashire' (p. 116); what is needed is 'victuals for childer, whose little voices are getting too faint and weak to cry aloud wi' hunger. [...] I've seen a father who had killed his child rather than let it clem before his eyes' (p. 220). John Barton's fury, like Nicholas Higgins's naïve empiricism, is an example of the novel exploring the excesses, as well as the good work, of the realist view: his execrations have all of the elements of Gaskell's detailism: the preoccupation with physical suffering and the symptoms of hunger, the attention to the testimonies provided by one's own eyes, and the fact that a frustrated resolve emerges from a perceived *right response* to facts. But after Harry's murder, the novel has no

---

[86] Gallagher, *Industrial Reformation*, p. 71.

sympathy for Barton's feelings. Soon after the act of violence, Mary encounters a starving Italian boy on the streets of Manchester. 'With his soft voice, and pleading looks, he uttered, in his pretty broken English, the word—"Hungry! so hungry"', to which Mary's reply is: 'Oh, lad, hunger is nothing—nothing!' (p. 270). It is a response that seems to go against the very grain of the novel's representations of starvation, yet it implies that hunger is insignificant when compared to the miseries caused by politically motivated crime. Excess, *Mary Barton* suggests, is every bit as problematic as dearth of feeling, yet both appear to stem from the same root cause: unreasoning or inflexible responses to material problems. Dickens's address to the Manchester Athenaeum in 1843 stated that although it is hard for the working-class man to 'keep the wolf—hunger—from his door, let him but once have chased the dragon—ignorance—from his hearth, and self-respect and hope are left him'.[87] The newly built Athenaeum gave Manchester workers access to a well-stocked library for a reasonable fee, and Dickens was likely to be thinking of ignorance as lack of book leaning, yet in Gaskell's work the type of ignorance to be kept at bay was the unreasoning reaction to the same wolf at the door. In some mitigation of the killing of Harry Carson, the narrator of *Mary Barton* says, emphatically, '*he did not know what he was doing*' (p. 434; italics in original); speaking to his victim's father, Barton corroborates, 'I did not know what I was doing' (p. 435). With wider reference to working-class activists, Gaskell says 'they know what they do' (p. 436). Ignorance does not, of course, absolve Barton of his crime, yet the meeting between him and Carson, during his last moments, is intended to parallel their experiences and have us realize that the wealthy characters are not to be absolved either: in drawing his sketch, Harry Carson knew not what *he* did, and he was also punished for his ignorance. The principal sin in the novel is not anger, then, but the lack of a reasoned and intelligence reaction— similar to that advocated, in varying ways, by Holland, Carpenter, and Kay.

In *North and South*, the most intense periods of hunger are the result of strike action. The condemnations of working-class violence that we see in *Mary Barton* are intensified in the later novel. Having been criticized by W. R. Greg (famously) and others for representing a one-sided picture of social problems in the earlier novel (it was alleged she was more in favour of the operative classes), Gaskell sought to set the balance right by presenting a more 'complete' picture.[88] What the author actually achieved was a sensitive portrait of the impressions of an outsider, Margaret Hale, whose sympathies were able to move from one class to another. Nevertheless, whereas in *Mary Barton* the graphic descriptions of starvation are an implicit criticism of the mill-owning class's intellectual and physical neglect of the workers, in *North and South* the most detailed accounts of hunger

---

[87] Charles Dickens, Speech to the Manchester Athenaeum, 5 October 1843, in *Speeches; Literary and Social* (London: John Camden Hotten, n.d.), pp. 74–81 (pp. 78–9) .

[88] See Easson, *Elizabeth Gaskell*, p. 82.

are intended to be a warning against strikes in which Workers' Unions risk becoming tyrannical. Prior to playing a part in the scene featuring the brooding combination of angry, striking workers, led by Boucher, Margaret witnesses the former telling Higgins that his wife 'cannot live long a' this 'n. Hoo's just sinking away—not for want o' meat hersel'—but because hoo cannot stand th' sight o' the little ones clemming. Ay, clemming!' (p. 154). Again, as in *Mary Barton* and the alleged encounter with the labourer later recorded in *The Gentleman's Magazine*, there is insistence upon the *actuality* of starving: Boucher repeats himself in order, it seems, for it to be understood that his use of the word 'clemming' is appropriate and not just a figure of speech. 'There's our lile Jack', he adds, 'lying a-bed, too weak to cry, but just every now and then sobbing up his heart for want of food' (p. 154). 'He lies clemming', he insists. Higgins 'looked up, with eyes brimful of tears, to Margaret, before he could gain courage to speak' (p. 154). This silent appeal to Margaret underscores her role as observer of the scene and arbiter, even, of the truth. Typical of Gaskell's way of writing, the most affecting parts of the scene rely upon an insistence on hardship as real, as a form of physical suffering requiring interpretation.

It is necessary that Boucher (and, by extension, the novel) insists upon the truth of his family's clemming because hunger, as we have seen, was easily denied, misunderstood, misidentified, and overlooked. Soon after the scene outlined above, Mr. Hale says to his daughter:

> I am not so convinced as you are about that man Boucher's utter distress; for the moment, he was badly off, I don't doubt. But there is always a mysterious supply of money from these Unions; and, from what you said, it was evidence the man was of a passionate, demonstrative nature, and gave strong expression to all he felt.   (p. 166)

Boucher's account of his family's distress is undermined by the fact that there is no physiological evidence to support what he says. Hale visits Boucher's home and finds his family enjoying the charitable donations made by other striking families; he assumes, then, that the labourer's claims must be exaggerated. This reaction from one of the novel's middle-class characters is, I argue, the kind of response that Gaskell's realism works hard to counterbalance. What is most troubling about Hale's suggestion is the vague sense he has of 'a mysterious supply of money' coming from somewhere. As arguments go, it is little better than Mr. Micawber's sense that 'something will come about', and is, in fact, spectacularly ill-suited to thinking about charity in the industrial world of Milton, where suffering comes with real rather than 'mysterious' consequences.

Nicholas Higgins's response to Boucher's poverty is, predictably, to blame the masters. The mill owners, Higgins says, 'tell us to mind our own business, and they'd mind theirs. Our business being, yo' understand, to take the bated wage, and be thankful; and their business to bate us down to clemming point, to swell their profits' (p. 134). Yet, the result of the strike is even worse clemming: 'O, father!' says Bessy, 'what have ye gained in striking? Think of that first strike when mother died—how we all had to clem—you worst of all' (p. 133). Boucher becomes 'weak wi' passion and clemming' after he has led the strikers into further action: he is 'that poor clemmed man', who will never get 'well o'er this clemming' (p. 201). And to underscore the *physical* nature of his hunger, Gaskell has the kindly physician Dr. Donaldson say to Thornton: 'Your bad weather, and your bad times, are my good ones. When trade is bad, there's more undermining of health, and preparation for death going on among you Milton men than you're aware of' (p. 213). Donaldson echoes what medical experts like D. J. Corrigan wrote about the links between poverty, starvation, and health during the Irish Famine (see Chapter 1); he simultaneously challenges the kind of assumptions we see in Mr. Hale where the hysterical poor, talking of hunger, are likely to know nothing of the real nature of what they say.

As in *Mary Barton*, Gaskell condemns working-class aggression in *North and South* because it is the result of clouded, rather than rational, judgement. What comes across in the novel's most scathing criticisms of the 'tyrannies' of trade unionism is an acknowledgement of the problems caused by the Union's lack of reason. For instance, Boucher says to Higgins:

> You know well, that a worser tyrant than e'er th' masters were says 'Clem to death, and see 'em a' clem to death, ere yo' dare go again th' Union.' [...] You may be kind hearts, each separate; but once banded together, yo've no more pity for a man than a wild hunger-maddened wolf.   (p. 155)

A hunger-maddened wolf is quite a different thing to a hunger-maddened worker; the latter does not necessarily see his thinking faculties pinched by his starvation, though it is—as the author shows—a key problem. It is when men gather together that the capacity for intellection and the search for rational solutions play truant and the driving principle is wolfish instinct. In Higgins's account of Boucher's ostracism from the union, he intimates that the wish to do good is what drives the alliance, though the means of going about it are far from delicate:

> It's a great power [the union]: it's our only power. I ha' read a bit o' poetry about a plough going o'er a daisy, as made tears come into my eyes [...]. Th' Union's the plough, making ready the land for harvest time. Such as Boucher [...] mun just make up their mind to be put out of the way. I'm sore vexed wi' him just now.
>   (p. 293)

The reference is to Robert Burns's 'To a Mountain Daisy' (1789), in which the narrator mourns the loss of a 'wee, modest, crimson-tipped flow'r' he overturns with his plough. Burns compares the flower's fate to that of the poet, and to mankind, whose subjectivities and brief lives are ravaged by the march of time. In its employment of the image, *North and South* has more in common with the theme as it is used in Tennyson's *In Memoriam* (1849), where the 'single life' is mourned against the savagery of a nature more 'careful of the type'. In her novel the daisy becomes a thinking, feeling subject, and the plough is the socialist project—careful of the union, yet careless of the single life. The implication is that trade unionism itself becomes a kind of machine, mindful of its overall aim, but fundamentally unable to take apart its work, and its own components, with the intention of thinking about them sensitively.

In *North and South*, as in *Mary Barton*, what is sought, then, or what is seen as the remedy that will unite the classes, is clarity of vision brought about by careful thought and perception. In the earlier novel, Carson comes to realize that 'a perfect understanding, and complete confidence and love, might exist between masters and men; that the truth might be recognized that the interests of the one were the interests of all, and, as such, required the consideration and deliberation of all' (p. 457). The key words here are 'perfect understanding' and 'consideration and deliberation'. Love and affection are only possible, it seems, through the spirit of good knowledge. Similarly, in *North and South* an understanding between Thornton and his workers is brought about when he ascertains the truth about Higgins's adoption of Boucher's children:

> Two hours of his hard penetrating intellectual, as well as bodily labour, did he give up to going about collecting evidence as to the truth of Higgins's story, the nature of his character, the tenor of his life. He tried not to be, but was convinced that all that Higgins had said was true.   (p. 325)

'I did not believe you', Thornton tells Higgins. 'But I know now that you spoke truth' (p. 326). This is the beginning of the mill-owner's plan to

> cultivat[e] some intercourse with the hands beyond the mere 'cash nexus' [...] Such intercourse is the very breath of life. A working man can hardly be made to feel and know how much his employer may have laboured in his study at plans for the benefit of his work people. [...] We should understand each other better, and I'll venture to say we should like each other more.   (p. 431–2)

Notice the way the last line of this quotation is arranged. *Mary Barton*'s optimistic idea of *love* between the classes has been modified to a *liking* here, yet the idea of *understanding* remains unchanged. Knowledge—or, at least, the will to understand the social and material challenge critically—is central to Gaskell's idea of poverty and its interpretations.

The Lancashire Cotton Famine and *Sylvia's Lovers*

Gaskell thus perceived the knowledge of poverty as strongest and most powerful when built using materialist, as well as emotional, tools. The later novel *Sylvia's Lovers* (1863) throws a good deal of light on this subject. It is, as Carol Lansbury has noted in her fine assessment of the story, a 'necessary preface to *Mary Barton* and *North and South*';[89] its setting in Monkshaven (based on Whitby in North Yorkshire) during the Napoleonic era allows the author to explore a perceived shift from a type of common logic 'typified by [...] lack of introspection and [an] inability to examine motives and intentions',[90] to a more critical, rationalizing response to external events. What makes this shift possible, I argue, is a change in focus from superstition, folklore, and tradition to physiology and starvation.

The novel begins with a portrait of the people of 1800 being a simpler folk than the people of the 1860s:

> In looking back to the last century, it appears curious to see how little our ances-
> tors had the power of putting two things together, and perceiving either the dis-
> cord or harmony thus produced. Is it because we are farther off from those
> times, and have, consequently, a greater range of vision? [...] It seems puzzling
> to look back on men such as our vicar, who almost held the doctrine that the
> King could do no wrong, yet were ever ready to talk of the glorious Revolution,
> and to abuse the Stuarts for having entertained the same doctrine, and tried to
> put it in practice. But such discrepancies ran through good men's lives in those
> days. It is well for us that we live at the present time, when everybody is logical
> and consistent.[91]

The last line is meant to be ironic, of course, given that many arguments for industrial reform were every bit as biased as the vicar's sense of radical politics; and yet the passage signifies a serious perception of cultural and epistemological changes between 1790 and 1860. In another passage, Gaskell identifies earlier agricultural communities as having 'little analysis' and a lack of 'self-consciousness':

> In the agricultural counties, and among the class to which these [...] persons
> belonged, there is little analysis of motive or comparison of characters and
> actions, even at this present day of enlightenment. Sixty or seventy years ago
> there was still less. [...] Taken as a general rule, it may be said that few knew
> what manner of men they were, compared to the numbers now who are fully

---

[89] Lansbury, *Elizabeth Gaskell*, p. 160.   [90] Ibid., p. 161.
[91] Elizabeth Gaskell, *Sylvia's Lovers*, ed. by Andrew Sanders (1863; Oxford: Oxford University Press 2008), p. 68. Subsequent references to this edition will be made in the text.

conscious of their virtues, qualities, failings, and weaknesses, and who go about comparing others with themselves—not in a spirit of Pharisaism and arrogance, but with a vivid self-consciousness that more than anything else deprives characters of freshness and originality.   (p. 74)

In this portrait of a sense of self-consciousness depriving people of 'freshness and originality' we see something of the nostalgia Gaskell felt for a declining way of life. Geoffrey Sharps observes that 'among the most salient features of nearly all the characters are their simplicity and spontaneity: they feel rather than reflect; they act rather than think; they look outwards rather than turn inwards.'[92] One of Gaskell's main sources when writing *Sylvia's Lovers* was George Young's *History of Whitby* (1817), which confirmed that the historic whaling community was comprised of men and women who had an 'ancient simplicity of manners'.[93] In another part of *Sylvia's Lovers*, Gaskell writes:

It is astonishing to look back and find how differently constituted were the minds of most people fifty or sixty years ago; they felt, they understood, without going through reasoning and analytic processes, and if this was the case among the more educated, of course it was still more so in the class to which Sylvia belonged.   (p. 318)

For all her wistful remembrances of a time gone by, Gaskell could never be happy with this sort of unexamined existence; the ideas she had explored in her industrial novels, combined with her Unitarian values, suggested that a more analytical approach was central to doing much of the good that needed to be done in the nineteenth century.

Turning to the material status of the people of Monkshaven, there are key differences to be observed between the whaling community of *Sylvia's Lovers* and the cotton communities of *Mary Barton* and *North and South*. Whereas the latter represent the working classes as badly served by local industry, the former portrays the Monkshaven poor as relatively well-provided for. The Robsons' kitchen has 'unusual plenty' (p. 85) at the start of the novel, and the heroine is first introduced to us while she is on her way to buy the material for a new cloak. These would be extraordinary luxuries for the Davenports or the Bouchers; *Alton Locke* (1850) shows us how new cloaks were extravagances reserved for the well-to-do in the London of the mid-nineteenth century; yet, in the whaling towns of the late eighteenth century, there was money enough for the humble to be well turned out. The only image we have of hunger at the start of *Sylvia's Lovers* is the 'half

---

[92] Sharps, *Observation and Invention*, p. 392.
[93] George Young, *A History of Whitby, and Streoneshalh Abbey, with a Statistical Survey of the Vicinity to the Distance of Twenty-five Miles*, 2 vols. (Whitby: Clark and Medd, 1817), vol. 2, p. 635.

starved' cattle with 'an odd, intelligent expression in their faces [...] which is seldom seen in the placidly stupid countenances of the well-fed animals' (p. 4). A pinched appetite leads to a piqued intelligence, reminding us of the way clemming is the basis of radical cunning in the 1848 novel. In *Sylvia's Lovers* there is many a sign that the well-fed inhabitants of Monkshaven lack the intelligence of their starving mid-nineteenth-century counterparts. The heroine, for instance, rejects her cousin Philip's attempts to teach her reading and writing: 'I'm none wanting to have learning', she tells him; 'what does reading and writing do for one?' (p. 93); it is an attitude Gaskell shows to be not out of place in Monkshaven.

Although they are more comfortably off than the poor workers of the industrial novels, the whaling people have their complaints and their causes of rebellion. The army's impressment of fishermen for the purpose of fighting the French exercises the whaling community against the state, leading to the storming of the press gang's rendezvous and the hanging of Daniel Robson, the heroine's father, for allegedly leading the mob. The novel opens with the press gang seizing members of a whaling crew and murdering a sailor named Darley. At his funeral, his father

> felt, in his sore perplexed heart, full of indignation and dumb anger, as if he must go and hear something which should exorcize the unwonted longing for revenge that disturbed his grief, and made him conscious of that great blank of consolation which faithfulness produces. And for the time he was faithless. How came God to permit such cruel injustice of man? Permitting it, He could not be good. Then what was life, and what was death, but woe and despair?   (p. 69)

There are three interlinking crises represented in the senior Darley's feelings: the rage he feels against the state for the unjust nature of his son's death; his loss of faith; and a failure of knowledge represented by a pair of rhetorical questions: 'what was life', 'what was death'? In Gaskell's philosophy, these three forms of perplexity are connected: tranquillity among the working classes relies upon the healthy exercise of logic, and an appreciation for that logic was, speaking Unitarianly, a God-given faculty.

Like the anger of Barton, Higgins, and Boucher, Daniel Robson's hatred of the press gang is characterized as a misguided response to real injustice. The presence of the King's men in the district leads to rumbling energies that have all the characteristics of a strike:

> A Yorkshire gentleman of rank said that his labourers dispersed like a covey of birds, because a press-gang was reported to have established itself so far inland as Tadcaster [...] No fish was caught, for the fishermen dared no venture out to sea; the markets were deserted, as the press-gangs might come down on any gathering of men; prices were raised, and many were impoverished; many others ruined. [...] The shops were almost deserted; there was no unnecessary

expenditure by the men; they dared not venture out to buy lavish presents for the wife or sweetheart or little children. The public-houses kept scouts on the look-out; while fierce men drank and swore deep oaths of vengeance in the bar—men who did not maunder in their cups, nor grow foolishly merry, but in whom liquor called forth all the desperate, bad passions of human nature.

Indeed, all along the coast of Yorkshire, it seemed as if a blight hung over the land and the people. Men dodged about their daily business with hatred and suspicion in their eyes, and many a curse went over the sea to the three fatal ships lying motionless at anchor three miles off Monkshaven.   (pp. 249–50)

The presence of the press gang is a crisis that requires all the language of an industrial turn-out: men grow angry, there are no luxuries for their sweethearts, poverty and ruin grow common. The passage also makes use of the language of famine—'a blight hung over the land'—and, similar to the anger caused by the clemming in the earlier novels, the reaction to the problem is 'desperate' and comprised of 'bad passions'.

Foremost among these 'bad passions' are Robson's obsessions:

Daniel Robson was [...] like one possessed. He could hardly think of anything else, though he himself was occasionally weary of the same constantly recurring idea, and would fain have banished it from his mind. [...] Since his wife's illness the previous winter he had been a more sober man until now. He was never exactly drunk, for he had a strong, well-seasoned head; but the craving to hear the last news of the actions of the press-gang drew him into Monkshaven nearly every day at this dead agricultural season of the year; and a public-house is generally the focus from which gossip radiates; and probably the amount of drink thus consumed weakened Robson's power over his mind, and caused the concentration of thought on one subject. This may be a physiological explanation of what afterwards was spoken of as a supernatural kind of possession, leading him to his doom.   (p. 253)

This description's use of physiology is likely to have been inspired by Carpenter's *Physiology of Temperance and Total Abstinence* (1853). Bearing in mind the connections between Carpenter and the Gaskells, as well as the fact that William Gaskell wrote a small collection of poems entitled *Temperance Rhymes* (1839), it is difficult to surmise how the author of *Sylvia's Lovers* could have not known Carpenter's ideas on the subject. 'Alcoholized blood on the brain', he noted, has a

direct tendency [...] to weaken the controlling power of the Will, whilst it augments the activity of the automatic of Impulse part of our nature; and wherever the lower feelings and passions have a constitutional or acquired predominance, they will manifest themselves in the conduct, as soon as, being themselves inflamed, they are left free, by the temporary annihilation of voluntary power, from the restraint under which they may have been previously kept.[94]

Carpenter's later *Principles of Mental Physiology* (1874) claimed that mental stimuli inscribed themselves onto the mind, creating channels that formed habits of automatic action independent of will.[95] Gaskell's explanation of Robson's obsession fits with the psychological context of the mid-nineteenth century, and yet the general impression that the character's feelings are a 'supernatural kind of possession' tallies more with the folkloric climate of the late eighteenth century. In the combination of one epistemological approach (the scientific) with another (the superstitious), the narrative voice is elevated to that of knowing onlooker; this echoes what Gaskell writes about the 'little analysis' that went with the agricultural counties of the previous century. The characters may be 'none wanting to have learning', but the novel appears to have the opposite feeling: it wishes to study these simpler people, to watch their passions develop, and to chart the results of an anti-empiricist response to perceived social problems. For Daniel Robson, of course, things turn out badly, which may seem to be a condemnation of his rebellion, but is actually a more complex insight into the links between thought (or the lack of it) and the responses people make to social wrongs.

The writing of *Sylvia's Lovers* was interrupted by the Lancashire Cotton Famine of 1862. According to Easson, 'relief committees were organized and Gaskell was active, whether cutting up calico for shirts to provide sewing for women or raising and dispensing money'.[96] Uglow believes that Gaskell worked herself 'almost to death' in the relief effort, and, as a result, the third volume of *Sylvia's Lovers* was turned into a 'spiritual allegory [...], a desperate search for belief in a better world'.[97] While the ending of the novel does indeed search for a better world, it is similar to the conclusions of *Mary Barton* and *North and South* in that it finds spiritual and moral solutions in a logical, material, and realist approach to the problems associated with extreme poverty.

In 1861, the MP for Manchester, Thomas Bazley, stood before the British Association for the Advancement of Science, during its conference in his city, and issued a warning about the over-reliance on imports of raw cotton from the Southern American States:

---

[94] William B. Carpenter, *The Physiology of Temperance and Total Abstinence being an Examination of the Effects of the Excessive, Moderate, and Occasional Use of Alcoholic Liquors on the Healthy Human System* (London: Henry G. Bohn, 1853), p. 46.

[95] For the best summary of this theory and Carpenter's contribution to it, see Jenny Bourne Taylor and Sally Shuttleworth (eds), *Embodied Selves: An Anthology of Physiological Texts, 1830–1890* (Oxford: Oxford University Press, 1998), pp. 95–101. On the topic of physiological psychology more generally, see Rylance, *Victorian Psychology*, pp. 70–109 and Jane Wood, *Passion and Pathology in Victorian Fiction* (Oxford: Oxford University Press, 2001).

[96] Easson, *Elizabeth Gaskell*, p. 170.   [97] Uglow, *Elizabeth Gaskell*, pp. 319, 504.

The wonder is that so large a supply of cotton could be procured from that one source, the United States [...] During the last year the consumption of cotton in Great Britain was 85 per cent from the United States [...] The present position of the trade is most precarious and dangerous.[98]

The Civil War in America led to a blockade being placed on exports and, as fore-warned by Bazley, the Lancashire mills suffered from want of raw material. In *Das Kapital* (1867), Marx suggested that the crisis was caused, to a large extent, by the development of more sophisticated apparatus which had had the effect of putting manual labourers out of work: 'more productive machinery on a larger scale was concentrated in the hands of a smaller number of capitalists'. Between 1861 and 1868, he claimed, 338 cotton factories had gone out of business—not because of the effects of the American war, but because fewer 'hands' were needed now that machines were doing most of the work.[99]

Notwithstanding, the 1862 cotton crisis became the centre of a great deal of discussion on the question of what constitutes famine and whether the present calamity qualifies as such. To some, the term *cotton famine* referred only to the shortage of cotton—Lancashire did not see a *food* famine, as such, but it did see a *cotton* famine in the literal sense.[100] In a letter to Vernon Lushington, however, Gaskell said: 'There is no doubt about the distress; bad enough in Manchester; infinitely worse at Blackburn and Preston: & in South Lancashire generally. [...] Some people say we have touched our worst as to the distress: but I fear not,—very much.'[101] Gaskell declined the offer to write an account of the crisis in *The Daily News*, saying that 'the new phases of life and character, which, doubtless, this sad crisis does call out, they are so varied, so indistinct, & so difficult to appreciate truly, that I, living here in Manchester, with the best opportunities, should shrink from the attempt to define them'.[102] According to this account, the famine had caused nothing short of a revolution in the 'life and character' of the Lancashire people. Gaskell could, of course, have been exaggerating in order to excuse herself from the *Daily News* work, but there is certainly enough support for what she says in other sources. In 1861, the Medical Officer for Health, Sir John Simon, asked the physician Edward Smith to investigate the nutritional health of the Lancashire operatives. Measuring carbon and nitrogen in the food

[98] Thomas Bazley, 'A Glance at the Cotton Trade', *Report of the Thirty-first Meeting of the British Association for the Advancement of Science* (London: John Murray, 1862), pp. 206–8 (p. 206).

[99] Karl Marx, *Das Kapital*, trans. as *Capital*, ed. by David McLellan (1867; Oxford: Oxford University Press, 2008), p. 266.

[100] Norman Longmate, *The Hungry Mills: The Story of the Lancashire Cotton Famine 1861–5* (London: Maurice Temple Smith, 1978), p. 71.

[101] Elizabeth Gaskell, letter to Vernon Lushington, ?15 April 1862, Gaskell Letters 2, pp. 237–9 (p. 238). In an earlier letter to Florence Nightingale, dated 22 January 1862, Gaskell says that she had discussed the matter with Bazley. See Gaskell Letters 2, p. 231.

[102] Elizabeth Gaskell, letter to unknown recipient, 7 February 1862, Gaskell Letters, p. 677.

that was most readily available in times of distress, Smith gauged that families were unable to maintain 'even minimal food requirements'.[103] Five years later, John Watts wrote in *The Facts of the Cotton Famine* that there were 'evidences of famine except fever and pestilence; and these were only prevented by the extraordinary liberality by which the universal public [...] met the cry of distress, and rushed to its relief'.[104] The lack of pestilence, or 'famine fever', was, according to Watts, the factor that prevented the Lancashire crisis from being as destructive as the Irish Hunger had been. It also meant that the suffering, 'great' and 'nobly borne', was less visible to the outside world.

Nevertheless, George Buchanan, physician to the London Fever Hospital, suggested that Lancashire had not escaped the fever. Fewer people died from the condition, he conceded, but there was an 'epidemic' of typhus nonetheless: 'I visited Preston first on the 29th of October, and found in the House of Recovery (the parish fever hospital) fifty-two cases of *bona-fide* typhus.'[105] In a five-week period during 1862, a total of 109 cases of typhus had presented themselves.[106] William Rayner, a surgeon based in Stockport, insisted in a letter to *The Lancet* that it was difficult to tell when a patient had been badly affected by the famine, as hunger predisposes the body to a series of conditions which may not be identified as actual starvation.[107] And yet there were a fair number of famine and fever deniers. John Beddoe, physician to the Bristol Royal Infirmary, accused Buchanan, in the *British Medical Journal*, of 'gross exaggeration'.[108] Another correspondent noted that Buchanan ought to be 'sharply criticised' because there was 'nothing like an epidemic of true typhus in Manchester'.[109] In his *History of the Cotton Famine* (1864), R. Arthur Arnold claimed: 'the numbers of the homeless were not so great as many be found upon any winter's night in London'.[110] Edwin Chadwick joined in the debate, writing in the *Manchester Daily Examiner and Times* that the famine had actually had a positive effect on the people;[111] as Arnold explains, the cotton famine encouraged operatives to go out into the open air more often; women were forced to take better care of their homes and their children; and working people were not able to overindulge themselves in food and drink.[112]

[103] Carleton B. Chapman, 'Edward Smith (?1818–1874): Physiologist, Human Ecologist, Reformer', *Journal of the History of Medicine and Allied Sciences*, 22:1 (1967), pp. 1–26 (p. 15).

[104] John Watts, *The Facts of the Cotton Famine* (London: Simpkin, et al., 1866), p. 230.

[105] George Buchanan, 'On Recent Typhus in Lancashire', *Lancet*, 14 February 1863, pp. 174–6 (p. 174).

[106] Buchanan, 'Typhus in Lancashire', p. 175.

[107] William Rayner, 'Letter to the Editor', *Lancet*, 6 December 1862, p. 632.

[108] John Beddoe, 'On the Death Rates in the Cotton Districts', *British Medical Journal*, 3 January 1863, pp. 8–9 (p. 9).

[109] Unsigned, 'Manchester', *British Medical Journal*, 7 March 1863, pp. 250–1 (p. 251).

[110] R. Arthur Arnold, *The History of the Cotton Famine* (London: Saunders et al., 1864), p. 112.

[111] W. O. Henderson, *The Lancashire Cotton Famine, 1861–1865* (Manchester: Manchester University Press, 1934), pp. 102–3.

[112] R. Arthur Arnold, *History*, pp. 156–58.

As a Lancashire sexton was reported to have said at the time, 'poverty seldom dees. There's far more kilt wi' o'er-heytin an' o'erdrinking nor wi' bein' pinched.'[113]

As one would expect, this perception (typical, as we have seen, of Chadwick's way of thinking) was far from being accepted universally. In an article for *All the Year Round*, it was reported that, among 'the Lancashire operatives [...] the average health was found to be below par whenever the quantity of food taken was pronounced by such a test to be inadequate'.[114] Physicians like Buchanan responded to doubts over the severity of the famine by stressing, in line with what Corrigan had said about the Irish Crisis, that it is often difficult to know when an individual has died from starvation, or whether he or she had succumbed to one of the secondary conditions linked to extreme hunger. Buchanan reported his findings to the Privy Council, insisting that the 'diagnosis' of starvation involved a careful interpretation of its 'giveaway' signs:

> Universal emaciation and pallor do not, indeed, at first strike a visitor to these towns. [...] But when the visitor penetrates into the houses of the poor, he observes a very different standard of health. There is a wan and haggard look about the people [...] Mothers, who most of all starve themselves, have got pale and emaciated. At Ashton was added the testimony that mothers have become weaker in childbirth, and faint readily from any excess of hæmorrhage at that time. Lactation has been noticed to be unwisely prolonged, the mother pleading inability to purchase food appropriate for a weaned child. [...] Intractable diarrhœa prevailed in the summer and autumn in Preston, but not elsewhere. A hæmorrhagic tendency has been witnessed in several towns; and actual scurvy has been seen among the cotton-workers in Stockport, Preston, and Salford.[115]

Buchanan's report is as much about ways of looking as it is about the subject being looked at. The observer needs to penetrate the hardest-hit areas and, once inside, he must come face to face with a range of inconsistent physiological symptoms. 'There can be little doubt', Buchanan therefore concludes, 'that under the present conditions of food, lodging, and clothing, the healthy-state of the unemployed operatives in Lancashire is gradually deteriorating.'[116]

Philip Hepburn's Body

Gaskell drew upon Buchanan's kind of social physiology not only to make her work more realistic, but also to underscore the importance of the material and

---

[113] Quoted in Longmate, *Hungry Mills*, p. 98.

[114] Unsigned, 'The Lives and Deaths of the People', *All the Year Round*, 12 (1864), pp. 198–205 (p. 200).

[115] Unsigned, 'Report on the Health of the Cotton Operatives', *Lancet*, 10 January 1863, pp. 43–4 (p. 43).

[116] Ibid., p. 44.

corporeal puzzle in the processes of thinking intelligently about famine. In the third volume of *Sylvia's Lovers*, specifically, reconciliation and atonement rely upon an interpretation of Philip Hepburn's anatomy, which is smashed and burned during the war against Bonaparte, then starved during the agricultural famine of 1800.

Soon after Hepburn rescues his love rival, the dashing harpooner Charlie Kinraid, during the Battle of Acre, the latter rejects tales of ghosts and visions when his doctor tries to convince him that it was the ghost of Hepburn that must have saved him. 'It was him', replies Kinraid, 'it was flesh and blood, and not a spirit' (p. 434). Afterwards, Philip imagines himself in the position of Sir Guy, Earl of Warwick, who in legend returns to his wife Phillis after a long period at war:

> In the small oblong of looking-glass hung against the wall, Philip caught the reflection of his own face, and laughed scornfully at the sight. The thin hair lay upon his temples in the flakes that betoken long ill-health; his eyes were the same as ever, and they had always been considered the best feature in his face; but they were sunk in their orbits, and looked hollow and gloomy. As for the lower part of his face, blackened, contracted, drawn away from his teeth, the outline entirely changed by the breakage of his jaw-bone, he was indeed a fool if he thought himself fit to go forth to win back that love which Sylvia had forsworn.
>
> (pp. 466–7)

As with Kinraid's rejection of the ghostly interpretation of his rescue, Hepburn's interest is in his own flesh and blood—his sunken eyes, blackened and contracted face, and broken jawbone. The fable of Guy and Phillis comes crashing about his ears because the later stages of the novel require the tools of modern physiology rather than myth and legend to create a plot resolution.

Foreshadowing what would occur during the Lancashire Cotton Famine, the war with the French at the turn of the nineteenth century caused an agricultural famine in Britain. Having come through the worst of the 1860s crisis, and finding time to sit down to her manuscript of *Sylvia's Lovers* again, Gaskell chose to set the closing scenes among the hardships felt by the rural communities of the early 1800s:

> It was the spring of 1800. Old people yet can tell of the hard famine of that year. The harvest of the autumn before had failed; the war and the corn laws had brought the price of corn up to a famine rate; and much of what came into the market was unsound, and consequently unfit for food, yet hungry creatures bought it eagerly, and tried to cheat disease by mixing the damp, sweet, clammy flour with rice or potato meal. Rich families denied themselves pastry and all unnecessary and luxurious uses of wheat in any shape; the duty on hair-powder was increased; and all these palliatives were but as drops in the ocean of the great want of the people.   (p. 481)

Gaskell's source for information on the 1800 famine was likely to have been volume 42 of the *Annual Register*, which William borrowed from the Portico Library.[117] Her choice of the 1800 famine is highly significant. Occurring two years after the publication of Malthus's *Essay on Population* (1798), it was seen as an opportunity for Malthus to 'prove' some of the principles of his theory. He published a pamphlet entitled *An Investigation of the Cause of the Present High Price of Provisions* (1800), claiming that the existing Poor Laws were driving up prices by providing for the most poor at the expense of others.[118] According to Harold A. Boner, 'the pamphlet attracted considerable attention, not only to itself, but to the *Essay on Population*'.[119] *Sylvia's Lovers* appears at first to confirm Malthus's view by focusing on the rise in prices. Living a short distance from Monkshaven, Philip starves 'as too many [did], for insufficiency of means to buy the high-priced food' (p. 488). Yet, his story also exposes how Malthus's argument was self-defeating: if all the alms are given to the worst off, then being close to starvation, Philip should qualify for assistance. Indeed, if the Poor Laws were supporting the poorest, there could be no famine, as hunger, before the New Poor Law, was the result of the most poverty-stricken receiving no social relief. Malthus's response to the 1800 famine was typical of his deductive reasoning: having formed an overarching theory, he hoped to find evidence to support it in individual cases or events. The alternative, inductive approach is showcased in Buchanan's writing and the final stages of *Sylvia's Lovers*, where material evidence becomes the basis of more considered interpretations.

In spite of his hunger, Philip manages to rescue his estranged daughter from the sea after he witnesses her being swept away by the tide. In so doing, he is fatally injured and is close to death by the time he is visited by his wife Sylvia, the woman he tricked into marriage by allowing her to believe that her true lover, Kinraid, was dead. Focusing on his starved and shattered body, Gaskell makes the point that the unequal distribution of food during the famine of 1800 (and, by implication, in 1862) was not the result of overfeeding the poor, as Malthus and his disciples believed, but of the imbalanced nature of industrial capitalism, which allowed some to prosper and others to starve. Following his accident, Sylvia finds Philip in a room that 'was dark, all except the little halo or circle of light made by a dip candle' (pp. 494–5); the 'dripping clothes [have been] cut off from the poor maimed body by the doctor's orders' (p. 495) and, while Sylvia appears 'spirit-like', 'white, noiseless, and upborne from earth' (p. 495), Philip guiltily turns 'his poor disfigured face to the wall, hiding it in shadow' (p. 495). Philip's death has plenty about it that is sentimental, to be sure, but there is also a clear determination to

---

[117] See Shirley Foster, *Elizabeth Gaskell: A Literary Life* (Basingstoke: Palgrave Macmillan, 2002), p. 157.

[118] Harold A. Boner, *Hungry Generations: The Nineteenth-Century Case against Malthusianism* (New York, NY: King's Crown Press, 1955), pp. 23–4.

[119] Ibid., p. 24.

focus on the dying man's disfigurements in spite of the melodramatic tragedy playing out: 'the [not *his*] poor maimed body' is contrasted with the angelic qualities of his wife who notices, in spite of all Hepburn has done to wrong her, 'he was short o' food [...] and we had plenty' (p. 493); while she had been 'living in [the] ease and comfort' of a modestly prosperous fishing port, 'her husband's daily life' in the country was 'a struggle with starvation' (p. 493).

In *Sylvia's Lovers*, we might ask whether the novel's weepy resolution could ever be realized without focus on its major character's physical sufferings. The novel always had an interest in putting the more modern, empirical approach alongside traditional, folkloric interpretations of events, but, following the cotton crisis of 1862, Gaskell appears eager to find spiritual and emotional solutions through physiological representation, which is not inconsistent with the way her industrial novels perceived the detailed description of bodies and environments as key to a more intelligent, and sympathetic, response to poverty.

4

Charles Dickens

'Nothink and Starwation'

Dickens had some sympathy with Kingsley's idea that the study of the natural world was a panacea for social ills. In his review of *The Poetry of Science, or Studies of the Physical Phenomena of Nature* (1848) by mineralogist, statistician, and Fellow of the Royal Society, Robert Hunt, Dickens wrote:

> To show that the facts of science are at least as full of poetry, as the most poetical fancies ever founded on an imperfect observation and a distant suspicion of them [...]; to show that [...] there is, in every forest, in every tree, in every leaf, and in every ring on every sturdy trunk, a beautiful and wonderful creation, always changing, always going on, always bearing testimony to the stupendous workings of Almighty Wisdom, and always leading the student's mind from wonder on to wonder, until he is wrapt and lost in the vast worlds of wonder by which he is surrounded from his cradle to his grave; it is a purpose worthy of the natural philosopher, and salutary to the spirit of the age.[1]

According to Michael Slater, this review shows how Dickens believed that 'Scientific discoveries, far from binding us "in stern utilitarian chains" like the poor Gradgrind children [...] should, in fact, become the successors to the fairy-tales of our early reading';[2] yet, the use of the word 'salutary' in this passage—a word favoured, as we have seen, by statisticians, social reformers, and political economists of the nineteenth century—suggests that Dickens sees a link between the natural sciences and social good. Dickens also had a good deal of sympathy with Gaskell's notion that the middle and working classes, men and masters especially, needed to find better ways of getting along. As Stephen Blackpool lay dying in *Hard Times* (1854), for instance, he says that

---

[1] Charles Dickens, Review of Robert Hunt, *The Poetry of Science, or Studies of the Physical Phenomena of Nature*, in Dickens Journalism 2, pp. 129–34 (p. 131).

[2] Michael Slater, *The Genius of Charles Dickens: The Ideas and Inspiration of Britain's Greatest Novelist* (London: Duckworth Overlook, 2011), p. 20. See also Adelene Buckland, '"The Poetry of Science": Charles Dickens, Geology, and Visual and Material Culture in Victorian London', *Victorian Literature and Culture*, 35 (2007), pp. 679–94.

The Science of Starving in Victorian Literature, Medicine, and Political Economy. Andrew Mangham,
Oxford University Press (2020). © Andrew Mangham.
DOI: 10.1093/oso/9780198850038.001.0001

if Mr. Bounderby had ever know'd me right—if he'd ever know'd me at aw—he would'n ha' took'n offence wi' me. [...] I ha' seen more clear, and ha' made it my dyin' prayer that aw th'wold may on'y coom together more, an get a better unnerstan'in o' one anther.[3]

Patrick Brantlinger has noted that 'the war between capital and labor', in Dickens's work, 'is simply an unfortunate mistake, to be corrected by better feeling on both sides'. More recently, Juliet John has suggested that the author emphasized 'connection between individuals and social groups, with the rejection of inwardly focused individualism and/or the tribal reliance on difference and separatism of party and protest politics'.[4] Dickens also put a great deal of energy into satirizing the problems he saw as the result of approaches to poverty which were crystallized in the New Poor Law of 1834. In this, Sally Ledger has shown Dickens to be inspired by political firebrands such as William Cobbett and Douglas Jerrold.[5] In the following chapter, I suggest that physiological ideas of starvation assisted Dickens in his own battles with the ideological and legislative systems which he saw as guilty of both simplifying the problems of poverty and creating catch-all measures that amounted to little more than state-sponsored neglect. Gail Turley Houston has suggested that the author's interest in hunger harks back to his 'own memories of [...] starving' in Warren's Blacking Factory: 'Dickens was psychologically working though his own transition from a lower-middle-class young man to a mature man of fame and means'.[6] Yet I do not agree that it is possible to reduce Dickens's complex portrayals of hunger to a single episode in his own life: while the Blacking Factory experience was acknowledged by Dickens to have had a formative effect on him, it is also true that his interest in starvation had larger cultural, political, and epistemological influences at the time of writing.

In suggesting that Dickens turned to science as a way of understanding the emotive question of poverty-related hunger, it may seem that we are going to face the obstacle of the author's famous view that 'there is a range of imagination in most of us, which no amount of steam-engines will satisfy, and which The-great-exhibition-of-the-works-of-industry-of-all-nations, itself, will probably leave unappeased'.[7] 'In an utilitarian age', Dickens said, 'it is a matter of grave

---

[3] Charles Dickens, *Hard Times*, ed. by Kate Flint (1854; London: Penguin, 2003), p. 264. Subsequent references to this edition will be given in the text.

[4] Patrick Brantlinger, 'Dickens and the Factories', *Nineteenth-Century Fiction*, 26:3 (1971), pp. 270–85 (p. 281); Juliet John, *Dickens and Mass Culture* (Oxford: Oxford University Press, 2010), p. 41. Italics in original.

[5] Sally Ledger, *Dickens and the Popular Radical Imagination* (Cambridge: Cambridge University Press, 2009).

[6] Gail Turley Houston, *Consuming Fictions: Gender, Class and Hunger in Dickens's Novels* (Carbondale and Edwardsville, IL: Southern Illinois University Press, 1994), p. 37.

[7] Charles Dickens, 'The Amusements of the People' (1), *Household Words*, 1 (1850), Dickens Journalism 2, pp. 179–85 (p. 181).

importance that Fairy tales should be respected.'[8] And 'do not let us', he concluded, 'in the laudable pursuit of the facts that surround us, neglect the fancy and the imagination which equally surround us as part of the great scheme'.[9] Dickens's insistence that our lives contain a vital need for poetry, imagination, and fantasy is signalled most forcefully in *Hard Times* (1854), where the effects of Gradgrind's Utilitarian philosophy, prescribed by Mr. M'Choakumchild in the schoolroom and Mr. Bounderby in the factory, is responsible for the tragic fates of Louisa Gradgrind and Stephen Blackpool, respectively: 'What do *I* know, father', says Louisa, 'of tastes and fancies; of aspirations and affections; of all that part of my nature in which such light things might have been nourished? What escape have I had from problems that could be demonstrated, and realities that could be grasped?' (p. 100; italics in original). 'Like Marx', Juliet John writes, Dickens was 'concerned that for the working classes, the hard, monotonous life of industrial labour', a thing he associates with a utilitarian experience, 'involved the dehumanization or "reification" of people who were expected to behave like cogs in a machine'.[10] Indeed, the view that *Hard Times* polarizes 'the competing philosophies of Mr. Gradgrind's Utilitarianism and the circus's traditional humanism'[11] is a common one in Dickens criticism. Patrick Brantlinger, following F. R. Leavis's thinking, claimed that 'the Sleary philosophy' that 'people mutht be amuthed' and that 'they can't alwayth a working, nor yet they can't be alwayth a learning' (p. 45) contains 'no profound revelations, no metaphysical alternative to materialism nor [...anything] close to socialism'.[12] For Chris Brooks, the circus and the fancy it represents furnish only a 'temporary relief from the inhumanities of Coketown'.[13] Yet the inhumanities of the fictional town are powerful, I argue, because of the predominant absence of fancy; we know from Dickens's sympathetic representations of working men such as Daniel Doyce and George Rouncewell's brother that he was not against industry in principle. Joel J. Brattin notes that Dickens creates an 'equivocal but generally positive figure of the Ironmaster' and 'paints an unambiguously positive figure of an industrial revolutionary: the engineer and inventor Daniel Doyce'.[14] In an important 1843 address to the Manchester Athenaeum he

[8] Charles Dickens, 'Frauds on Fairies', *Household Words*, 8 (1853), Dickens Journalism 3, pp. 166–74 (p. 168).
[9] Charles Dickens, Speech to the Annual Meeting of the Institutional Association of Lancashire and Cheshire (3 December 1858), in *Speeches Literary and Social by Charles Dickens* (London: Camden Hotten, n.d.), pp. 157–66 (p. 166).
[10] John, *Dickens and Mass Culture*, p. 41.
[11] Patricia E. Johnson, '*Hard Times* and the Structure of Industrialism: The Novel as Factory', *Studies in the Novel*, 21:2 (1989), pp. 128–37 (p. 129).
[12] Brantlinger, 'Dickens and the Factories', p. 282.
[13] Chris Brooks, *Signs for the Times: Symbolic Realism in the Mid-Victorian World* (London: George Allen and Unwin, 1984), p. 67.
[14] Joel J. Brattin, 'Three Revolutions: Alternative Routes to Social Change in *Bleak House*', in *Charles Dickens as an Agent of Change*, ed. by Joachim Frenk and Lena Steveker (New York, NY: AMS Press, 2015), pp. 20–31 (pp. 19, 21).

praised the northern metropolis as a 'little world of labour',[15] and suggested that the will to advancement offered the workers and masters a potential 'commonwealth of Utopia', where there could be no 'knowledge of party difficulties, or public animosities between side and side, or between man and man'.[16] In apparent contradiction to what he would write about the oppressiveness of the Gradgrind children's various 'ologies' and their 'conchological cabinet, [...] metallurgical cabinet, [...] mineralogical cabinet', and 'specimens [...] arranged and labelled' (p. 17), Dickens went on to criticize, in his Athenaeum speech, the 'large class of men' who suggest that 'a little learning is a dangerous thing':

> I should be glad to hear such people's estimate of the comparative danger of 'a little learning' and a vast amount of ignorance; I should be glad to know which they consider the most prolific parent of misery and crime. Descending a little lower in the social scale, I should be glad to assist them in their calculations, by carrying them into certain gaols and nightly refuges I know of, where my own heart dies within me, when I see thousands of immortal creatures condemned, without alternative or choice, to tread, not what our great poet calls the 'primrose path' to the everlasting bonfire, but one of jagged flints and stones, laid down by brutal ignorance, and held together, like the solid rocks, by years of this most wicked axiom.[17]

The seeming inconsistency between this message, delivered in the cotton industry's capital, and the alleged 'anti-intellectualism' of *Hard Times*[18] is no inconsistency at all, but evidence, I argue, of Dickens's fundamental belief in the need for balance. Sleary's philosophy is that people can't *always* be working, or *always* learning; he offers no '*alternative* to the mechanisation of labour and the philosophy of utilitarianism', nor any 'metaphysical *alternative* to materialism' because labour, philosophy, and materialism do not need alternatives, they needed counterweights. What makes Coketown a monotonous modern nightmare is not the presence of mechanical labour and positivist approaches to learning, but the *absence* of the fairy abstractions that make these forms of progress bearable. Indeed, in a letter to Henry Cole Dickens said of Mr. Gradgrind 'that there is reason and good intention in much that he does—in fact, in all that he does—but that he over-does it'.[19]

The interpretation of a polarization between fact and fancy in Dickens, and the assumption that he celebrates the latter as an alternative to the former, obscures a more complex relationship between those two energies in his work. The truth of the matter is summed up neatly in Juliet John's *Dickens and Mass Culture* (2010),

---

[15] Charles Dickens, Speech to the Manchester Athenaeum, 5 October 1843, in *Speeches*, pp. 74–81.
[16] Ibid., p. 74.   [17] Ibid., pp. 77–8.   [18] Brantlinger, 'Dickens and the Factories', p. 282.
[19] Charles Dickens, letter to Henry Cole, 17 June 1854, Dickens Letters 7, p. 354.

where she features a quote from Dickens's 1869 address to the Birmingham and Midland Institute:

> It is commonly assumed—much too commonly—that this age is a material age, and that a material age is an irreligious age. I confess [...] that I do not understand this much-used and much-abused phrase, a 'material age', I cannot comprehend— if anyone can: which I very much doubt—its logical signification. [...] Do I make a more material journey to the bedside of my dying parents or my dying child, when I travel there at the rate of sixty miles an hour, than when I travel thither at the rate of six? Rather, in the swift case, does not my agonized heart become over-fraught with gratitude to that Supreme Beneficence from whom alone can have proceeded the wonderful means of shortening my suspense?

' "Material" inventions', John observes, 'enhance the spiritual dimension of life'.[20] In Dickens's 'Preliminary Word' (1850), the preface he writes for the first issue of *Household Words*, it is suggested that spiritual dimensions appear *within* ordinary material life: 'in all familiar things, even in those which are repellent on the surface, there is Romance enough, if we will find it'.[21] In the closing paragraph of *The Chimes* (1844), Dickens rewrote *A Midsummer Night's Dream*'s 'If we shadows have offended' epilogue:

> Had Trotty dreamed? Or are his joys and sorrows, and the actors in them, but a dream; himself a dream; the teller of this tale a dreamer, waking but now? If it be so, O listener, dear to him in all his visions, try to bear in mind the stern realities from which these shadows come.[22]

Where Shakespeare's comedy aims to dispel any 'realities' by stressing the fictive nature of his drama, Dickens highlights how the dreams of *The Chimes*, like those of *A Christmas Carol* (1843), emerge out of the real world rather than any alternative, fantastic dimension. The 'Preliminary Word' makes it apparent that understanding the spiritual aspects of familiar things is an important social responsibility:

> We seek to bring into innumerable homes, from the stirring world around us, the knowledge of many social wonders, good and evil, that are not calculated to render any of us less ardently persevering in ourselves, less tolerant of one another, less faithful in the progress of mankind, less thankful for the privilege of living in

[20] John, *Dickens and Mass Culture*, p. 174.
[21] Charles Dickens, 'A Preliminary Word', *Household Words*, 1 (1853), Dickens Journalism 2, pp. 175–9 (p. 177).
[22] Charles Dickens, *The Chimes* in *Christmas Books*, ed. by Ruth Glancy (1844; Oxford: Oxford University Press, 1988), pp. 93–182 (p. 182). Subsequent references to this edition will be given in the text.

this summer-dawn of time. [...Our aim is to] teach the hardest workers at this whirling wheel of toil, that their lot is not necessarily a moody, brutal fact, excluded from the sympathies and graces of imagination; to bring the greater and the lesser in degree, together, upon a wide field, and mutually dispose them to a better acquaintance and a kinder understanding [...] The mightier inventions of this age are not, to our thinking, all material, but have a kind of souls in their stupendous bodies which may find expression in Household Words.[23]

Were we to focus on evidence of the author's belief in fancy as a richer alternative to reality in this passage, we would set about highlighting the terms 'fact', 'hard workers', 'wheel of toil', 'wonder', 'imagination', and 'soul'. Doing so, however, might cause us to overlook the words 'knowledge' and 'understanding', and miss the important evidence that, as in the Athenaeum speech, Dickens envisaged a world where the classes were brought together not by the mechanics of the age's industrialism, nor even by fancy, but by the *knowledge* that each of those energies make possible when they are in balance. In 'On Strike' (1854), the article he wrote in response to the Preston turn-out, he notes:

> I believe [...] that into the relations between employers and employed, as into all the relations of this life, there must enter something of feeling and sentiment; something of mutual explanation, forbearance, and consideration; something which is not to be found in Mr. McCulloch's dictionary, and is not exactly state-able in figures; otherwise those relations are wrong and rotten at the core and will never bear sound fruit.[24]

Sitting in between McCulloch's dictionary and figures, on one side of the scale, and feeling and sentiment, on the other, is 'explanation, forbearance, and consideration'. In Dickens's social thought, knowledge (or, as we shall see, the kind of thinking that *leads to* accurate knowledge—that which we might call patient, detailed, or ruminative) is the pivot that balances and fastens fact and fancy together. Hence, rather than favouring the spiritual dimension over the material, Dickens saw careful and intelligent responses to reality as the means of creating the sympathies and affections that were crucial to social questions.

Nothink

It made sense, then, that Dickens was angered by interpretations of social problems that he perceived to be too simplistic. We see a powerful example of this

[23] Dickens, 'Preliminary Word', p. 177.
[24] Charles Dickens, 'On Strike', *Household Words*, 8 (1854), Journalism 3, pp. 196–210 (p. 199).

in an early piece of journalism he wrote for *Bell's Life in London* entitled 'The Streets—Night' (1836):

> [A] wretched woman with [an] infant in her arms, round whose meagre form the remnant of her own scanty shawl is carefully wrapped, has been attempting to sing some popular ballad, in the hope of wringing a few pence from the compassionate passer-by. A brutal laugh at her weak voice is all she has gained. The tears fall thick and fast down her own pale face; the child is cold and hungry, and its low half stifled wailing adds to the misery of its wretched mother, as she moans aloud, and sinks despairingly down on a cold damp doorstep.
>
> Singing! How few of those who pass such a miserable creature as this think of the anguish of the heart, the sinking of soul and spirit, which the very effort of singing produces. Bitter mockery! Disease, neglect, and starvation, faintly articulating the words of the joyous ditty, that has enlivened your hours of feasting and merriment, God knows how often! It is no subject of jeering. The weak tremulous voice tells a fearful tale of want and famishing; and the feeble singer of this roaring song may turn away, only to die of cold and hunger.[25]

Janis McLarren Caldwell notes that, in descriptions such as these, Dickens 'demands his readers attend and see';[26] yet, what I would argue is that 'The Streets—Night' illustrates how the problem is that passers-by already see, they just do not see well. Their fault, as Dickens points out, is that few of them 'think' about what the feebleness of voice indicates; their sensitivity is a fleeting, momentary vision, approaching nothing like the kind of careful perception of reality that the woman's 'disease, neglect and starvation' necessitate. The solution, the author suggests, is not only to see, but to see *intelligently*—to use the interpretive strategies that we see exemplified in the way the description itself unpacks the scene: the weak tremulous voice tells a tale of want and famishing; it is an indication of a sad physiological reality.

More broadly, Dickens's social-problem writing, like Kingsley's and Gaskell's, sought to expose the ways in which questions of poverty had been ill-considered by those who meant well, but whose unconsidered trust in laissez faire prevented them from seeing the full gravity of the matter. For example, *The Chimes*, according to Michael Slater, is 'the most overtly Radical fiction [Dickens] ever wrote',[27] with the text's main political opponent being the statistical brainwashing of

---

[25] Charles Dickens, 'The Streets—Night', Bell's Life in London, 17 January 1836, Journalism 1, pp. 55–60 (pp. 58–9).

[26] Janis McLarren Caldwell, 'Illness, Disease and Social Hygiene', in Sally Ledger and Holly Furneaux (eds.), *Charles Dickens in Context* (Cambridge: Cambridge University Press, 2011), pp. 343–9 (p. 347) .

[27] Michael Slater, *Charles Dickens* (2009; New Haven and London, 2011), p. 229. Ledger similarly notes that 'The Chimes is perhaps the most avowedly radical of Dickens's works of fiction' (*Radical Imagination*, p. 130).

political economists. Yet, lumped in with such evils are the hypocrisies of the 'Poor Man's Friend', Lord Joseph Bowley, and the arrant stupidity of Alderman Cute. The latter, as Slater and Ledger discuss, was based on Sir Peter Laurie, 'a well-known Middlesex magistrate who was celebrated for his bluff jocularity and his ability (as he saw it) to talk to offenders in their own language'.[28] In his previous role as London Mayor, Laurie had expressed his determination to "put down" suicide', a resolve that Dickens turns into Alderman Cute's intention to 'put down Starvation':

> 'You see, my friend,' pursued the Alderman, 'there's a great deal of nonsense talked about Want—"hard up," you know; that's the phrase, isn't it? ha! ha! ha!— and I intend to Put it Down. There's a certain amount of cant in vogue about Starvation, and I mean to Put it Down. That's all!'   (p. 112)

In a letter to his brother-in-law Henry Austin, Dickens called Laurie 'that incarnation of a Vulgar Soul and a thoroughly mean and sordid spirit'; to his friend Douglas Jerrold he had called all such 'city aristocracy' 'sleek, slobbering, bow-paunched, overfed, apoplectic, snorting cattle'.[29] In 1841 Jerrold himself aimed a number of savage criticisms at Laurie in *Punch*, concluding that 'Sir Peter has, very justly, no compassion for the famishing wretch stung and goaded "to jump the life to come." Why should he? Sir Peter is of that happy class of men who have found this life too good a thing to leave'.[30] Similarly, in *The Chimes*, Dickens suggests that Cute's comfortable life gives *him* a limited view of what starvation actually involves:

> Remember, Justice, your high moral boast and pride [of 'putting down']. Come, Alderman! Balance those scales. Throw me into this, the empty one, no dinner, and Nature's founts in some poor woman, dried by starving misery and rendered obdurate to claims for which her offspring *has* authority in holy mother Eve. Weigh me the two, you Daniel, going to judgment, when your day shall come! Weigh them, in the eyes of suffering thousands, audience (not unmindful) of the grim farce you play. Or supposing that you strayed from your five wits—it's not so far to go, but that it might be—and laid hands upon that throat of yours, warning your fellows (if you have a fellow) how they croak their comfortable wickedness to raving heads and stricken hearts.   (p. 152)

[28] Ledger, *Radical Imagination*, p. 126. See also Michael Slater, 'Carlyle and Jerrold into Dickens: A Study of *The Chimes*', *Nineteenth-Century Fiction*, 24:4 (1970), pp. 506–26 (pp. 524–5).
[29] Charles Dickens, letter to Henry Austin, 21 March 1850, Dickens Letters 6, pp. 69–70 (p. 70) and letter to Douglas Jerrold, 3 May 1843, Dickens Letters 3, pp. 481–3 (p. 482).
[30] 'Q' [Douglas Jerrold], 'Sir Peter Laurie on Human Life', *Punch, or the London Charivari*, 1 (1841), p. 210.

Against the croaking of men like Cute, we are given the material reality identified also in 'The Streets—Night': a starving mother and child. The reference to the scale underscores the fact that the hunger question is, essentially, a matter of flesh, real and complex in its physicality rather than simple and arbitrary. The core of the problem, according to Dickens, can be glimpsed in the suggestion that the Alderman has only five wits: combined with his croaking, his lack of intelligence is figured as dangerous. A similar position is reproduced in the satirical dismissal of Mrs. Pardiggle's 'philanthropy' in *Bleak House* (1852--3): 'I am incapable of fatigue', she says about her good works: 'I am never tired, and I mean to go on until I have done.'[31] Her sense that her work might be done is similar to Laurie's view that a problem as complex as suicide can be 'put down'. Esther Summerson tries to decline Mrs. Pardiggle's invitation to accompany her on her charitable rounds:

> I had not that delicate knowledge of the heart which must be essential to such a work. That I had much to learn, myself, before I could teach others, and that I could not confide in my good intentions alone. For these reasons I thought it best to be as useful as I could, and to render what kind services I could to those immediately about me, and to try to let that circle of duty gradually and naturally expand itself.   (p. 117)

'You are wrong, Miss Summerson', replies Mrs. Pardiggle. The narrative implies, of course, that Esther is correct; she sees the problem as requiring more delicacy of thought than the methods of the bullish do-gooder Mrs. Pardiggle can give it.

Jo the crossing sweeper, Mrs. Jellyby's children, and the figurative Tom of Tom-All-Alone's are *Bleak House*'s symbols of the results of unmindful philanthropy. What Jo knows, he tells Woodcourt, is 'nothink and starwation' (p. 669). Pam Morris has suggested that the boy's frequent refrain 'I know nothink' (no-think) refers to the boy's ignorance, and his inability to construct a subjective self.[32] Yet, for me, the oxymoronic suggestion that the boy *knows* no-think connotes that the boy's experiences entail a lack of thinking by those who *ought* to be thinking about his condition: the 'no-thinks' of Jo's world are the Pardiggles, Jellybys, and Chadbands, and they are, along with his starvation, the only things he knows. We see an example of this when he is dragged, by a police officer, into an audience with the well-fed Mr. Chadband:

> 'This boy', says the constable, 'although he's repeatedly told to, won't move on—'
>
> 'I'm always a-moving on, sar', cries the boy, wiping away his grimy tears with his arm. 'I've always been a-moving and a-moving on, ever since I was born. Where can I possibly move to, sir, more nor I do move!'

---

[31] Charles Dickens, *Bleak House*, ed. by Stephen Gill (1852–3; Oxford: Oxford University Press, 2008), pp. 116–17. Subsequent references to this edition will be given in the text.

[32] Pam Morris, *Dickens's Class Consciousness: A Marginal View* (London: Macmillan, 1991), p. 96.

'He won't move on,' says the constable calmly, with a slight professional hitch of his neck involving its better settlement in his stiff stock, 'although he has been repeatedly cautioned, and therefore I am obliged to take him into custody. He's as obstinate a young gonoph as I know. He WON'T move on.'

'Oh, my eye! Where can I move to!' cries the boy, clutching quite desperately at his hair and beating his bare feet upon the floor of Mr. Snagsby's passage.

'Don't you come none of that or I shall make blessed short work of you!' says the constable, giving him a passionless shake. 'My instructions are that you are to move on. I have told you so five hundred times.'

'But where?' cries the boy.

'Well! Really, constable, you know,' says Mr. Snagsby wistfully, and coughing behind his hand his cough of great perplexity and doubt, 'really, that does seem a question. Where, you know?'

'My instructions don't go to that,' replies the constable. 'My instructions are that this boy is to move on.'

Do you hear, Jo? It is nothing to you or to any one else that the great lights of the parliamentary sky have failed for some few years in this business to set you the example of moving on. The one grand recipe remains for you—the profound philosophical prescription—the be-all and the end-all of your strange existence upon earth. Move on! You are by no means to move off, Jo, for the great lights can't at all agree about that. Move on!   (pp. 284–5)

Woodcourt considers it strange that ' "in the heart of a civilised world this creature in human form should be more difficult to dispose of than an unowned dog". But it is none the less a fact because of its strangeness', adds the narrator, 'and the difficulty remains' (p. 664). That Jo's case is replicated at the doors of workhouses all over London is of little consequence to *Bleak House*'s constable; his instructions are to move vagrants on, to work without questioning the broader picture. His determination to shuffle Jo along, then, represents the mindless form of social work that is derided in much of Dickens's writing about poverty. The author's ironic, alliterative reference to the 'profound philosophical prescription' of moving on suggests that the measures put in place by parliament have been decidedly unprofound and unphilosophical—a stinging criticism of a social system that had prided itself on its foundations in the philosophies of Malthus and Bentham.

In the long quotation above, Dickens's main targets are the 'thinkers' of the Peter Laurie School. There is an oblique reference to Laurie in the injunction 'you are by no means to move off, Jo, for the great lights can't at all agree about that', suggesting, sardonically, that such 'great lights' are anything but great or luminous.

Similarly, the problem with Mr. Gradgrind's social philosophy is not only the fact-based principles it imposes, but the way it is unwilling to pull material evidence apart and analyse it carefully. In the chapter 'Never Wonder', it is related how

'Louisa had been overheard to begin a conversation with her brother one day, by saying "Tom, I wonder"—upon which Mr. Gradgrind, who was the person over-hearing, stepped forth into the light, and said, "Louisa, never wonder!"' (p. 52). Wonder, like fancy, is one of the abstractions that Dickens explores against utili-tarian logic in the novel; yet the word 'wonder' is used, in this context, as a verb and, as such, it relates more to a form of thinking than it does to that which might be deemed wonderful. Louisa is not indulging in a moment's dreamlike wonder, in fact, but is prefacing an enquiry: 'I wonder if it will rain tomorrow', perhaps. The narrator adds: 'by means of addition, subtraction, multiplication, and div-ision, settle everything somehow and never wonder' (p. 52). There is a library in Coketown where 'Gradgrind is greatly tormented' by the 'melancholy fact, that [...] readers persisted in wondering. They wondered about human nature, human passions, human hopes and fears, the struggles, triumphs and defeats, the cares and joys and sorrows, the lives and deaths of common men and women!' (p. 53). Although Gradgrind is troubled by the idea that labourers 'sometimes, after fif-teen hours' work, sat down to read mere fables' (p. 53), thus appearing to show more interest in fiction than facts, he is also concerned that they, like Louisa, approach knowledge in a way that is ruminative rather than guided by system or statistics; they will persist in taking Defoe, author of stories in which people wan-der off course, 'to their bosoms, instead of Euclid', inventor of a geometrical sys-tem of rigorous mathematical proof (p. 53). Dickens says that 'herein lay the spring of the mechanical art and mystery of educating the reason without stop-ping to the cultivation of the sentiments and affections' (p. 52). The main problem with Gradgrind and M'Choakumchild's stifling the sentiments and affections is its discouragement of the kind of intellection that is crucial to their development.

Seeing Dogmatically

When Ebenezer Scrooge is invited to make a donation to a seasonal collection for the poor, he says of the workhouse that 'those who are badly off must go there', to which it is objected, 'many can't go there; and many would rather die.' Scrooge's famous reply is: '"If they would rather die [...] they had better do it, and decrease the surplus population. Besides—excuse me—I don't know that." "But you might know it," observed the gentleman.'[33] In Scrooge's character we find the two, inter-linking mindsets that Dickens seemed keen to hold to account for his age's social problems: the wish not to know of pauperism in any detail, and the mindless sub-scription to what E. P. Thompson called the 'ideological dogma' of new reform.[34]

---

[33] Charles Dickens, *A Christmas Carol*, in *Christmas Books*, pp. 1–90 (pp. 11–12). Subsequent refer-ences to this edition will be given in the text.

[34] E. P. Thompson, *The Making of the English Working Class* (New York, NY: Vintage, 1966), p. 267.

In *Sartor Resartus* (1834), Thomas Carlyle satirized followers of Malthus in the character of Hofrath Heuschrecke, author of a pamphlet entitled *Institute for the Repression of Population*:

> Enough for us to understand that Heuschrecke is a disciple of Malthus; and so zealous for the doctrine, that his zeal almost literally eats him up. A deadly fear of Population possesses the Hofrath; something like a fixed-idea; undoubtedly akin to the more diluted forms of Madness. Nowhere, in that quarter of his intellectual world, is there light; nothing but a grim shadow of Hunger; open mouths opening wider and wider; a world to terminate by the frightfullest consummation: by its too dense inhabitants, famished into delirium, universally eating one another.[35]

For Dickens, political economy was a major nuisance, not only because of the legislative measures it had encouraged,[36] but also because of the ways it gave the solvent class a mandate for thinking about poverty in simple and uncritical ways. As Southey put it in 1803, Malthus might be known for his 'patient research', but such was not apparent in his *Essay on the Principle of Population* (1798); in 1812 he renewed his attack by saying that political economy had positively encouraged 'a colliquative diarrhoea of the intellect, arising from its strong appetite and weak digestion'.[37] In a review of Harriet Martineau's *Illustrations of Political Economy*, John Stuart Mill complained, in less scatological terms, that early adoptions of Malthus's science had

> take[n] for granted the immutability of arrangements of society, many of which [were] in their nature fluctuating or progressive, and enunciate[d] with as little qualification as if they were universal and absolute truths, propositions which are perhaps applicable to no state of society except the particular one in which they happened to live.[38]

To be fair, Malthus's *Essay* had warned against hasty and untested hypotheses: 'an untried theory cannot fairly be advanced as probable, much less as just, till all the

---

[35] Thomas Carlyle, *Sartor Resartus: The Life and Opinions of Herr Teufelsdröckh*, ed. by Kerry McSweeney (1834; Oxford: Oxford University Press, 2008), p. 172.

[36] On the influence Malthus had on the 1834 poor law, see Mitchell Dean, *The Constitution of Poverty: Toward a Genealogy of Liberal Governance* (London: Routledge, 1990), pp. 100–5 and Geoffrey Gilbert, Introduction, in R. Malthus, *An Essay on the Principle of Population*, ed. by Geoffrey Gilbert (1798; Oxford: Oxford University Press, 1993, 2008), p. xxiii.

[37] Reprinted in Robert Southey, *Essays, Moral and Political* (1832). Quoted in Donald Winch, *Riches and Poverty: An Intellectual History of Political economy in Britain, 1750–1834* (Cambridge: Cambridge University Press, 1996), p. 293.

[38] John Stuart Mill, 'On Miss Martineau's Summary of Political Economy,' *The Monthly Repository*, 8 (1834), pp. 318–22 (p. 319).

arguments against it have been maturely weighed, and clearly and consistently refuted'.[39] Yet, political economy is the means by which Ebenezer Scrooge lets himself off the hook when it comes to giving any sustained thought, or money, to those in need: 'it is not my business [...] It's enough for a man to understand his own business, and not to interfere with other people's' (p. 12). In an 1843 letter to Jerrold, Dickens had had political economy in mind when he wrote: 'I vow to God that I think the Parrots of Society are more intolerable and mischievous than its Birds of Prey'.[40] A species of 'that Devil Cant',[41] political economy is, he added in a speech in Boston, Massachusetts, a 'mole-eyed philosophy which loves the darkness, and winks and scowls in the light'.[42] Echoing Southey's suggestion that Malthus sought to 'starve the poor into celibacy', Dickens accused political economy of holding by a 'principle that a surplus of population must and ought to starve'.[43]

In his article 'On Strike', however, Dickens conceded that 'Political Economy [is] a great and useful science in its own place', but one should 'not transplant [one's] definition of it from the Common Prayer Book, and make it a great king above all gods'.[44] In 'A Nightly Scene in London' (1856), a piece he wrote for *Household Words*, he added:

> I know that the unreasonable disciples of a reasonable school, demented disciples who push arithmetic and Political Economy beyond all bounds of sense [...] and hold them to be all-sufficient for every case, can easily prove that such things ought to be, and that no man has any business to mind them. Without disparaging those indispensable sciences in their sanity, I utterly renounce and abominate them in their insanity.[45]

Political economy had become, for Dickens, a creed which solicited a mindless form of devotion from its followers. A *disciple* is, by definition, one who takes another as his or her teacher and leader; it involves, in Dickens's use of the term, the resignation of one's ability to think and decide for oneself—hence why he identifies political economy's disciples as 'unreasonable' and 'demented'. Malthusian theory was, in the Carlylean terms Dickens found compelling, a sign

---

[39] Malthus, *Essay*, p. xxiii.

[40] Charles Dickens, letter to Douglas Jerrold, 3 May 1843, Dickens Letters 3, pp. 481–3 (pp. 481).

[41] Ibid., p. 482.

[42] Charles Dickens, speech delivered in Boston, 1 February 1842, *Speeches*, pp. 57–62 (p. 59);

[43] Robert Southey, 'Review of *An Essay on the Principle of Population*, by T. R. Malthus', Annual Review, 2 (1803), pp. 292–301 (p. 300); Letter to John Forster, 24 and 25 August 1846, Dickens Letters 4, pp. 608–9 (p. 609).

[44] Dickens, 'On Strike', p. 198.

[45] Charles Dickens, 'A Nightly Scene in London', *Household Words*, 13 (1856), Dickens's Journalism 3, pp. 346–51 (p. 351).

that the age had 'grown mechanical in head and in heart'.[46] Mr. Filer, the long-faced statistician in *The Chimes*, informs Meg Veck that her wish to get married is 'ignorance of the first principles of political economy' and evidence of her class's larger 'improvidence [and] wickedness' (p. 113). Those of the Vecks' order of life 'have no right or business to be married' as, indeed, 'they have no earthly right to be born. And *that* we know they haven't. We reduced it to a mathematical certainty' (p. 114; italics in original). They have no right to be fed either, it seems. Looking at the tripe that Trotty is having for his supper, Filer says 'tripe is without an exception the least economical, and the most wasteful article of consumption that the markets of this country can by possibility produce' (p. 109). Filer then gives a mind-boggling breakdown of the economics of tripe consumption and production, which, whether true or false, has no direct bearing on Trotty's dinner. Nor, indeed, need the forbidding statistics about marriage and population growth have much of an impact on Meg's decision to wed, yet Filer's sermon is successful, as were the arguments of Charles Trevelyan during the Irish Hunger, in converting wider social and political questions into burdens to be carried by individuals within the humbler classes. Alderman Cute forecasts the life of misery that Meg will have if she marries. Trotty then has a dream about what his daughter's future life will be if she does *not* marry, effectively challenging the prognostications of the 'Parrots of Society'. The fact that Trotty's alternative picture of his daughter's future appears in a dream does nothing to weaken the negation of Filer's and Cute's predictions; Dickens's strategy seems to involve complicating matters in order to suggest that the 'mathematical certainties', decided 'long ago', will fail to gauge the immediate and material bearings of social problems in any great depth.

All a Muddle

A good example of the ability to see social problems in all their complicated reality is to be found in Stephen Blackpool's famous idea of the 'muddle' in *Hard Times*. Speaking to Mr. Bounderby he says:

> We are in a muddle, sir. Look round town—so rich as 'tis—and see the numbers o' people as has been broughten into bein heer, fur to weave, an' to card, an' to piece out a livin', aw the same one way, somehows, 'twixt their cradles and their graves. Look how we live, an' wheer we live, an' in what numbers, an' by what chances, and wi' what sameness; and look how the mills is awlus a goin, and how they never works us no nigher to ony dis'ant object—ceptin awlus, Death. Look how you considers of us, and writes of us, and talks of us, and goes up wi' yor

---

[46] Thomas Carlyle, 'Signs of the Times', *Edinburgh Review*, 49 (1829), pp. 439–59 (p. 444).

deputations to Secretaries o' State 'bout us, and how yo are awlus right, and how we are awlus wrong, and never had'n no reason in us sin ever we were born. Look how this ha growen an' growen, sir, bigger an' bigger, broader an' broader, harder an' harder, fro year to year, fro generation unto generation. Who can look on 't, sir, and fairly tell a man 'tis not a muddle?   (pp. 147–8)

Stephen's reference to workers' numbers is mistakenly understood by the dim-witted Mr. Bounderby as a threat of workers' combination. Yet, the weaver's sense of the industrial situation being a muddle is, arguably, his most significant idea: Coketown and its multitude of workers, he implies, have problems of such intricacy that the deputations of secretaries of state, and so on, will be ill-qualified to make sense of the real state of affairs. In a conversation between Sissy Jupe and Louisa Gradgrind about the former's inability to get on at Mr. M'Choakumchild's school, Sissy says:

Mr. M'Choakumchild said he would try me again. And he said, This schoolroom is an immense town, and in it there are a million of inhabitants, and only five-and-twenty are starved to death in the streets, in the course of a year. What is your remark on that proportion? And my remark was—for I couldn't think of a better one—that I thought it must be just as hard upon those who were starved, whether the others were a million, or a million million. And that was wrong, too.   (p. 60)

This example echoes the conflict between Edwin Chadwick and William Farr (discussed in Chapter 1), where the former implied, though not so directly, that the relatively small number of starvations was a marker of the New Poor Law's success. Like Sissy, Farr argued that a handful of deaths from starvation, how-ever small, is still a tragedy. Yet, in the world of statistics and averages, this obvious truth loses it punch. According to Lesa Scholl, 'Sissy's response [...] exposes the tensions between statistics and the human face in the economic vision, and emphasises that communities are made of individuals'.[47] This ten-sion highlights how, according to *Hard Times*, numbers create social blind spots; the laws of averages encourage us to discount exceptions, no matter what they suggest about the shortcomings of the statistical method. *Hard Times* is particularly powerful in highlighting how the mathematical marginalization of some cases belongs to a larger, more problematic tendency to follow preformed channels of interpretation which barely acknowledges the muddled territories that needed to be chartered.

---

[47] Lesa Scholl, *Hunger Movements in Early Victorian Literature: Wants, Riots, Migration* (London: Routledge, 2016), p. 133.

Louisa Gradgrind's education at the hands of M'Choakumchild and her father results in her feelings of surprise when she sees the material realities of Stephen's and Rachael's lives:

> For the first time in her life Louisa had come into one of the dwellings of the Coketown Hands; for the first time in her life she was face to face with anything like individuality in connection with them. She knew of their existence by hundreds and by thousands. She knew what results in work a given number of them would produce in a given space of time. She knew them in crowds passing to and from their nests, like ants or beetles. [...]

> Something to be worked so much and paid so much, and there ended; something to be infallibly settled by laws of supply and demand; something that blundered against those laws, and floundered into difficulty; something that was a little pinched when wheat was dear, and over-ate itself when wheat was cheap; something that increased at such a rate of percentage, and yielded such another percentage of crime, and such another percentage of pauperism; something wholesale, of which vast fortunes were made; something that occasionally rose like a sea, and did some harm and waste (chiefly to itself), and fell again; this she knew the Coketown Hands to be. But, she had scarcely thought more of separating them into units, than of separating the sea itself into its component drops.

> (p. 155)

The living quarters of Stephen introduce Louisa to a world more complex than her facts and figures have allowed her to fathom. Although she is her father's pride for the extent of her knowledge, Louisa is profoundly ignorant when it comes to the working world that pulsates alongside her own. Earlier in the novel Dickens writes:

> So many hundred Hands in this Mill; so many hundred horse Steam Power. It is known, to the force of a single pound weight, what the engine will do; but, not all the calculators of the National Debt can tell me the capacity for good or evil, for love or hatred, for patriotism or discontent, for the decomposition of virtue into vice, or the reverse, at any single moment in the soul of one of these its quiet servants, with the composed faces and the regulated actions. There is no mystery in it; there is an unfathomable mystery in the meanest of them, for ever.— Supposing we were to reverse our arithmetic for material objects, and to govern these awful unknown quantities by other means!   (p. 71)

The 'other means' are not identified here, but the easy interpretation is that Dickens had in mind something like emotional, moral, fanciful, or poetic force as an alternative to measures and statistics. His purpose in *Hard Times*, however, is to complicate the subject, not recolour it. Reflected in the ponderous sentence structure, the good, the evil, the love and hatred, and so on, are simultaneously, and confusingly, not mysterious, yet full of mystery, 'for ever'. The failures of figures and measurements are exposed by a complexity that the passage leaves unchallenged; the 'muddle' requires a kind of mental strategy that the Gradgrind philosophy fails to deliver.

In the Christmas Books, Dickens had adapted the worlds of fantasy and dreaming to suit the view that social questions needed to be perceived as complicated and shifting—a direct contradiction of the way some political economists sought to subject social phenomena to a limited number of solid 'natural' laws. *The Chimes*, for example, paints a phantasmagorical picture of the lower classes figured as goblins, sprites, and elves, in a range of bewildering visualizations. According to Eleanor Courtemanche, the story underlines 'the vast gulf between the social scientist's facts and laws and the real unpredictability of experience':[48]

> [Totty Veck] saw the tower, whither his charmed footsteps had brought him, swarming with dwarf phantoms, spirits, elfin creatures of the Bells. [...] He saw them, of all aspects and all shapes. He saw them ugly, handsome, crippled, exquisitely formed. He saw them young, he saw them old, he saw them kind, he saw them cruel, he saw them merry, he saw them grim; he saw them dance, and heard them sing; he saw them tear their hair, and heard them howl. He saw the air thick with them. He saw them come and go, incessantly. He saw them riding downward, soaring upward, sailing off afar, perching near at hand, all restless and all violently active. Stone, and brick, and slate, and tile, became transparent to him as to them. He saw them in the houses, busy at the sleepers' beds. He saw them soothing people in their dreams; he saw them beating them with knotted whips; he saw them yelling in their ears; he saw them playing softest music on their pillows; he saw them cheering some with the songs of birds and the perfume of flowers; he saw them flashing awful faces on the troubled rest of others, from enchanted mirrors which they carried in their hands.
>
> He saw these creatures, not only among sleeping men but waking also, active in pursuits irreconcilable with one another, and possessing or assuming natures the most opposite. He saw one buckling on innumerable wings to increase his speed; another loading himself with chains and weights, to retard his. He saw some putting the hands of clocks forward, some putting the hands of clocks backward, some endeavouring to stop the clock entirely. He saw them representing, here a marriage ceremony, there a funeral; in this chamber an election, in that a ball; he saw, everywhere, restless and untiring motion.   (pp. 140–1)

---

[48] Eleanor Courtemanche, ' "Naked Truth is the Best Eloquence": Martineau, Dickens, and the Moral Science of Realism', ELH, 73:2 (2006), pp. 383–407 (p. 400).

Although a fantastic scene, this episode is closer to reality than the measurements or prognostications of political economists such as Mr. Filer. It transfigures, in fact, the challenge that life presents to any single observer. Trotty becomes 'bewildered by the host of shifting and extraordinary figures' (p. 141) because they are 'restless', 'untiring', 'irreconcilable', and they assume 'natures the most opposite'. Despite the repetition of 'he saw', the passage gives a sense that we cannot entirely trust what Trotty sees: 'stone, and brick, and slate, and tile, become transparent to him as to them'. Terms like 'restless' and 'violently active' give a warning of the insurgent potential of the masses, but this is given some context by the picture of their extraordinary variedness. Looking forwards, perhaps, to the opening of *A Tale of Two Cities* (1859), where we are informed that the late eighteenth century is the best of times, and the worst, we see a pulsating phenomenological contradiction in *The Chimes*'s phantoms: some go to the good, and some go to the bad. In either case, it is difficult to see how any one-size-fits-all rule would make sense of them all. In a rare example of Dickens talking about the social function of fiction outside of his novels, he wrote in a letter to the American publisher Henry Carey:

> To interest and affect the general mind in behalf of anything that is clearly wrong—to stimulate and rouse the public soul to a compassionate or indignant feeling that it *must not be*—without obtruding any pet theory of cause or cure, and so throwing off allies as they spring up—I believe to be one of Fiction's highest uses. And this is the use to which I try to turn it.[49]

While this comment might seem to be about making people *see* social problems, it also notes that a significant part of approaching the truth of public injustice is the avoidance of 'pet theory'. Throwing off such dogmatic thinking, *The Chimes* and *Hard Times* suggest, is essential to countering simplification and obfuscation of truth, both of which, it seems, had the effect of sanctioning donothingism.

We know of Dickens's descriptions of Tom-All-Alone's that there had been 'much mighty speech-making' (p. 654) about the slum conditions of London, and yet little that had come to any good. Early in *Bleak House* we get a glimpse of why this might be:

> Now, these tumbling tenements contain, by night, a swarm of misery. As on the ruined human wretch vermin parasites appear, so these ruined shelters have bred a crowd of foul existence that crawls in and out of gaps in walls and boards; and coils itself to sleep, in maggot numbers, where the rain drips in; and comes and goes, fetching and carrying fever and sowing more evil in its every footprint

[49] Charles Dickens, letter to Henry Carey, 24 August 1854, in Dickens Letters 7, pp. 404–5 (p. 405). Italics in original.

than Lord Coodle, and Sir Thomas Doodle, and the Duke of Foodle, and all the
fine gentlemen in office, down to Zoodle, shall set right in five hundred years—
though born expressly to do it.   (p. 236)

As with the minutiae of the Jarndyce case, and the swarming number of phantoms in *The Chimes*, there seems to be too much misery for Coodle, Doodle,
and Foodle (parodies of government commissioners) to deal with. When I say
too much misery I mean too great in number rather than too miserable in
nature. Although the latter is no insignificant fact for Dickens, the former is
more in-keeping with his sense that poverty is too muddled an issue for commissioner's creeds and hobby-horse theories to make sense of. The omniscient
narrator portrays the crossing sweeper as a means of stripping back the usual
chatter that surrounds Tom-All-Alone's and to get at what it is really like to live
in the slum:

> It must be a strange state to be like Jo! To shuffle through the streets, unfamiliar
> with the shapes, and in utter darkness as to the meaning, of those mysterious
> symbols, so abundant over the shops, and at the corners of streets, and on the
> doors, and in the windows! To see people read, and to see people write, and to see
> the postmen deliver letters, and not to have the least idea of all that language—to
> be, to every scrap of it, stone blind and dumb! It must be very puzzling to see the
> good company going to the churches on Sundays, with their books in their hands,
> and to think (for perhaps Jo DOES think at odd times) what does it all mean, and
> if it means anything to anybody, how comes it that it means nothing to me? To
> be hustled, and jostled, and moved on; and really to feel that it would appear to
> be perfectly true that I have no business here, or there, or anywhere; and yet to
> be perplexed by the consideration that I AM here somehow, too, and everybody
> overlooked me until I became the creature that I am! It must be a strange state,
> not merely to be told that I am scarcely human [...] but to feel it of my own
> knowledge all my life! To see the horses, dogs, and cattle go by me and to know
> that in ignorance I belong to them and not to the superior beings in my shape,
> whose delicacy I offend! Jo's ideas of a criminal trial, or a judge, or a bishop, or a
> government, or that inestimable jewel to him (if he only knew it) the Constitution,
> should be strange! His whole material and immaterial life is wonderfully strange;
> his death, the strangest thing of all.   (pp. 236–7)

I have argued in a previous book that a large part of Dickens's realist strategy is
the 'making strange' of people, places, and subjects using a form of corporeal
materialism.[50] In this extract from *Bleak House* it appears that to get some reliable

---

[50] Andrew Mangham, *Dickens's Forensic Realism: Truth, Bodies, Evidence* (Columbus, OH: Ohio
University Press, 2016).

sense of Jo's reality, the narrative must render signs, information, and language obscure. In a moment of free indirect style, the text shows how the boy has a sense of what would 'appear to be perfectly true', and yet he is simultaneously 'perplexed' by the disconnection between the opinions of others and his own material reality. Mr. Chadband's failure to reform Jo is remarkable, in my view, for the way it misses the obvious, material indications of the boy's poverty. As he says to Allan Woodcourt, just before he dies: 'Mr. Chadbands [...] wos a prayin wunst at Mr. Sangsby's and I heerd him, but he sounded as if he wos a speakin' to his-self, and not to me. He prayed a lot, but *I* couldn't make out nothink on it' (p. 676). Again, we have the reference to 'no-think' and to Jo's inability to understand the language of others. Chadband's prayer (or sermon) is so much gibberish to the boy because, Dickens implies, the minister's self-important blather is doled out without thought, without observation, and without careful consideration. Chadband first encounters the boy in a chapter in which he (the minister) has been particularly well fed by the Snagsbys:

> There is excellent provision made of dainty new bread, crusty twists, cool fresh butter, thin slices of ham, tongue, and German sausage, and delicate little rows of anchovies nestling in parsley, not to mention new-laid eggs, to be brought up warm in a napkin, and hot buttered toast. For Chadband is rather a consuming vessel—the persecutors say a gorging vessel—and can wield such weapons of the flesh as a knife and fork remarkably well.   (p. 281)

Chadband then shows, rather unexpectedly, some awareness of the physiology of food assimilation:

> 'My friends,' says he, 'what is this which we now behold as being spread before us? Refreshment. Do we need refreshment then, my friends? We do. And why do we need refreshment, my friends? Because we are but mortal, because we are but sinful, because we are but of the earth, because we are not of the air. Can we fly, my friends? We cannot. Why can we not fly, my friends? [...] Is it because we are calculated to walk? It is. Could we walk, my friends, without strength? We could not. What should we do without strength, my friends? Our legs would refuse to bear us, our knees would double up, our ankles would turn over, and we should come to the ground. Then from whence, my friends, in a human point of view, do we derive the strength that is necessary to our limbs? Is it,' says Chadband, glancing over the table, 'from bread in various forms, from butter which is churned from the milk which is yielded unto us by the cow, from the eggs which are laid by the fowl, from ham, from tongue, from sausage, and from such like? It is. Then let us partake of the good things which are set before us!'
>
> (p. 283)

Chadband is at a good distance from the point where his ankles might turn over for want of nutrition, yet it would make sense for his understanding of the one thing needful in himself to translate into to a perception of Jo's material needs. Such is not the case, however. In 'Snoring for the Million' (1842), a satirical article written for *The Examiner*, Dickens caricatured the government's setting up of singing classes for the poor which were intended to distract them from 'vicious indulgences'—presumably alcohol, sex, and radical politics.[51] Dickens undis-guisedly hated the initiative, writing:

> The Privy Council teaches the people to be vocal. The Government seeing the million with their mouths wide open, naturally think that they must want to sing; for it only recognizes two kinds of forks, the silver fork and the tuning fork, between which opposite extremes there is nothing. [...] 'John', says the Government to its starving servant, 'when you ramble up and down the market-places, dying of hunger, be careful, above all things, to sing perpetually'.[52]

Lack of material intervention is linked, in this piece of journalism, to a flatulent social idea. It is a species of air-headed thinking that Dickens saw to be the prob-lem leading to inadequate, and often pernicious, social measures.

Where for the Privy Council the tonic is to be found in singing, for Chadband it is to be found in praying. It remains for Snagsby and his servant Guster to remember that Jo might be hungry: 'Mr Snagsby loads him with some broken meats from the table, which he carries away, hugging in his arms' (p. 290);

> 'Here's something to eat, poor boy,' says Guster.
> 'Thank'ee, mum,' says Jo.
> 'Are you hungry?'
> 'Jist!' says Jo. (p. 383)

Dickens went through a good deal of ink in forming criticisms against the social reformers whose pet remedies were anything but practical. I have already dis-cussed how his disparagement of Gradgrind's literalism in *Hard Times* is driven by a view that the MP takes his philosophy too far. In the chapter where Louisa charges her father with the wilful starvation of her fancy, we are reintroduced to Gradgrind as follows:

> Although Mr. Gradgrind did not take after Blue Beard, his room was quite a blue chamber in its abundance of blue books. Whatever they could prove (which

---

[51] John Pyke Hullah, *Wilhem's Method of Teaching Singing Adapted to English Usage* (1841), quoted in Michael Slater's introduction to Charles Dickens, 'Snoring for the Million', *The Examiner*, 24 December 1842, Dickens Journalism 2, pp. 51–5 (p. 52).

[52] Dickens, 'Snoring for the Million', p. 53.

is usually anything you like), they proved there, in an army constantly strengthening by the arrival of new recruits. In that charmed apartment, the most complicated social questions were cast up, got into exact totals, and finally settled—if those concerned could only have been brought to know it. As if an astronomical observatory should be made without any windows, and the astronomer within should arrange the starry universe solely by pen, ink, and paper, so Mr. Gradgrind, in his Observatory (and there are many like it), had no need to cast an eye upon the teeming myriads of human beings around him, but could settle all their destinies on a slate, and wipe out all their tears with one dirty little bit of sponge.   (p. 95)

Dickens was not against blue books and the work that they did, as we shall see. His point in this passage was that Gradgrind has relied too much upon such reports, and not enough on the evidence available to his own eyes. In the ironic image of an observatory without windows, it is suggested that those most concerned with looking are the ones least likely to see. Certainly in Gradgrind's case, the problem is a failure to 'cast an eye upon the teeming myriads of human beings around him'—a failure which leads to, and stems from, the oversimplification of social questions with facts and measures.

The Tooting Disease and the New Poor Law

On 5 January 1849, Richard Grainger, surgeon and member of the newly established Central Board of Health, was sent to Tooting, eight miles southwest of London, to inspect a Juvenile Pauper Asylum run by a man named Bartholomew Drouet. For the fee of four shillings and sixpence per week per child, Drouet had been taking young boys from a number of London Poor-Law Unions whose workhouses had become too overburdened. Although there could have been exceptions, these boys were neither orphans, like Oliver Twist, nor unwanted children, like the inhabitants of Dotheboys Hall: they were likely to have been separated from their parents when their family had entered the workhouse. (To control the destitute class's cycles of endless reproduction, it was thought expedient to separate husbands from wives and children from parents.)

In the winter of 1848–9 several of Drouet's charges contracted cholera, with one child dying on 29 December. What Grainger found when he arrived six days later is summarized by A. W. C. Brice and K. J. Fielding in the 1968 article 'Dickens and the Tooting Disaster':

The children were overcrowded, undernourished, and thinly clad; the buildings were poor, and the whole place was surrounded by open sewers. It was insufficiently staffed for such an emergency, and the doctor in charge was only twenty-five; he was inexperienced, had been there two months, and he was paid for his full time service just fifty pounds a year. [...] Children died in cold, dark, crowded rooms, three or more in a bed, inevitably crying and vomiting, with only the most primitive sanitation, and sometimes cared for only by other children whose lives were endangered because there was no one else at first to help.[53]

One of these unfortunate children, Joseph Andrews, later testified that it was standard practice for 'a tub [to be] placed in the [dormitory] for the purposes of nature, which smelt very disagreeably, and after it was emptied in the morning water was placed in it for the purpose of scrubbing out the room.'[54] Nothing could have been more accommodating to the spread of cholera; as Pamela K. Gilbert has noted, cholera 'is a waterborne disease caused by a comma-shaped bacillus, or vibrio, which is generally transmitted between humans via the fecal-oral route. It enters the human body through ingestion of contaminated water or food, and multiplies in the gut.'[55] Grainger urged the Board of Guardians to transport all the sick children from Drouet's home to the Royal Free Hospital in London. When the children arrived at the hospital, staff noticed that they had the symptoms not only of cholera, but of starvation too. Grainger reported:

Their general appearance was unhealthy; a great many of them had a wasting of the limbs, and some were suffering from what is commonly known as pot-belly. Many were also suffering from itch [scabies] and other disorders. Their pulses were very weak, and there was every indication of a feeble system of body. In my opinion the appearance of the children denoted neglect, and that they were underfed.[56]

Grainger's diagnosis was confirmed by a number of his colleagues, including W. B. Whitfield, medical officer of the Holborn Union; Arthur Farr, medical professor at King's College; A. B. Garrod, physician at the University College Hospital; and T. C. Jackson, resident surgeon at the Royal Free. The latter admitted that the Tooting children's symptoms were so uniform (and consistent with the famine conditions they had experienced at Drouet's place) that 'their complaint was called "the Tooting disease".'[57] Another surgeon at the same hospital, W. Marsden,

[53] A. W. C. Brice and K. J. Fielding, 'Dickens and the Tooting Disaster', *Victorian Studies*, 12:2 (1968), pp. 227–44 (pp. 230–31).
[54] Unsigned, 'Trial of Mr. Drouet', *The Times*, 14 April 1849, p. 7.
[55] Pamela K. Gilbert, *Cholera and Nation: Doctoring the Social Body in Victorian England* (Albany, NY: State University of New York Press, 2008), p. 2.
[56] Unsigned, 'Trial of Mr. Drouet', *The Times*, 15 April 1849, p. 7.
[57] Unsigned, Untitled Report, *The Examiner*, 27 January 1849, pp. 57–8 (p. 57) .

made a comparison between the Tooting patients and some healthy Welsh school boys he had treated:

> I contrasted twenty-five of them with twenty-five of the Welsh School boys. I had them weighed. The weight of the Tooting children was 1,339lbs. 8oz.; of the Welsh children, 1,516lbs. 12oz.; giving a balance in favour of the Welsh boys of 177lbs. 4oz. Measuring across the chick part of the arms, the Tooting boys gave an aggregate of 161¾ inches, the Welsh children 179¾, giving 18 inches in favour of the Welsh children. The next part of the measurement is of the greatest importance. The Tooting boys measured in the aggregate 595 inches around the abdomen, while the Welsh children measured only 567½.[58]

In total, 126 Tooting boys died from cholera. The first child to do so in hospital was James Andrews, brother of the Joseph mentioned above. Whitfield had found the boy in a 'state of complete collapse'[59] and Mary Harris, a nurse at the hospital, said that

> he seemed very tired [when] I set him by the fire and gave him some supper. I gave him some bread and milk, and he said, "Oh, nurse, what a big piece of bread this is." [...] I put him to bed, and I observed as I undressed him, that he was very thin and emaciated.[60]

After he died, James was given a post-mortem examination by Garrod; he found numerous indicators of starvation: 'The body of the child was very much emaciated, and the appearance of the teeth denoted that he was a child of infirm constitution, and that he had not arrived at proper maturity. There was a total absence of fat even on those parts where it was generally thickest.'[61]

Thomas Wakley, coroner for Middlesex and long-term editor of *The Lancet*, officiated at the inquest into the boys' death. He knew that there was no way for the Crown Prosecution to convict Drouet for all the fatalities, so he chose to stress the probable manslaughter of James Andrews. Wakley's management of the inquest was characteristically thorough. He had a good deal of respect for the Board of Health which, in 1849, consisted of Grainger, Southwood Smith, Chadwick, and Dickens's brother-in-law, Henry Austin.[62] For the Poor Law Board, however, presided over at the time by the Whig Member of Parliament Charles Buller, he had little tolerance. In *The Examiner*, the newspaper edited by

---

[58] Ibid.   [59] Ibid.   [60] 'Trial of Mr. Drouet', 15 April, p. 7.   [61] Ibid.
[62] Wakley praised the board for its 'energy, vigour, and ability in the Tooting catastrophe', 27 January 1849, p. 103. Dickens had experienced Wakley's meticulousness first-hand at the 1840 inquest on a case of infanticide, for which Dickens had acted as a jury member. See Mangham, *Dickens's Forensic Realism*, pp. 1–20 and Claire Tomalin, *Charles Dickens: A Life* (London: Viking, 2011), pp. xxxix–xlii.

John Forster, Wakley's address to the jury during the Andrews inquest is recorded as follows:

> Parochial children, in point of law, were entitled to the same amount of protection as the children of the rich. [...] In 1834 the poor laws were changed, and a commission was appointed, which was to set everything right. This was not the occasion to criticise the circumstances which led to such an establishment, but it was impossible to omit referring to what had been the acts of that board as to Mr. Drouet's establishment. [...] It was a shocking, an odious, an abominable system, and it was an abomination to the character of this country that such a thing should ever have endured. Infant pauper children, dependent on the guardians, had an inefficient diet. What were the results? Early disease and early and lasting decrepitude. By this description of diet you created consumptive persons, you gave them diseased joints, and you imposed on the parishes lasting burdens.[63]

The jury retired for about an hour and then returned with the following verdict:

> We, the jury impanelled to inquire touching the death of James Andrews, unanimously agree to the following verdict, which is, that Bartholomew Peter Drouet is guilty of manslaughter, and that the guardians of the Holborn union have acted most negligently in their engagement with Mr. Drouet [...] We regret that the Poor Law Act is insufficient for the purposes for which it was intended, and hope the time is not far distant when the necessity for such establishments as Mr. Drouet's will entirely cease.

Wakley added 'I should flinch from my duty if I were to refrain from expressing my opinion that your verdict is strictly just, and that, if I were a juryman, my verdict would have been the same.'[64]

There are obvious similarities between the Tooting Asylum and *Nicholas Nickleby*'s Dotheboys Hall. *The Northern Star*, in fact, suggested that Wackford Squeers's infamous asylum for unwanted children was 'a perfect type of the now equally famed—perhaps we should say much more infamous—Tooting Purgatory'.[65] A more fitting comparison, however, would be with Mrs. Mann's baby farm in *Oliver Twist* (1838–9):

> The parish authorities magnanimously and humanely resolved, that Oliver should be 'farmed,' or, in other words, that he should be dispatched to a branch-workhouse some three miles off, where twenty or thirty other juvenile offenders against the poor-laws, rolled about the floor all day, without the inconvenience

---

[63] *Examiner*, 27 January 1849, p. 57.   [64] Ibid., p. 58.

[65] Unsigned, 'The Verdict on "Do-the-Boys-Hall"', The Northern Star, 27 January 1849, p. 5.

of too much food or too much clothing, under the parental superintendence of an elderly female, who received the culprits at and for the consideration of sevenpence-halfpenny per small head per week. Sevenpence-halfpenny's worth per week is a good round diet for a child; a great deal may be got for sevenpence-halfpenny, quite enough to overload its stomach, and make it uncomfortable. [...] It cannot be expected that this system of farming should produce any very extraordinary or luxuriant crop. Oliver Twist's ninth birthday found him a pale thin child, somewhat diminutive in stature, and decidedly small in circumference.[66]

Like the Tooting home for boys, Mrs. Mann's farm paints a damning portrait of poor children under the new legislative regime. According to Malthusian theory, pauper children were the very symbols of social disorder: products of the working-class inability to control its own numbers, their hunger was the manifestation of a destructive drain on resource. Mrs. Sowerberry, expecting the 'very small' Oliver to grow 'on our victuals and our drink', sees 'no saving in parish children [...]; for they always cost more to keep than they're worth' (p. 30). In *Bleak House*, Harold Skimpole says, about the crossing sweeper's appetite:

He is no doubt born with an appetite—probably, when he is in a safer state of health, he has an excellent appetite. Very well. At our young friend's natural dinner hour, most likely about noon, our young friend says in effect to society, 'I am hungry; will you have the goodness to produce your spoon and feed me?' Society, which has taken upon itself the general arrangement of the whole system of spoons and professes to have a spoon for our young friend, does NOT produce that spoon; and our young friend, therefore, says 'You really must excuse me if I seize it.'   (p. 455)

According to Michael Slater, the characterization of Jo had been inspired by a visit Dickens made to a Ragged School dormitory for men and boys in 1852.[67] The author also wrote about his visit in 'A Sleep to Startle Us', an article published in *Household Words* that same year. So scanty were the provisions in the school, Dickens reports, that it 'would scarcely be regarded by MR CHADWICK himself as a festive or uproarious entertainment'.[68] Looking into the dietaries of a number of workhouses, and, comparing them with mortality figures, Chadwick had argued in the years leading up to the coordination of the New Poor Law Bill that 'heavier diets, however much they might be wished for by those who were struggling for an independent existence outside the [work]house, were along the least

---

[66] Charles Dickens, *Oliver Twist*, ed. by Stephen Gill (1837–8; Oxford: Oxford University Press, 2008), pp. 4–5. Subsequent references to this edition will be given in the text.
[67] Slater, *Charles Dickens*, p. 342.
[68] Charles Dickens, 'A Sleep to Startle Us', *Household Words*, 9 (1852), Dickens Journalism 3, pp. 49–57 (p. 54).

healthy', and that 'an increase in the average amount of sickness bore a direct pro-portion to the amount of diet'.[69] Chadwick was horrified to find, on a trip to the Lawrence Workhouse in Reading, that

> the bread was good, the table beer pronounced 'excellent' [...] One inmate, a hale-looking man of sixty-three, had with his wife been on the parish more than forty years. On the whole the inmates were better off than the labourers, and better off than one-half of the ratepayers of the place out of the House; for they were well fed, had little work, and no responsibility.[70]

When he became the 'leading spirit' of the 1834 statute, Chadwick recommended that the workhouse should be a place where residents are 'starved into working; a place for the support of those who would do well and a terror to those who would do ill'.[71] According to Christopher Hamlin, Chadwick 'is reputed to have said that there was no such thing as an innocent pauper'.[72]

It was opinions such as these that convinced Dickens to cast Chadwick as the 'unnamed villain of *Oliver Twist*'.[73] Although the author would get to know the social reformer in the 1840s, and would praise his plans for a charitable kitchen in 1866, he consistently expressed ambivalent feelings towards Chadwick. In an 1851 speech to the Metropolitan Sanitary Association, he said that he had learned a great deal from the writings of the reformer. However, when the latter approached Dickens through Austin, asking for the endorsement of his *Report on the Sanitary Condition of the Labouring Population of Great Britain* (1842), Dickens promised to read the report 'with great interest and attention', though 'I do differ from him, to the death, on his crack topic, the new Poor Law'.[74] In a sideways dig at Chadwick, Dickens describes Mrs. Mann in *Oliver Twist* as

> a woman of wisdom and experience; she knew what was good for children; and she had a very accurate perception of what was good for herself. So, she appro-priated the greater part of the weekly stipend to her own use, and consigned the rising parochial generation to even a shorter allowance than was originally pro-vided for them. Thereby finding in the lowest depth a deeper still; and proving herself a very great experimental philosopher.   (p. 4)

---

[69] Benjamin Ward Richardson, *The Health of Nations: A Review of the Works of Edwin Chadwick*, 2 vols (London: Longman, Green, 1887), vol. 1, pp. 66–7.

[70] Ibid., vol. 2, p. 331.   [71] Ibid., vol. 2, p. 353; vol. 1, p. xxxii.

[72] Christopher Hamlin, *Public Health and Social Justice in the Age of Chadwick: Britain, 1800–1854* (Cambridge: Cambridge University Press, 1998), p. 23.

[73] Joseph W. Childers, 'Politicized Dickens: The Journalism of the 1850s', in *Palgrave Advances in Charles Dickens Studies*, ed. by John Bowen and Robert I. Patten (Basingstoke: Palgrave Macmillan, 2006), pp. 198–215 (p. 200).

[74] See Dickens, *Speeches*, pp. 315–18 (pp. 315–16) and letters to George Russell and Henry Austin, respectively 25 September 1842 and 5 March 1866, Dickens Letters 3 and 11, p. 330 and pp. 285–6.

A similar philosophy pervades over the running of the Mudfog workhouse:

> The members of this board were very sage, deep, philosophical men; and when they came to turn their attention to the workhouse, they found out at once, what ordinary folks would never have discovered—the poor people liked it! [...] So, they established the rule, that all poor people should have the alternative [...] of being starved by a gradual process in the house, or by a quick one out of it. [...] For the first six months after Oliver Twist was removed, the system was in full operation. It was rather expensive at first, in consequence of the increase in the undertaker's bill, and the necessity of taking in the clothes of all the paupers, which fluttered loosely on their wasted, shrunken forms, after a week or two's gruel. But the number of workhouse inmates got thin as well as the paupers; and the board were in ecstasies. [...] Oliver Twist and his companions suffered the tortures of slow starvation for three months: at last they got so voracious and wild with hunger, that one boy, who was tall for his age, and hadn't been used to that sort of thing (for his father had kept a small cook-shop), hinted darkly to his companions, that unless he had another basin of gruel *per diem*, he was afraid he might some night happen to eat the boy who slept next him, who happened to be a weakly youth of tender age.   (pp. 10–12)

This last reference to cannibalism is not as exaggerated as it may seem. Dickens's acquaintance, John Elliotson, noted in his *Human Physiology* (1835) that 'men and women were then living, who had destroyed and fed upon the bodies of their own families, to prevent starvation in very severe seasons'.[75] The one damning difference between such starving unfortunates and workhouse inmates is that the latter were famished deliberately. When Oliver attacks Noah Claypole for insulting his mother, Mr. Bumble tells Mrs. Sowerberry that she has overfed him:

> 'It's Meat.'
>
> 'What?' exclaimed Mrs. Sowerberry.
>
> 'Meat, ma'am, meat,' replied Bumble, with stern emphasis. 'You've over-fed him, ma'am. You've raised a artificial soul and spirit in him, ma'am unbecoming a person of his condition: as the board, Mrs. Sowerberry, who are practical philosophers, will tell you. What have paupers to do with soul or spirit? It's quite enough that we let 'em have live bodies. If you had kept the boy on gruel, ma'am, this would never have happened'
>
> 'Dear, dear!' ejaculated Mrs. Sowerberry, piously raising her eyes to the kitchen ceiling: 'this comes of being liberal!'   (pp. 50–1)

[75] John Elliotson, *Human Physiology* (London: Longman et al., 1835), p. 54.

Mrs. Sowerberry is anything but liberal. The meat she gives Oliver is offcuts intended for the dog and 'the worst end of the neck' (pp. 31, 43). Nonetheless, the philosophy of Bumble and the Board corresponds with the theory of Chadwick, who had suggested that the lower orders were 'injuriously affected by the "meat", that is to say, the animal food with which they were regaled'.[76]

The Examiner carried, as we have seen, a full report on the inquest into the death of James Andrews from the Tooting Academy. Dickens himself contributed no fewer than four articles on the Tooting catastrophe in the same newspaper. It was extremely unusual for Dickens to write a series of non-fictional articles after his initial sorties into journalism in the 1830s. In 1848 he had written a review of Catherine Crowe's *The Night-Side of Nature* (1848), with the intention of coming back to the topic in a later edition, yet the second piece never appeared. A year later, however, we see the Tooting incident holding Dickens's attention for an unusually long period of time. Two articles by him appeared around the time of James Andrews's inquest ('The Paradise at Tooting', 20 January; 'The Tooting Farm', 27 January), and two more were published when Drouet was put on a charge of manslaughter for the unlawful killing of Andrews ('A Recorder's Charge', 3 March; 'The Verdict for Drouet', 1 April). In the same issue of *The Examiner* that featured Wakley's summing-up of the inquest, Dickens noted that 'The New Poor Law, as it stands, be not efficient for the prevention of such inhuman evils'.[77] He made it absolutely clear, in all four *Examiner* articles, that he considered there to be a link between the children's cholera and their starvation:

> [Drouet] has a weakness in respect of leaving the sick to take care of themselves, surrounded by every offensive, indecent, and barbarous circumstance that can aggravate the horrors of their condition and increase the dangers of infection. [...] The dietary of the children is so unwholesome and insufficient, that they climb secretly over palings, and pick out scraps of sustenance from the tubs of hog-wash. [...] They are 'very lean and emaciated'.[78]

The links between the children's hunger and cholera exposed what Thomas W. Laqueur calls, in a different context, 'the lineaments of causality and of human agency [...] Someone or something did something that caused pain, suffering, or death and that could, under certain circumstances, have been avoided or mitigated'.[79] Because the loss of the Tooting boys was linked to cholera, there was

---

[76] Richardson, *Health of Nations*, vol. 1, p. 71.

[77] [Charles Dickens], 'The Tooting Farm', The Examiner, 27 January 1849, pp. 49–50 (p. 50).

[78] Charles Dickens, 'The Paradise at Tooting', The Examiner, 20 January 1849, Dickens Journalism 2, pp. 147–56 (pp. 150–1).

[79] Thomas W. Laqueur, 'Bodies, Details and the Humanitarian Narrative', in *The New Cultural History*, ed. by Lynn Hunt (Berkeley, Los Angeles, CA. and London: University of California Press, 1989), pp. 176–204 (p. 178).

the danger that their deaths might be chalked up to an Act of God rather than human agency. *The Satirist* insisted 'it is not the *nature of things*, but the *misconduct of persons*, that is answerable for the hideous havoc which death has made among those defenseless infant pensioners of legal charity'.[80] Similarly, the *Northern Star* praised Wakley for presiding over an inquest which did not resort to 'the disgusting verdict—"Died by the Visitation of God," when it was "as notorious as the sun at noon-day" that the subject of the inquiry had *died by the wickedness of his fellow men*'.[81]

Linked to rejections of the 'Visitation of God' idea was the association of commissions of cruelty with active neglect; as in some responses to the Irish Famine, where it was felt that the lack of English intervention had made England as culpable as the potato blight for the deaths of many hundreds of thousands, commentators on the Tooting Disaster saw Drouet's neglect of the children as tantamount to an act of murder. More broadly, ideas and linguistic strategies appropriated from a materialist, scientific understanding of starving allowed Dickens to demonstrate, in contradiction to the argument focusing on perceived 'Acts of God', or laws of nature, that the famines and fevers of the poorer classes could be forestalled and alleviated by the right kind of social interpretation. In the powerful article 'To Working Men' (1854), for example, which he wrote five years after his pieces on the Tooting epidemic, he drew a connection between the neglect of the working classes and wilful harm. The article was written in response to a new outbreak of cholera which had killed more than 100,000 people in 1854. Dickens anticipated the working man's thoughts as follows:

> Walking and sleeping, I and mine are slowly poisoned. Imperfect development and premature decay are the lot of those who are dear to me as my life. I bring children into the world to suffer unnaturally, and to die when my Merciful Father would have them live. [...] Shameful deprivation of the commonest appliances, distinguishing the lives of human beings from the lives of beasts, in my inheritance. My family is one of tens of thousands of families who are set aside as good for pestilence.[82]

The twin horsemen, Famine and Pestilence, represent no acts of God. They are, Dickens suggests, aberrations of the wishes of the 'Merciful Father' and 'unnatural'. The language is decidedly anti-Malthusian, and it conflicts with any absolution of human responsibility for the distresses of the poor. The link between poverty and

---

[80] Unsigned, 'The Tooting Catastrophe', The Satirist, 27 January 1849, p. 38. Italics in original.

[81] "Do-the-Boys-Hall", p. 5. Italics in original.

[82] Charles Dickens, 'To Working Men', *Household Words*, 10 (1854), Dickens Journalism 3, pp. 225–9 (p. 228).

disease in famine fever converts omission into commission ('I and mine are slowly poisoned').

The connections between hunger and disease appear to have been solidified in Dickens's mind through his acquaintanceship with Thomas Southwood Smith. The two men met in 1840 when the latter established 'The Sanatorium', a hospital for the treatment of nervous complaints, just across the road from where Dickens lived. In her biography of Southwood Smith, his granddaughter Gertrude Lewes (also the daughter-in-law of George Henry Lewes), recalled:

> When the building fund [for the Sanatorium] was opened, [Dickens] and several other literary men and artists came forward and gave for its benefit the first of those amateur performances which they repeated at a later period. They acted Ben Jonson's "Every Man in his Humour," at St. James's Theatre, on November 15, 1845, both audience and actors being brilliant. Charles Dickens, Douglas Jerrold, John Forster, Mark Lemon, Frank Stone, and others took part. I remember seeing them, as I peeped down from a side-box.[83]

Soon after the Tooting catastrophe, Dickens would become a frequent visitor to the office of the Board of Health, the same board which had sent Grainger to investigate Drouet's asylum in 1849. Dickens shared Chadwick's, Southwood Smith's, and Henry Austin's interest in the need for new city internment sites—an interest that would inform the representation of Nemo's inglorious place of burial in *Bleak House*.[84] He was 'perfectly stricken down' by Southwood Smith's *Report of the Parliamentary Commission on Children's Employment* ('Trades and Manufactures') and, as Slater records, 'he writes to [Southwood] Smith on 6 March, of publishing [...] "a very cheap pamphlet, called 'An appeal to the People of England, on behalf of the Poor Man's Child' " '.[85] The pamphlet never got written, but his letters to Southwood Smith suggest that the project was integrated into *A Christmas Carol*. Dickens also wrote a fiery defence of Southwood Smith's report in *The Morning Chronicle* in 1842. In response to the physician's findings, there had been a 'widespread support of Lord Ashley's Bill, one of the main provisions of which was to outlaw the employment underground of children under thirteen and of women, and it passed the Commons on 5 July'.[86] In the House of Lords, however, the bill was opposed by the Marquess of Londonderry, owner of a number of coalfields in County Durham. In his open letter to Lord Ashley,

---

[83] Gertrude Hill Lewes, *Dr Southwood Smith: A Retrospect* (Edinburgh and London: William Blackwood, 1898), pp. 83–4.

[84] See Charles Dickens, letter to Henry Austin, 21 January 1852, Dickens Letters 6, pp. 580–1.

[85] Slater, *Charles Dickens*, p. 213.

[86] Michael Slater, introduction to Charles Dickens, Review of *A Letter to Lord Ashley, MP, On the Mines and Collieries Bill* by C.W. Vane, Marquess of Londonderry, GCB', *Morning Chronicle*, 20 October 1842, Dickens Journalism 2, pp. 44–51 (p. 44).

Londonderry summarily dismissed Southwood Smith as 'another commissioner and a Unitarian'. It was an observation, Dickens sardonically wrote, 'full of generous point and purpose'.[87] As was in the character of the man who had ridiculed the shallow thinking of Sir Peter Laurie, Dickens attacked the Marquess for his lack of intelligent reflection: the letter 'has [not] one thought, or argument, or line of reasoning, in its whole compass'.[88]

The same could hardly be said of the work of Southwood Smith, however, which succeeded in linking the materialism of physiological research with a larger enterprise for thinking critically. In his aptly titled *Philosophy of Health* (1834), for instance, it was argued: 'Nothing would seem a fitter study for man than the nature of man in this [physiological] sense of the term. A knowledge of the structure and functions of the body is admitted to be indispensable'.[89] What is more, 'exertions of this kind beget in those for whom, and towards those by whom, they are made, benignant feelings—respect, veneration, gratitude, love'.[90] Here, the layman with an understanding of physiology makes a marked contrast to the Marquess of Londonderry in Dickens's estimation—a man who, with the intention of protecting his own investments in the mining industry, had made ill-considered arguments about the employment of women and children.

While working at the London Fever Hospital in the 1820s and 1830s, Southwood Smith had set about understanding the laws of epidemic disease. He helped Bentham set up the *Westminster Review* and contributed a number of articles which would eventually be expanded into the *Treatise on Fever* (1830). In both the articles and the treatise, he claimed that 'epidemics commence, spread, and cease in a manner perfectly peculiar. They arise, for example, in some particular quarter of town, and do not attack the other districts which happen to be the nearest it'.[91] Fever attacks certain areas, in other words, because those districts are predisposed to infection: '*Penury*', he added, '*can thus, at any time and in any place, create a mortal plague*.'[92] Such views are what informed Dickens's sense, in 'To Working Men', that 'deprivation of the common appliances' expose thousands of families as 'food for pestilence'. That such was the case in Tooting appeared to have been confirmed by the fact that 'Mr. Drouet's establishment was the only place in the parish where cholera appeared'.[93] The Angel of Death had not flown

---

[87] Dickens, Review of *A Letter to Lord Ashley*, p. 47.   [88] Ibid.

[89] Thomas Southwood Smith, *The Philosophy of Health; or, An Exposition of the Physical and Mental Constitution of Man, with a view to the Promotion of Human Longevity and Happiness*, 2 vols (1834; London: C. Cox, 1847), vol. 1, p. 4.

[90] Ibid., p. 97.

[91] [Thomas Southwood Smith], 'Contagion and Sanitary Laws', *Westminster Review*, 3 (1825), pp. 134–67 (p. 145).

[92] Thomas Southwood Smith, *A Treatise on Fever* (London: Longman et al, 1830), p. 324. Italics in original. Christopher Hamlin shows that by the time of Southwood Smith's 1838 report on the prevalence of fever, conducted under the auspices of the Commission, he cast 'doubt on the claim that fever reflected want'. *Public Health and Social Justice*, p. 118.

[93] 'Trial of Mr. Drouet', 14 April, p. 7.

over indiscriminately; 'the diet [of the children] was not sufficient to give them that strength which would have been necessary to enable them to resist [the] prejudicial influences' of infection.[94] When Wakley asked one boy what he thought had brought the cholera to Drouet's, he answered, 'want of enough grub'.[95]

In his *Examiner* articles, Dickens alleged that 'a kick, which would be nothing to a child in sound health, becomes, under Mr. Drouet's course of management, a serious wound. Boys who were intelligent before going to Mr. Drouet, lose their animation afterwards (so swears a Guardian) and become fools'.[96] The Guardian in question was Mr. Goodrich, a man 'who had remarked, after the examination of a boy named JOHN THOMAS, that he was a very intelligent boy before he went to Tooting, but now he appeared to have lost all his animation, and seemed nearly a fool'. According to the *Northern Star*, this made the boy 'a reproduction of "SMIKE," the victim of the celebrated "Mr. SQUEERS" '.[97] Dickens took the story of John Thomas, however, and created Guster in *Bleak House*. She is described as

> a lean young woman from a workhouse (by some supposed to have been chris-
> tened Augusta) who, although she was farmed or contracted for during her
> growing time by an amiable benefactor of his species resident at Tooting, and
> cannot fail to have been developed under the most favourable circumstances,
> 'has fits,' which the parish can't account for.   (p. 144)

Guster is left with a long-term condition which appears to belong to the same family of psychosomatic conditions as John Thomas's. She reminds us of the material nature of poverty—its long-term effects and physiological repercussions. As such, she embodies evidence that opposes the mindless and dogmatic prattle that surrounds social reform in the novel.

Anticipating the complex social explorations of *Bleak House*, Dickens sug-gested in the *Examiner* pieces that the Tooting tragedy had not been considered with the in-depth analysis it required. Specifically, the Board of Guardians whose job it was to inspect Drouet's asylum had done so very shoddily. *The Northern Star* argued that 'the Guardians well deserved thrashing for keeping the children at DROUET'S den, long after they became aware of the infamous system carried on at that establishment'.[98] Six months before the outbreak of cholera a report had been sent to the guardians stating that a number of the children had run away from the place because they had been 'insufficiently fed, and otherwise badly treated'.[99] On 22 August, the same guardians received another report detailing the 'brutal treatment, and consequent illness, of two children'.[100] Six days later, Mr. Robinson, the Workhouse Surgeon, and Mr. Johnson, who had been deputed

---

[94] *The Examiner*, 27 January, p. 57.   [95] 'Do-The-Boys-Hall', p. 5.
[96] Dickens, 'Paradise at Tooting', p. 151.   [97] 'Do-The-Boys-Hall', p. 5.
[98] 'Do-The-Boys-Hall', p. 5.   [99] Ibid.   [100] Ibid.

to visit Drouet's 'farm', reported that fifty-eight children were suffering with 'general debility, sore eyes, wasting of the limbs, &c.'.[101] The symptoms, they said, were 'decidedly characteristic of bad food, or an insufficiency of food'.[102] Still, the guardians permitted Drouet to continue running his asylum. Dickens argued: 'the Board of Guardians concerned are grossly in the wrong. The plain truth is, that they took for granted what they should have thoroughly sifted and ascertained.'[103] The basis upon which he criticized the Board of Guardians was the same upon which he praised Wakley's inquest; in contrast to the former's insufficient sifting of the evidence was the coroner's detailed study of the 'physical deterioration of the surviving children'.[104] The jurymen's conclusion that Drouet was guilty of manslaughter and the Board guilty of wilful negligence thus pleased Dickens as much as it did Wakley.

Yet, when Drouet came to criminal trial in the following months, the winds had changed in his favour. The Court Recorder at the Old Bailey, the staunch Tory Charles Ewan Law, set a tone at the start of proceedings which eventually lead to the defendant's acquittal. Reported by Dickens in one of the later *Examiner* articles, the Recorder's charge was that Drouet

> *was accused of having caused the deaths of no less than four children* [although Drouet was on trial for the death of only one, James Andrews], *by a degree of criminal neglect, in not giving them proper food, by crowding them together in an unwholesome atmosphere, and a general inattention to those precautions which were necessary to preserve a number of children, placed together under such circumstances, in a state of ordinary bodily health.* [...] The important question, however, was, what act had been done by the defendant that had conduced to the death of the deceased.[105]

This last sentence formed the 'technicality' that got Drouet acquitted; what act *had* he actually committed? Also, had the chain of causation between James Andrews's death and Drouet's mistreatment been broken, essentially, by the cholera? Mr. Ballantine, speaking in Drouet's defence, said:

> Suppose A was to strike B a violent blow, which might for a time make him very susceptible of injury, and while in this state C was to inflict another blow upon B, which added to the blow of A, inflicted some time before, caused death, was it to be said that A was guilty of manslaughter? It was very similar here. Mr. Drouet might represent A, and the cholera C.[106]

[101] Ibid.   [102] Ibid.   [103] Dickens, 'Tooting Farm', p. 50.   [104] Ibid., p. 49.
[105] [Charles Dickens], 'A Recorder's Charge', The Examiner (3 March 1849), pp. 129–30 (p. 129) . Italics in original.
[106] 'Trial of Mr. Drouet', 15 April 1849, p. 7.

When the jury returned a verdict of 'not guilty', there was 'a burst of applause' in the courtroom.[107] (Drouet's freedom was to be short-lived, as he died the following July from heart failure.) At the time of the acquittal *The Times* featured an editorial in which it observed:

> We cannot see that Mr. BALLANTINE materially, or at all, varied the argument. That learned person, indeed, by way of doing something new, adopted the system in use amongst itinerant lecturers. He had recourse to the letters of the alphabet in order to illustrate the position which was sufficiently clear as it stood. Thus, the spirit of the Cholera Morbus was represented by C; the little unfortunate, JAMES ANDREWS, was idealized away into B; and the tender-hearted, child-loving Drouet was spoken of as A. [...] The analogy between the letters of the alphabet and the actors in the Tooting tragedy may perhaps be drawn a little closer. Let A be represented as holding B's head under water for four minutes' space, then let C relieve guard, and continue the enforced immersion for one minute more. At the end of the fifth minute let B be taken out drowned, and if no evidence be adducted to show that he was fresh and well at the end of the fourth minute A is acquitted. [...] There is something indescribably sickening about the report of this trial. [...] When [the doctors and nurses at the Free Hospital] examined the unfortunate creatures they found their skins covered with loathsome diseases—there were pallid cheeks and flushed cheeks—their bellies were swollen and bloated from the unwholesome nature of their diet. In the midst of such a state of facts comes the Cholera—"big C," as Mr. BALLANTINE playfully calls it—and sweeps away 130 of these children within the space of a few days.[108]

The absence of a single act leading to the death of James Andrews was interpreted by the court as evidence of the defendant's lack of culpability. Yet, for both *The Times* and Dickens, the question was much more complicated, and hinged on the physical evidence which suggested a much longer and more intricate system of neglect. In *The Times*'s rejection of Ballantine's A, B, C argument, we see a similarity to the objections raised, in Dickens's work, to statistical whitewashing. The alternative strategy, showcased by *The Times* editorial, is to suggest that the issue is simultaneously more complex and *physical* than Ballantine had made it. Dickens added in one of his *Examiner* pieces:

> The question is, *what act has been done* by the defendant to conduce to the death of the deceased! Is it? Or does the question extend itself into a series of acts, no one among them in itself perhaps involving the terrible catastrophe so widely

---

[107] Ibid.   [108] Unsigned, Untitled Report, The Times, 15 April 1849, pp. 4–5 (p. 4).

known, but all, taken together, involving that degree of gross neglect of ordinary precaution for the safety of human life, which constitutes one form of manslaughter?[109]

He then quotes from the *Journal of Public Health*:

'Let us set aside all the inhumanity and brutal indifference which have been brought out in evidence'—on this Tooting case—'the hunger and thirst, the cold, the ill-treatment, the uncleanliness, the diseases of filth and neglect, the itch, scald heads, the sore eyes, the running tetters, the scrofulous affections of the joints, and abscesses, the thin shanks and pot bellies, the diseased bowels, the foundation for the consumption of coming years, which were inflicted on these much-abused children.'[110]

Physical symptoms are, for Dickens, a way of complicating the question of whether Drouet could be responsible for killing Andrews by omission. What the Tooting catastrophe offered was an example of role of physiological evidence in questioning individual and social responsibility. As with medicine's complications of the 'Act of God' argument, writ large in the work of Thomas Southwood Smith, Dickens saw corporeal evidence as the starting point of a more complex and thorough investigation into the causes of, and possible solutions to, the social problem.

Seeing Intelligently

Offering an alternative, more powerful system of social thinking to what he called the 'Indifferents' and the 'Incapables',[111] Dickens, like Gaskell, stressed the need to see poverty as a set of physical signs and processes that required careful and intelligent consideration. Hunger was an important image and tool for him because of the way it was difficult to diagnose and pin down. For example, when drawing our attention to the complexity of meaning, in the mystery surrounding Nemo's corpse in *Bleak House*, he uses the language of famine:

Mr. Tulkinghorn [...] comes to the dark door on the second floor. He knocks, receives no answer, opens it, and accidentally extinguishes his candle in doing so. [...] In the rusty skeleton of a grate, pinched at the middle as if poverty had gripped it, a red coke fire burns low. In the corner by the chimney stand a deal table and a broken desk, a wilderness marked with a rain of ink. In another corner a ragged old portmanteau on one of the two chairs serves for cabinet or

[109] Dickens, 'A Recorder's Charge', p. 129. Italics in original.   [110] Ibid., p. 130.
[111] Dickens, 'To Working Men', p. 228.

wardrobe; no larger one is needed, for it collapses like the cheeks of a starved man. The floor is bare, except that one old mat, trodden to shreds of rope-yarn, lies perishing upon the hearth. No curtain veils the darkness of the night, but the discoloured shutters are drawn together, and through the two gaunt holes pierced in them, famine might be staring in—the banshee of the man upon the bed.   (p. 151)

Gordon Bigelow has suggested that 'the image of Ireland' is invoked here to condense anxieties over

the failure of the representative sign. The linguistic failure that characterises Chancery is depicted here as a total breakdown of all the analogous systems in the novel: the sign, the patronymic, the commodity. All crash in Nemo's writing without meaning, his affiliation without the proper name, his hollow housekeeping, his addictive eating (of opium) without nourishment. Ireland comes to stand for the chaos of circulation.[112]

What I would add to this convincing premise is the idea that 'the failure of the representative sign' relies upon the construction (also at work, as I have argued, during the Irish Hunger) of the starving body as a complex, potentially misleading subject. What is uppermost in Dickens's description of Nemo's corpse is neither the scribe's writing nor the linguistic failures of Chancery, but combinations of objects with physical descriptions (broken desk, ragged portmanteau, bare floor, discoloured shutters, gaunt holes), all of which reflect the medical strategy of seeing bodies through pathological states (collapsing cheeks, starved man, poisoned man, dead man). In *Oliver Twist*, when the protagonist is taken with Mr. Sowerberry to collect the corpse of a starved woman, we are informed that the streets of the district are 'stagnant and filthy. The very rats, which here and there lay putrefying in its rottenness, were hideous with famine' (p. 38). The woman's husband and mother fare little better:

The man's face was thin and very pale; his hair and beard were grizzly; his eyes were bloodshot. The old woman's face was wrinkled; her two remaining teeth protruded over her under lip; and her eyes were bright and piercing. [...] They seemed so like the rats he had seen outside.   (p. 38)

Again, there is the combination of pathological adjective and corporeal noun, which is central to any symptomatology: thin face, pale face, wrinkled face, grizzly hair, bloodshot eyes, protruding teeth, piercing eyes. In the later novel, Nemo's

---

[112] Gordon Bigelow, *Fiction, Famine, and the Rise of Economics in Victorian Britain and Ireland* (Cambridge: Cambridge University Press, 2003), p. 92.

cadaver is discovered after the light of the candle carried by Tulkinghorn is extinguished, leaving him in obscurity. Similarly, the pauper woman in *Oliver Twist* dies 'in the dark—in the dark' (p. 39). In both cases it seems that light is extinguished in order to preclude a hasty reading of poverty's symptoms. The detailed view, exemplified by the way in which the narrative itself indulges in excessive, listing descriptions, has to be a careful one—a gaze that is aware of its flaws and its partial-sightedness.

In 'A Nightly Scene in London', Dickens indicates that such a mode of looking was needed to counterbalance the way 'disciples [of] arithmetic and political economy' had fooled themselves, and others, into believing that they can 'easily prove' things.[113] He interviews one of the five female paupers he sees outside the Whitechapel workhouse. 'Gaunt with want, and foul with dirt', he asks her:

'What have you had to eat?'

'Nothing.'

'Come!' said I. 'Think a little. You are tired and have been asleep, and don't quite consider what you are saying to us. You have had something to eat today. Come! Think of it!'

'No, I haven't. Nothing but such bits as I could pick up about the market. *Why, look at me!*'

She bared her neck, and I covered it up again.[114]

This dialogue has something in common with Gaskell's alleged conversation with the poor labourer who asks her 'have ye ever seen a child clemmed to death?'; Dickens is similarly confronted by the poor woman's bodily evidence of hunger. His reaction, as we have seen, was to renounce the 'demented disciples' of political economy. He praised those who, by contrast, 'mind such things, and who think them infamous in our streets'.[115] It is significant, I argue, that he uses the words 'mind' and 'think', instead of 'notice' and 'see'. The problem is not that people did not see, but that, like political economists as he perceived them, they saw without much critical thought.

It would be wrong to suggest, however, that Dickens criticized only the political economists for their sheep-like approaches to poverty. In 'A Sleep to Startle Us', he anticipates *Bleak House*'s 'Dead, my lords and gentlemen' passage by dismissing a host of religious doctrinaires, followers of 'Gorham controversies, and Pusey controversies and Newman controversies, and twenty other edifying controversies', for not 'com[ing] out of the controversies for a little while' in order to

[113] Dickens, 'A Nightly Scene in London', p. 351.
[114] Dickens, 'A Nightly Scene', pp. 249–50; italics in original.   [115] Ibid., p. 351.

think about the destitute starving around them.[116] The article describes the condition of the hungry paupers of Field Lane School, including a 'lame old man' who goes missing:

> Everybody had seen the male old man upstairs asleep, but he had unaccountably disappeared. What he had being doing with himself was a mystery, but, when the inquiry was at its height, he came shuffling and tumbling in, with his palsied head hanging on his breast an emaciated drunkard, once a compositor, dying of starvation and decay. He was so near death, that he could not be kept there, lest he should die in the night.[117]

The old man's lameness endows him with an obvious, troublesome physicality, and yet he is, for all that, mysterious, itinerant, unaccountable, and disappearing. In his former life as a compositor, he would have been tasked, like Nemo, with creating texts and meaning; he would have specialized in making sense of signs and symbols, and yet here he is, inarticulate and impermanent. He is typical of Dickens's ability to stress the ironic vagueness or mystery of a subject by focusing on the complex nature of its materiality. Like the hunger he experiences at Field Lane, and how it is described by medical and physiological experts, the old compositor becomes a signifier both of want and absence and a troublesome, present corporeality. Simple yet complex, he comes and goes like hunger—he is found and lost again. It is therefore difficult to imagine how any simple observation could account for the old man in 'A Sleep to Startle Us', as it would be difficult, indeed, for Lord Coodle, Sir Thomas Doodle, the Duke of Foodle, and all the fine gentlemen in office, down to Zoodle, to make sense of Tom-All-Alone's.

In *A Christmas Carol*, Scrooge's spectral journeys into the past, present, and future allow him and his theories of political economy to be brought face-to-face with the miserable and complex realities of abjection. His witnessing of a 'wretched woman with an infant' on the street soon after the visitation of Jacob Marley is a parable of the futility of economic theory. The spirits of the dead seek to interfere for good 'in human matters', but they have lost the power to do so because, like Marley, they never moved 'beyond the narrow limits' of their own selfish aims and beliefs when they lived (pp. 24, 21). The Ghost of Christmas Present shows Scrooge the infant embodiments of ignorance and want: 'wretched, abject, frightful, hideous, miserable' (p. 66). 'Have they no refuge or resource?' Scrooge asks, ' "Are there no prisons?" said the Spirit, turning on him [...] with his own words. "Are there no work-houses?" ' (p. 67). Although they are allegories, the spirit's children are bestowed with physical attributes: 'Yellow, meagre, ragged, scowling, wolfish; [and] prostate too in their humility. Where graceful youth

---

[116]   Dickens, 'A Sleep to Startle Us', p. 57.   [117]   Ibid., p. 56.

should have filled their features out, and touched them with its freshest tints, a stale and shrivelled hand, like that of age, had pinched, and twisted them, and pulled them to shreds' (p. 67). It is clear from this description that *A Christmas Carol* was written, in part, as a response to Southwood Smith's research on the conditions of labouring children. The reformer had himself observed how the lack of 'good and sufficient food', combined with 'warm and decent clothing', resulted in children's ' "bodily health" [being] seriously and generally injured; they are for the most part stunted in growth, their aspect being pale, delicate, and sickly, and they present altogether the appearance of a race which has suffered general physical deterioration'.[118] That a whole race could suffer general physical deterioration is supported by a late piece of Dickens journalism, which stated that 'starvation in the second and third generation takes a pinched look'.[119] Following Laqueur's idea of a new 'humanitarian narrative' based, in the nineteenth century, on 'unprecedented quantities of fact, on minute observations' and the 'reality effect',[120] Mike Sanders has argued that the 'most powerful symbol of the harm wreaked on working-class bodies [by industrial culture was] that of the figure of the malnourished factory-child, deformed or exhausted as a result of unnatural labour'.[121] This certainly appears to be true of Southwood Smith's working children.

Against definitions of starvation as a physical, congenital, and chronic condition, Dickens sets the abstract notions of political economy. In linking Tiny Tim's frailties to his present, poverty-stricken condition, the text draws a link, similar to Southwood Smith's, between want of food and bad health: 'If these shadows remain unaltered by the Future', says the ghost, 'the child will die'. As in *The Chimes* and the visions of 'Want' and 'Ignorance', Scrooge's sense of the future is nothing like the prognostications of political economists because it focuses on physiology. What if Tiny Tim should die, asks the Spirit:

'What then? If he be like to die, he had better do it, and decrease the surplus population.'

Scrooge hung his head to hear his own words quoted by the Spirit, and was overcome with penitence and grief.

'Man,' said the Ghost, 'if man you be in heart, not adamant, forbear that wicked cant until you have discovered What the surplus is, and Where it is. Will you decide what men shall live, what men shall die? It may be that, in the sight of Heaven, you are more worthless and less fit to live than millions like this poor

[118] Thomas Southwood Smith, *The Physical and Moral Condition of the Children and Young Persons Employed in Mines and Manufactures* (London: John W. Parker, 1843), p. 149.
[119] Charles Dickens, 'A Small Star in the East', *All The Year Round* (New Series), 1 (1868), Dickens Journalism 4, pp. 352–64 (p. 360).
[120] Laqueur, 'Humanitarian Narrative', p. 177.
[121] Mike Sanders, 'Manufacturing Accident: Industrialism and the Worker's Body in Early Victorian Fiction', *Victorian Literature and Culture*, 28:2 (2000), pp. 313–29 (p. 316).

man's child. Oh God! to hear the Insect on the leaf pronouncing on the too much life among his hungry brothers in the dust!'.   (pp. 55–6)

Dickens aims to do in narrative what William Farr had attempted to do with a more critical interpretation of Chadwick's statistics. Scrooge's spirit encounter with Tiny Tim (specifically the boy's ailing body) shows 'What' and 'Where' poverty is. Against the statistical abstractions created by Chadwick and taught by the likes of Mr. McChoakumchild, we have, counterbalanced, a more nuanced picture of the realities of poverty.

Conclusion

In *The Victorian Social-Problem Novel* (1996), Josephine M. Guy writes:

> The Victorians' understanding of society is certainly naïve, and their proposed solutions to, say, unemployment, inequality of wealth, and so on, are woefully inadequate. Indeed, social-problem novels can tell us almost nothing about how we might resolve our own social problems (and we should be surprised and perhaps alarmed if they could, or if any critic seriously proposed that they could).[1]

I am prepared to surprise, and perhaps alarm, by being that critic who seriously proposes that the Victorians tell us a great deal about our own social problems. Indeed, it is a hope of mine that, as readers worked their way through this book, they have noticed the occasional similarity between the Victorian world and our own. That I expect to see more of a kinship with the nineteenth century than Guy has much to do, I am sure, with the twenty-odd years that separates my writing from hers. She was writing in the optimistic 1990s, on the cusp of a new dawn in British politics, and as America was enjoying its prosperous Clinton years. It would be years before the major financial crisis of 2007–8 taught us all a hard lesson about international economics.

In the wake of that financial crisis there was, according to hundreds of news reports, a resurgence of 'Victorian' medical conditions. In the summer of 2014, a Health and Social Care Information Centre report showed that there were 86,870 hospital admissions for gout between 2013–14 in the UK, an increase of 78 per cent on 2009–10 (48,720); new notifications of tuberculosis remained high, with 8,751 cases reported in 2012; hospital admissions for scarlet fever doubled, from 403 to 845; and there was a 71 per cent increase in admissions for malnutrition, from 3,900 in 2009–10 to 6,690 in 2013–14.[2] According to John Middleton, writing in *The Guardian*, we should be concerned about this return of 'Victorian diseases'. 'Official figures showing a rise in diseases linked to poverty, such as gout, TB [tuberculosis], measles, malnutrition and whooping cough are a barometer of failure and neglect'. They are the result of 'a period of enforced deprivation, with

---

[1] Josephine M. Guy, *The Victorian Social-Problem Novel* (London and Basingstoke: Macmillan, 1996), p. 11.

[2] John Middleton, 'Why We Should be Concerned about the Return of Victorian Diseases', *The Guardian*, 8 August 2014, https://www.theguardian.com/healthcare-network/2014/aug/08/return-victorian-diseases-gout-tb-measles-malnutrition [accessed April 2018].

The Science of Starving in Victorian Literature, Medicine, and Political Economy. Andrew Mangham,
Oxford University Press (2020). © Andrew Mangham.
DOI: 10.1093/oso/9780198850038.001.0001

the biggest cut in average wages since Dickens's era'.[3] 'Victorian diseases have come back to haunt us', corroborates The Telegraph's health editor Laura Donnelly, reacting to the same report; yet 'experts [have] said the increasing cases of gout [she overlooks tuberculosis, measles, malnutrition, and whooping cough] are likely to reflect rising obesity levels, with two-thirds of adults now overweight or obese, and are also associated with excessive drinking'.[4] There are two important questions to be asked here. Firstly, what is it that makes gout, tuberculosis, measles, malnutrition, and whooping cough 'Victorian'? All these conditions existed, to a greater degree in fact, in earlier periods in history. As James Vernon notes, 'standards of living—as measured by a combination of diet, health, and income— had actually improved' in the nineteenth century, even if the gap between rich and poor had become more pronounced.[5] Indeed, what my study suggests is that, while there is nothing to identify these conditions as quintessentially Victorian, the interdisciplinary discussion of them as linked to poverty is a distinct feature of the era. The nineteenth century explored, through medicine and physiology, the connections between social conditions and pathologies that related, directly or indirectly, to malnutrition. The novel, as we have seen, explored and popularized this material focus, often drawing on science for its plots and characterizations, and sharing the wish to anatomize hunger and its attendant maladies—to turn social-reform narratives inside out and to peer at their workings. Although poverty, starvation, and their secondary conditions have been the curse of humankind since the dawn of civilization, we associate them with the nineteenth century not simply because it is a period that closely precedes our own, but because the Victorians laid the ground for our critical understandings of hunger as a scientific, material, philosophical, and social event.

The second point to come from a comparison of Middleton's and Donnelly's articles is the parallel that may be drawn between their varying senses of causality and nineteenth-century constructions of the same. These opposing forms of thought have been with us since the eighteenth century and show no signs of leaving. Donnelly links a pathological 'event'—in this case, the increase of gout— to the behaviours of individuals, identifying the main problem to be people eating and drinking too much.[6] Nothing could be more Malthusian: first, because of its selective focus on the evidence; and, second, because of its interpretation of social problems as the result of individuals' actions. Middleton, meanwhile, opts for guarded scepticism: 'Interpreting the figures, we should be a little cautious about

[3] Ibid.

[4] Laura Donnelly, 'Victorian Diseases have Come Back to Haunt Us', The Telegraph, 23 July 2014, https://www.telegraph.co.uk/news/health/news/10985260/Victorian-diseases-have-come-back-to-haunt-us.html [accessed April 2018].

[5] James Vernon, Hunger: A Modern History (Cambridge MS and London: Belknap Press of Harvard University Press, 2007), p. 6.

[6] Florian Schui has made a link between Malthusian thinking and austerity in Austerity: The Great Failure (New Haven and London: Yale University Press, 2014), pp. 147–9.

the impact of hospital coding—there has been upward pressure to code everything in the patient's discharge summary for hospitals to pull in maximum pay-
ment by results.'[7] Using the same kind of logic employed by a number of scientists,
medics, and authors I have discussed in the preceding chapters, he moves the
issue away from the supposedly immoderate behaviours of individuals towards 'a
picture of neglect—by government with its active impoverishment of poorer
parts of our society and with its complacent neglect of public health nutrition.'[8]

The key word here is *complacent*, meaning an uncritical satisfaction with one's
way of interpreting things. Since 2010 the British government's way of going
about things has been overshadowed by the dangerous idea of austerity. According
to Mark Blyth:

> Austerity is a form of voluntary deflation in which the economy adjusts through
> the reduction of wages, prices, and public spending [especially on the 'welfare
> state'] to restore competitiveness, which is (supposedly) best achieved by cutting
> the state's budget, debts, and deficits. Doing so, its advocates believe, will inspire
> 'business confidence' since the government will neither be 'crowding-out' the
> market for investment by sucking up all the available capital through the issu-
> ance of debt, nor adding to the nation's already 'too big' debt.

Blyth makes a compelling case for why we should see austerity as a 'zombie economic idea'; although 'it has been disproven time and again, [...] it just keeps
coming.'[9] While it is beyond the remit of this study to argue a case for or against
austerity, it is worth noting the similarities it bears, in theory, to providential
political economy. It seeks to shift responsibility for civic failure onto the shoulders of individuals. As Blyth notes, it was the banks and big businesses who
caused the global financial crisis of 2007–8, yet it is the taxes of individuals left
footing the bill. Since the 1980s, large companies have been dominant in the
wealth of the West because of the neoliberal strategies that overshadow global
economics. According to David Harvey:

> Neoliberalism is in the first instance a theory of political economic practices that
> proposes that human well-being can best be advanced by liberating individual
> entrepreneurial freedoms and skills within an institutional framework character-
> ised by strong private property rights, free markets, and free trade. [...] State
> interventions in markets (once created) must be kept to a bare minimum because,
> according to the theory, the state cannot possibly possess enough information to
> second-guess market signals (prices) and because powerful interest groups will

---

[7] Middleton, 'Why We Should be Concerned'.   [8] Ibid.
[9] Mark Blyth, *Austerity: The History of a Dangerous Idea* (Oxford: Oxford University Press, 2013),
p. 2, 10.

inevitably distort and bias state interventions (particularly in democracies) for their own benefit. [...] It holds that the social good will be maximized by maximizing the reach and frequency of market transactions, and it seeks to bring all human action into the domain of the market.[10]

We are now feeling the repercussions of these ideas; the spirit of entrepreneurialism has not trickled down through all ranks of society, and uneven conditions mean that the welfare state has a more vital role than ever. Under the twin scourges of neoliberalism and austerity, however, welfare has been cut back. The problem, we have been told, is a drain on resources caused by state pensions, disability living allowances, the National Health Service (in the UK), public libraries, universities, and the wages of doctors, nurses, and school teachers. At fault is immoderate spending at lower levels. In the nineteenth century, conservative political economy offered a convenient method of attributing poverty to the immoderate behaviours of the lower classes rather than showing how sovereign wealth had been deposited within a class whose lack of social responsibility ensured it would never benefit the many as opposed to the few. It is astonishing how little has changed.

I am not meaning to argue that we have much to learn from the history and literature of the nineteenth century because its people were *like* us, but, rather, because they *are* us. Neoliberalism and austerity are iterations of a conservative way of thinking that has been with us at least as far back as the New Poor Law— intellectual historians might trace it back to John Locke through Bentham, Malthus, and Adam Smith.[11] Kingsley, Gaskell, and Dickens, like their physiological and medical contemporaries, teach us much about the ways we understand poverty, because they react to a pattern of thinking that remains influential. Through a range of narratives, images, and case studies, they explore how the complication of an issue, particularly through medicine's insistence on the fallibilities of perception and the shifting nature of matter, allows us to question the convenient stories whose conclusions have become *complacent*. They create a picture of reality not through the rejection of feeling or sentiment, but by creatively capturing how reality is itself a construct, full of conflict, prevarication, and complexity. If we live in a neoliberal, neo-Malthusian world, we must also find our place in a neo-materialist, neo-historicist one, where the ability to look at bodies and how they suffer, in Victorian novels and in the world around us, allows a more intelligent interpretation of how, in the words of Marx and Engels, we are 'measured not by the power of separate individuals but by the power of society'.[12]

---

[10] David Harvey, *A Brief History of Neoliberalism* (Oxford: Oxford University Press, 2005), pp. 2–3. See also William Davies, *The Limits of Neoliberalism: Authority, Sovereignty and the Logic of Competition* (California: Sage, 2014).

[11] See Blyth, *Austerity*.

[12] Karl Marx and Friedrich Engels, *The Holy Family, or Critique of Critical Critique* (1845; Moscow: Foreign Languages, 1956), p. 176.

Bibliography

Primary Sources

Carlyle, Thomas. *Sartor Resartus: The Life and Opinions of Herr Teufelsdröckh*, ed. by Kerry McSweeney (1834; Oxford: Oxford University Press, 2008).

Dickens, Charles. *The Chimes* in *Christmas Books*, in *Christmas Books*, ed. by Ruth Glancy (1844; Oxford: Oxford University Press, 1988), pp. 93–182.

Dickens, Charles. *A Christmas Carol* (1844), in *Christmas Books*, ed. by Ruth Glancy (Oxford: Oxford University Press, 1988), pp. 1–90.

Dickens, Charles. 'The Amusements of the People' (1), *Household Words*, 1 (1850), Dickens Journalism 2, pp. 179–85.

Dickens, Charles. *Bleak House*, ed. by Stephen Gill (1852–3; Oxford: Oxford University Press, 2008).

Dickens, Charles. 'Frauds on Fairies', *Household Words*, 8 (1853), Dickens Journalism 3, pp. 166–74.

Dickens, Charles. *Hard Times*, ed. by Kate Flint (1854; London: Penguin, 2003).

Dickens, Charles. 'A Nightly Scene in London', *Household Words*, 13 (1856), Dickens Journalism 3, pp. 346–51.

Dickens, Charles. *Oliver Twist*, ed. by Stephen Gill (1837–8; Oxford: Oxford University Press, 2008).

Dickens, Charles. 'On Strike', *Household Words*, 8 (1854), Journalism 3, pp. 196–210.

Dickens, Charles. 'The Paradise at Tooting', *The Examiner*, 20 January 1849, Dickens Journalism 2, pp. 147–56.

Dickens, Charles. 'A Preliminary Word', *Household Words*, 1 (1853), Dickens Journalism 2, pp. 175–9.

Dickens, Charles. 'A Recorder's Charge', *The Examiner* (3 March 1849), pp. 129–30.

Dickens, Charles. 'A Sleep to Startle Us', *Household Words*, 9 (1852), Dickens Journalism 3, pp. 49–57.

Dickens, Charles. 'A Small Star in the East', *All The Year Round (New Series)*, 1 (1868), Dickens Journalism 4, pp. 352–64.

Dickens, Charles. Speech delivered in Boston, 1 February 1842, *Speeches; Literary and Social* (London: John Camden Hotten, n.d.), pp. 57–62.

Dickens, Charles. Speech to the Annual Meeting of the Institutional Association of Lancashire and Cheshire (3 December 1858), in *Speeches Literary and Social by Charles Dickens* (London: Camden Hotten, n.d.), pp. 157–66.

Dickens, Charles. Speech to the Manchester Athenaeum, 5 October 1843, in *Speeches; Literary and Social* (London: John Camden Hotten, n.d.), pp. 74–81.

Dickens, Charles. Review of Robert Hunt, *The Poetry of Science, or Studies of the Physical Phenomena of Nature* (1849), in Dickens Journalism 2, pp. 129–34.

Dickens, Charles. 'The Streets—Night', *Bell's Life in London*, 17 January 1836, Journalism 1, pp. 55–60.

Dickens, Charles. 'The Tooting Farm', *The Examiner*, 27 January 1849, pp. 49–50.

Dickens, Charles. 'To Working Men', *Household Words*, 10 (1854), Dickens Journalism 3, pp. 225–9.

Gaskell, Elizabeth. *Mary Barton*, ed. by Edgar Wright (1848; Oxford: Oxford University Press, 1998).

Gaskell, Elizabeth. *North and South*, ed. by Angus Easson (1854–5; Oxford: Oxford University Press, 1998).

Gaskell, Elizabeth. *Sylvia's Lovers*, ed. by Andrew Sanders (1863; Oxford: Oxford University Press, 2008).

Gillies, Mary. 'A Labourer's Home', *Howitt's Journal*, 1 (1847), pp. 61–4.

Gillies, Mary. 'Recent Novels', *Fraser's Magazine* 39 (1849), pp. 417–32.

Kingsley, Charles. 'The Agricultural Crisis', *North British Review*, 14 (1850), pp. 85–121.

Kingsley, Charles. *Alton Locke, Tailor and Poet: An Autobiography*, ed. by Elizabeth A. Cripps (1850; Oxford: Oxford University Press, 1983).

Kingsley, Charles. *Cheap Clothes and Nasty* (1849; London: William Pickering, 1850).

Kingsley, Charles. 'Cholera, 1866', in *The Water of Life and other Sermons* (London: Macmillan, 1879), pp. 189–202.

Kingsley, Charles. 'The Church *versus* Malthus', *The Christian Socialist*, 15 February 1851, p. 121 and 29 March 1851, p. 170.

Kingsley, Charles. 'First Sermon on the Cholera', *Sermons on National Subjects* (London: Macmillan, 1880), pp. 134–43.

Kingsley, Charles. 'Froude's History of England, vols VII and VIII', *Macmillan's Magazine*, 9 (1863–4), pp. 211–24.

Kingsley, Charles. *Health and Education* (1874; New York, NY: D. Appleton, 1893).

Kingsley, Charles. 'Human Soot' (1870), *All Saints' Day and other Sermons*, ed. by W. Harrison (London: Macmillan, 1909), pp. 302–11.

Kingsley, Charles. *Glaucus, or the Wonders of the Shore* (1855) in *The Water-Babies and Glaucus* (London: Dent, 1949).

Kingsley, Charles. 'Letters to the Chartists I', *Politics for the People*, 6 May 1848, pp. 28–30.

Kingsley, Charles. 'A Mad World My Masters', *Fraser's Magazine*, 57 (1858), pp. 133–42.

Kingsley, Charles. 'Old and New' (1848), *Poems by Charles Kingsley* (New York, NY: J. F. Taylor, 1908), p. 258.

Kingsley, Charles. 'A Parable from Liebig' (1848), *Poems by Charles Kingsley* (New York, NY: J. F. Taylor, 1908), p. 257.

Kingsley, Charles. 'The Poetry of a Root Crop' (1845), *Poems by Charles Kingsley* (New York, NY: J. F. Taylor, 1908), p. 232.

Kingsley, Charles. 'The Physician's Calling' in *The Water of Life and other Sermons* (London: Macmillan, 1879), pp. 14–26.

Kingsley, Charles. *The Water-Babies*, in *The Water-Babies and Glaucus* (London: Dent, 1949).

Kingsley, Charles. *The Water of Life and other Sermons* (London: Macmillan, 1879).

Kingsley, Charles. *Yeast: A Problem* (1848; Dover, NH: Alan Sutton, 1994).

Martineau, Harriet. *Illustrations of Political Economy: Selected Tales*, ed. by Deborah Anna Logan (1832; Ontario: Broadview Press, 2004).

Pope, Alexander. *Essay on Man* (1734) in *The Works of Alexander Pope*, 8 vols. (London: Longman et al., 1847), vol. 4, pp. 1–160.

Trollope, Anthony. *Castle Richmond*, ed. by Mary Hamer (1860; Oxford: Oxford University Press, 1989).

Wordsworth, William. *The Prelude*, ed. by J. C. Maxwell (1805–6/1850; London: Penguin, 1982).

Medical and General Scientific Sources

Abercrombie, John. *Inquiries Concerning the Intellectual Powers and the Investigation of Truth* (1830; New York, NY: Harper and Brothers, 1840).

Abernethy, John. *An Enquiry into the Probability and Rationality of Mr. Hunter's Theory of Life* (London: Longman et al., 1814).

Beaumont, William. *Experiments and Observations on the Gastric Juice, and the Physiology of Digestion*, ed. by Andrew Combe (1833; Edinburgh, Maclachlan and Stewart, 1838).

Beddoe, John. 'On the Death Rates in the Cotton Districts', *British Medical Journal*, 3 January 1863, pp. 8–9.

Bernard, Claude. *Introduction à l'Étude de la Médecine Expérimentale*, trans. by Henry Copley Greene as *An Introduction to the Study of Experimental Medicine* (1865; New York, NY: Dover Publishing, 1957).

Bichat, Xavier. *Anatomie Générale: appliquée à la Physiologie et à la Médecine*, trans. by George Hayward as *General Anatomy, applied to Physiology and Medicine* (Boston, MS: Richardson and Lord, 1822).

Buchanan, George. 'On Recent Typhus in Lancashire', *The Lancet*, 14 February 1863, pp. 174–6.

Budd, William. 'On Intestinal Fever', *The Lancet*, 2 (1859), pp. 131–3.

Carpenter, William B. *Nature and Man: Essays Scientific and Philosophical*, ed. by J. Estlin Carpenter (New York, NY: D. Appleton, 1889).

Carpenter, William B. 'Physiology for the People I', *Howitt's Journal*, 1 (1847), pp. 100–2.

Carpenter, William B. 'Physiology for the People II', *Howitt's Journal*, 1 (1847), pp. 132–4.

Carpenter, William B. 'Physiology for the People IV', *Howitt's Journal*, 1 (1847), pp. 198–201.

Carpenter, William B. *The Physiology of Temperance and Total Abstinence being an Examination of the Effects of the Excessive, Moderate, and Occasional Use of Alcoholic Liquors on the Healthy Human System* (London: Henry G. Bohn, 1853).

Carpenter, William B. *Principles of Human Physiology*, ed. by Henry Power (1842; Philadelphia: Henry C. Lea, 1876).

Carpenter, William B. *Principles of Mental Physiology, with their Applications to the Training and Discipline of the Mind, and the Study of Its Morbid Conditions* (London: Henry S. King, 1874).

Cheyne, George. *The English Malady: or, a Treatise of Nervous Diseases of all Kinds* (London: G. Strahan, 1733).

Combe, Andrew. *The Physiology of Digestion Considered with Relation to the Principles of Dietetics* (1836; Boston, Marsh, Capen, Lyon and Webb, 1840).

Corrigan, D. G. *On Famine and Fever as Cause and Effect in Ireland* (Dublin: J. Fannin, 1846).

Darwin, Erasmus. *The Temple of Nature; or, the Origin of Society* (London: J. Johnson, 1803).

De Réaumur, René Antoine Ferchault. *Observations sur la Digestion des Oiseaux* (Paris: De L'Imprimerte Royale, 1752).

Elliotson, John. *Human Physiology* (London: Longman et al., 1835).

Foster, Michael. *Lectures on the History of Physiology* (1901; New York, NY: Dover, 1970).

Gillespie, A. Lockheart. *The Natural History of Digestion* (London: Walter Scott, 1898).

Graves, Robert J. 'On the Progress of Asiatic Cholera', *The Dublin Quarterly Journal of Medical Science*, 2 (1846), pp. 289–316.

Guy, William A. *Principles of Forensic Medicine* (London: Henry Renshaw, 1845).

Guy, William A. *Public Health: A Popular Introduction to Sanitary Science* (London: Henry Renshaw, 1870).

Harrison, James Bower. *The Medical Aspects of Death and the Medical Aspects of the Human Mind* (London: Longman et al., 1852).

Holland, Henry. 'Materialism as a Question of Science and Philosophy', in *Fragmentary Papers on Science and Other Subjects* (London: Longman et al., 1875), pp. 206–13.

Holland, Henry. 'The Progress and Spirit of Physical Science' (1858), in *Essays on Scientific and Other Subjects contributed to the Edinburgh and Quarterly Reviews* (London: Longman et al., 1862), pp. 1–49.

Howard, Richard Baron. *An Inquiry into the Morbid Effects of Deficiency of Food, Chiefly with Reference to their Occurrence amongst the Destitute Poor* (London: Simpkin, Marshall, et al., 1839).

Hunter, John. *Lectures on the Principles of Surgery* (1786–7; Philadelphia: Haswell et al., 1839).

Hunter, John. *Observations on Certain Parts of the Animal Œconomy* (1786; Philadephia: Haswell et al., 1840).

Ingram, J. K. 'Presidential Address', *Report of the Forty-Eighth Meeting of the British Association for the Advancement of Science; Held at Dublin in August 1878* (London: John Murray, 1879), pp. 641–58.

Keill, James. *Essays on Several Parts of the Animal Oeconomy* (London: George Strahan, 1717).

Lewes, George Henry. *Comte's Philosophy of the Sciences: Being an Exposition of the Principles of the Cours de Philosophie Positive of Auguste Comte* (London: Henry G. Bohn, 1853).

Lewes, George Henry. *The Physiology of Common Life*, 2 vols. (London: William Blackwood and Sons, 1859).

Lewes, George Henry. *The Problems of Life and Mind*, 3 vols. (1877; Boston, MA and New York, NY: Houghton Mifflin, 1891).

Lhotsky, Johann. *On Cases of Death by Starvation, and Extreme Distress among the Humbler Classes* (London: John Ollivier, 1844).

Liebig, Justus von. *Familiar Letters on Chemistry, and its Relation to Commerce, Physiology, and Agriculture* (Philadelphia: James M. Campbell, 1843).

Liebig, Justus von. 'Lectures on Organic Chemistry, number 10', *The Lancet*, 22 June 1844, pp. 395–8.

Murchison, Charles, *A Treatise on the Continued Fevers of Great Britain* (1862; London: Longman et al., 1884).

Ottley, Drewry, *The Life of John Hunter in The Works of John Hunter, F.R.S.*, ed. by James F. Palmer, 5 vols. (London: Longman et al., 1835), vol. 1, pp. 1–198.

Paris, John. *A Treatise on Diet: with a View to Establish, on Practical Grounds, a System of Rules for the Prevention and Cure of the Diseases Incident to a Disordered State of the Digestive Functions* (1826; London: Sherwood, Gilbert and Piper, 1837).

Playfair, Lyon. 'Professor Liebig's Report on "Organic Chemistry applied to Physiology and Pathology', *Report of the Twelfth Meeting of the British Association for the Advancement of Science* (London: John Murray, 1843), pp. 42–54.

Popham, John. 'Notes on the Climate and Diseases of the City of Cork', *The Dublin Quarterly Journal of Medical Science*, 15 (1835), pp. 290–308.

Prout, William. 'Inquiry into the Origins and Properties of Blood', *Annals of Medical Surgery*, 1 (1816), 10–26.

Purefoy, Thomas. 'Observations on Remittent Fever in Ireland', *Dublin Quarterly Journal of Medical Science*, 16 (1853), pp. 318–31.

Rayner, William. 'Letter to the Editor', *The Lancet*, 6 December 1862, p. 632.

Southwood Smith, Thomas. 'An Address to the Working Classes of the United Kingdom, on their Duty in the Present State of the Sanitary Question', *Howitt's Journal*, 1 (1847), pp. 3–4.

Southwood Smith, Thomas. 'Contagion and Sanitary Laws', *Westminster Review*, 3 (1825), pp. 134–67.

Southwood Smith, Thomas. *The Philosophy of Health; or, An Exposition of the Physical and Mental Constitution of Man, with a view to the Promotion of Human Longevity and Happiness*, 2 vols. (1834; London: C. Cox, 1847).

Southwood Smith, Thomas. *The Physical and Moral Condition of the Children and Young Persons Employed in Mines and Manufactures* (London: John W. Parker, 1843).

Southwood Smith, Thomas. *A Treatise on Fever* (London: Longman et al., 1830).

Spallanzani, Lazzaro. *Dissertations Relative to the Natural History of Animals and Vegetables*, trans. by anon., 2 vols. (1780; London: John Murray, 1784).

Spallanzani, Lazzaro. *Memoirs on Respiration*, ed. by John Senebier (London: Thomas Cox, 1805).

Spencer, Herbert. 'A Theory of Population, Deduced from the General Law of Animal Fertility', *Westminster Review*, 57 (1852), pp. 468–501.

Spencer, Herbert. 'The Ultimate Laws of Physiology', *The National Review*, 5 (1857), pp. 332–55.

Thackrah, Charles Turner. *The Effects of the Arts, Trades, and Professions and of the Civic States and Habits of Lining, on Health and Longevity* (London: Longman et. al, 1832).

Thackrah, Charles Turner. *Lectures on Digestion and Diet* (London: Longman et al., 1824).

Unsigned, 'Manchester', *British Medical Journal*, 7 March 1863, pp. 250–1.

Unsigned. 'Report on the Health of the Cotton Operatives', *The Lancet*, 10 January 1863, pp. 43–4.

General Eighteenth- and Nineteenth-Century Sources

Alison, William Pulteney. *The Management of the Poor in Scotland and its Effects on the Health of the Great Towns* (Edinburgh: William Blackwood and Sons; London: Thomas Cadell, 1840).

Alison, William Pulteney. *Reply to the Pamphlet entitled 'Proposed Alteration of the Scottish Poor Law Considered and Commented on, by David Monypenny, Esq. of Pitmilly'* (Edinburgh: William Blackwood and Sons; London: Thomas Cadell, 1840).

Arnold, R. Arthur. *The History of the Cotton Famine* (London: Saunders et al., 1864).

Banks, P. W. 'Touching Opinion and Evidence', *Fraser's Magazine*, 41 (1850), pp. 237–49.

Bazley, Thomas, 'A Glance at the Cotton Trade', *Report of the Thirty-first Meeting of the British Association for the Advancement of Science* (London: John Murray, 1862), pp. 206–8.

Carlyle, Thomas. *Chartism* (1839; London: James Fraser, 1840).

Carlyle, Thomas. 'Corn-Law Rhymes', *Edinburgh Review*, 55 (1832), pp. 338–61.

Carlyle, Thomas. *Past and Present* (New York: William H. Colyer, 1843).

Carlyle, Thomas. 'Signs of the Times', *Edinburgh Review*, 49 (1829), pp. 439–59.

Chalmers, Thomas. *The Christian Economy of Large Towns* (Glasgow: Chalmers and Collins, 1823).

Chalmers, Thomas. *On Political Economy in Connection with the Moral State and Moral Prospects of Society* (New York, NY: Appleton, 1832).

Chalmers, Thomas. 'Political Economy of a Famine', *North British Review*, 13 (1847), pp. 247–90.

Drouet, Bartholomew (criminal case). Unsigned, Untitled Report, *The Examiner*, 27 January 1849, pp. 57–8; Unsigned, 'The Verdict on "Do-the-Boys-Hall"', *The Northern Star*, 27 January 1849, p. 5; Unsigned, 'The Tooting Catastrophe', *The Satirist*, 27 January 1849, p. 38; Unsigned, 'Trial of Mr. Drouet', *The Times*, 14 April 1849, p. 7; Unsigned, Untitled Report, *The Times*, 15 April 1849, pp. 4–5; Unsigned, 'Trial of Mr. Drouet', *The Times*, 15 April 1849, p. 7.

Engels, Friedrich. *The Condition of the Working Class in England*, ed. by Victor Kiernan (1845; London: Penguin, 1987).

Gaskell, William, 'Unitarian Christians Called to Bear Witness to the Truth: A Sermon Preached Before the Supporters of the British and Foreign Unitarian Association at their Annual Meeting, in Essex-Street Chapel, London, June 11, 1862' (London: Edward T. Whitfield, 1862).

Grahame, James. *An Inquiry into the Principle of Population (1816)*, cited in *Population: Contemporary Responses to Thomas Malthus*, ed. by Andrew Pyle (Bristol: Thoemmes Press, 1994).

Hazlitt, William. *A Reply to the Essay on Population by the Rev. T. R. Malthus*, in *The Complete Works of William Hazlitt*, ed. by P. P. Howe, 21 vols. (1807; London and Toronto: J. M. Dent, 1830), vol. 1, pp. 177–364.

Hawkins, F. Bisset. *Elements of Medical Statistics* (London: Longman et al., 1829).

Howitt, William. 'The Fast and the Famine', *Howitt's Journal*, 1 (1847), pp. 181–2.

Howitt, William and Mary Howitt. 'William and Mary Howitt's Address to their Friends and Readers', *Howitt's Journal*, 1 (1847), pp. 1–2.

Jerrold, Douglas. 'Sir Peter Laurie on Human Life', *Punch, or the London Charivari*, 1 (1841), p. 210.

Leigh, Percival. 'Address from an Undertaker to the Trade', *Household Words*, 1 (1850), pp. 301–4.

Lewes, George Henry, 'Realism in Art: Recent German Fiction'in *Westminster Review*, 70 (1858), pp. 488–518.

Lloyd, Walter. *The Story of Protestant Dissent and English Unitarianism* (London: Philip Green, 1899).

Malthus, T. R. *An Essay on the Principle of Population*, ed. by Geoffrey Gilbert (1798: Oxford University Press, 2008).

Malthus, T. R. *An Essay on the Principle of Population* [1806 edition], ed. by Patricia James, 2 vols. (1806; Cambridge: Cambridge University Press, 1989).

Marx, Karl. Letter to Heinrich Marx, November 1837, in *Writings of the Young Marx on Philosophy and Society*, trans. and ed. by Loyd D. Easton and Kurt H. Guddat (1967; Indianapolis, IN: Hackett, 1997), pp. 39–50.

Marx, Karl. *Das Kapital*, trans. as *Capital*, ed. by David McLellan (1867; Oxford: Oxford University Press, 2008).

Marx, Karl, and Friedrich Engels. *The Holy Family, or Critique of Critical Critique* (1845; Moscow: Foreign Languages, 1956).

Marx, Karl, and Friedrich Engels. *The German Ideology* (1846), in *Writings of the Young Marx on Philosophy and Society*, trans. and ed. by Loyd D. Easton and Kurt H. Guddat (1967; Indianapolis, IN: Hackett, 1997), pp. 403–73.

Marx, Karl, and Friedrich Engels. *The Communist Manifesto*, ed. by Gareth Stedman Jones (1848; London: Penguin, 2002).

Mill, John Stuart. 'On Miss Martineau's Summary of Political Economy', *The Monthly Repository*, 8 (1834), pp. 318–22.

Mill, John Stuart. 'On the Definition of Political Economy; and on the Method of Investigation Proper to It', (1836) in *The Collected Works of John Stuart Mill*, ed. John M. Robson, 33 vols. (Toronto: University of Toronto Press, London: Routledge and Kegan Paul, 1967), vol. 4, pp. 309–39.

Mill, John Stuart. *Principles of Political Economy*, ed. by Donald Winch (1848; London: Penguin, 1985).

Mill, John Stuart. *Utilitarianism*, ed. by Mary Warnock (1861; London: Fontana, 1971).

Newman, John Henry. *Apologia Pro Vita Sua*, ed. by Ian Ker (1864; London: Penguin, 1994).

Newman, John Henry. 'The Tamworth Reading Room', in *Discussions and Arguments on Various Subjects* (London: Basil Montagu Pickering, 1872), pp. 254–305.

Newman, John Henry. 'Wisdom and Innocence', in *Sermons Bearing on the Subjects of the Day* (London: J. G. F. and J. Rivington, 1843).

O'Rourke, John. *The Great Irish Famine* (1874; Dublin: Veritas, 1989).

Priestley, Joseph. *Disquisitions Relating to Matter and Spirit* (London: J. Johnson, 1777).

Richardson, Benjamin Ward. *The Health of Nations: A Review of the Works of Edwin Chadwick*, 2 vols. (London: Longman, Green, 1887).

Shuttleworth, James Kay. *The Moral and Physical Condition of the Working Classes Employed in the Cotton Manufacture in Manchester* (London: James Ridgeway, 1832).

Shuttleworth, James Kay. *Thoughts and Suggestions on Certain Social Problems* (London: Longman et al., 1873).

Smythe, George Sydney, Speech to the Manchester Athenaeum, in *Athenaeum Addresses 1843–1848* (Manchester: Manchester City News, 1875), pp. 31–7.

Southey, Robert. 'Review of *An Essay on the Principle of Population*, by T. R. Malthus', *Annual Review*, 2 (1803), pp. 292–301.

Spencer, Herbert. *The Proper Sphere of Government* (London: W. Brittain, 1843).

Stevenson, William. 'The Political Economist I', *Blackwood's Edinburgh Magazine*, 15 (1824), pp. 522–31.

Trevelyan, Charles. *The Irish Crisis* (London: Longman et al., 1848).

Unsigned. 'As the Famine which brought the Israelites', *The Times*, 16 September 1856, p. 6.

Unsigned. 'Dreadful Case of Starvation', *Morning Chronicle*, 25 February 1828, p. 4.

Unsigned. 'Famine in the South of Ireland', *Fraser's Magazine*, 35 (1847), pp. 491–504.

Unsigned. 'The Lives and Deaths of the People', *All the Year Round*, 12 (1864), pp. 198–205.

Unsigned. 'Metamorphosis of Food', *All the Year Round*, 5 (1861), pp. 6–9.

Unsigned. 'Mrs. Gaskell', *Gentleman's Magazine*, 279 (1895), pp. 124–38.

Unsigned. 'Poverty', *All the Year Round*, 13 (1865), pp. 512–15.

Unsigned. Review of *Culina Famulatrix Medicinæ* by Ignatius, *Edinburgh Review*, 6 (1805), pp. 350–7.

Unsigned. Review of *Mary Barton*, *British Quarterly Review*, 9 (1849), pp. 117–36.

Unsigned. 'Preservation of Ann Martin', *Kirby's Wonderful and Eccentric Museum; or Magazine of Remarkable Characters*, 6 vols. (London: R. S. Kirby, 1820), vol. 6, pp. 143–4.

Vansittart, Charles. *A Sermon on Famine: the Expediency of a Public Fast, and the Duty of Personal Abstinence in the Present Time of Dearth* (London: James Burns, 1847).

Watts, John. *The Facts of the Cotton Famine* (London: Simpkin, et al., 1866).

Young, George. *A History of Whitby, and Streoneshalh Abbey, with a Statistical Survey of the Vicinity to the Distance of Twenty-five Miles*, 2 vols. (Whitby: Clark and Medd, 1817).

Zola, Emile. *The Experimental Novel and Other Essays*, trans. by Belle M. Sharman (New York, NY: Cassell, 1893).

Secondary Sources

Abberley, Will, 'Animal Cunning: Deceptive Nature and Truthful Science in Charles Kingsley's Natural Theology', *Victorian Studies*, 58:1 (2015), pp. 34–56.

Abrams, Philip. *The Origins of British Sociology: 1834–1914* (Chicago and London: Chicago University Press, 1968).

Akiyama, Yuriko. *Feeding the Nation: Nutrition and Health in Britain before World War One* (London: Taurus, 2008).

Anger, Suzy. *Victorian Interpretation* (Ithaca, NY and London: Cornell University Press, 2005).

Armstrong, Nancy. *Desire and Domestic Fiction: A Political History of the Novel* (Oxford: Oxford University Press, 1987).

Bashford, Alison, and Joyce E. Chaplin. 'Malthus and the New World', in Robert J. Mayhew (ed.), *New Perspectives on Malthus* (Cambridge: Cambridge University Press, 2016), pp. 105–27.

Betensky, Carolyn. *Feeling for the Poor: Bourgeois Compassion, Social Action, and the Victorian Novel* (Charlottesville, VA and London: University of Virginia Press, 2010).

Bigelow, Gordon. *Fiction, Famine, and the Rise of Economics in Victorian Britain and Ireland* (Cambridge: Cambridge University Press, 2003).

Billington, Josie. *Faithful Realism: Elizabeth Gaskell and Leo Tolstoy: a Comparative Study* (London: Associated University Presses, 2002).

Blyth, Mark. *Austerity: The History of a Dangerous Idea* (Oxford: Oxford University Press, 2013).

Bodenheimer, Rosemary. *The Politics of Story in Victorian Social Fiction* (1988; Ithaca, NY and London: Cornell University Press, 1991).

Boner, Harold A. *Hungry Generations: The Nineteenth-Century Case against Malthusianism* (New York, NY: King's Crown Press, 1955).

Bourke, Austin. *The Visitation of God: The Potato and the Great Irish Famine* (Dublin: Lilliput Press, 1993).

Bowen, John, and Robert I. Patten. *Palgrave Advances in Charles Dickens Studies* (Basingstoke: Palgrave Macmillan, 2006).

Boyce, Charlotte. 'Representing the "Hungry Forties" in Image and Verse: The Politics of Hunger in Early-Victorian Illustrated Periodicals', Victorian Literature and Culture, 40 (2012), pp. 421–49.

Brake, Laurel, and Marysa Demoor (eds.). *Dictionary of Nineteenth-Century Journalism in Great Britain and Ireland* (Gent: Academia Press, 2009).

Brantlinger, Patrick. 'Dickens and the Factories', *Nineteenth-Century Fiction*, 26:3 (1971), pp. 270–85.

Brattin Joel J. 'Three Revolutions: Alternative Routes to Social Change in *Bleak House*', in *Charles Dickens as an Agent of Change*, ed. by Joachim Frenk and Lena Steveker (New York, NY: AMS Press, 2015), pp. 20–31.

Brice, A. W. C., and K. J. Fielding. 'Dickens and the Tooting Disaster', *Victorian Studies*, 12:2 (1968), pp. 227–44.

Brill, Barbara, and Alan Shelston. 'Manchester: "A Behindhand Place for Books": The Gaskells and the Portico Library', *Gaskell Society Journal*, 5 (1991), pp. 27–36.

Brock, W. H. *From Prolyte to Proton: William Prout and the Nature of Matter* (Bristol and Boston, MA: Adam Hilger, 1985).

Brooks, Chris. *Signs for the Times: Symbolic Realism in the Mid-Victorian World* (London: George Allen and Unwin, 1984).

Buckland, Adelene. '"The Poetry of Science": Charles Dickens, Geology, and Visual and Material Culture in Victorian London', *Victorian Literature and Culture*, 35 (2007), pp. 679–94.

Bynum, W. F., and Roy Porter. *William Hunter and the Eighteenth-Century Medical World*, ed. by W. F. Bynum and Roy Porter (1985; Cambridge: Cambridge University Press, 2002).

Caldwell, Janis McLarren. 'Illness, Disease and Social Hygiene', in Sally Ledger and Holly Furneaux (eds.), *Charles Dickens in Context* (Cambridge: Cambridge University Press, 2011) pp. 343–9.

Camporesi, Piero. *Il Pane Salvaggio*, trans. as *Bread of Dreams: Food and Fantasy in Early Modern Europe* by David Gentilcore (1980; Chicago, IL: University of Chicago Press, 1989).

Carpenter, Kenneth J. *Protein and Energy: A Study of Changing Ideas in Nutrition* (Cambridge: Cambridge University Press, 1994).

Carroll, David. *George Eliot and the Conflict of Interpretations: A Reading of the Novels* (Cambridge: Cambridge University Press, 1992).

Cazamian, Louis. *The Social Novel in England, 1830–1850*, trans. by Martin Fido (1903; London: Routledge and Kegan Paul, 1973).

Chapman, Carleton B. 'Edward Smith (?1818–1874): Physiologist, Human Ecologist, Reformer', *Journal of the History of Medicine and Allied Sciences*, 22:1 (1967), pp. 1–26.

Childers, Joseph W. *Novel Possibilities: Fiction and the Formation of Early Victorian Culture* (Philadelphia: University of Pennsylvania Press, 1995).

Childers, Joseph W. 'Politicized Dickens: The Journalism of the 1850s', in *Palgrave Advances in Charles Dickens Studies*, ed. by John Bowen and Robert I. Patten (Basingstoke: Palgrave Macmillan, 2006), pp. 198–215.

Chitty, Susan. *The Beast and the Monk: A Life of Charles Kingsley* (London: Hodder and Stoughton, 1974).

Cleere, Eileen, *The Sanitary Arts: Aesthetic Culture and the Victorian Cleanliness Campaigns* (Columbus, OH: Ohio State University Press, 2014).

Connell, Philip. *Romanticism, Economics and the Question of 'Culture'* (Oxford: Oxford University Press, 2005).

Coole, Diana, and Samantha Frost. *New Materialisms: Ontology, Agency, and Politics* (Durham, NC: Duke University Press, 2010).

Courtemanche, Eleanor. '"Naked Truth is the Best Eloquence": Martineau, Dickens, and the Moral Science of Realism', *ELH*, 73:2 (2006), pp. 383–407.

Cross, Stephen J. 'John Hunter, the Animal Oeconomy and Late Eighteenth-Century Physiological Discourse', *Studies in History of Biology*, 5 (1981), pp. 1–110.

Cunningham, Valentine. 'Soiled Fairy: *The Water-Babies* in its Time', *Essays in Criticism*, 35:2 (1985), pp. 121–48.

Cvetkovich, Ann. *Mixed Feelings: Feminism, Mass Culture, and Victorian Sensationalism* (New Brunswick, NJ: Rutgers University Press, 1992).

Dames, Nicholas. *The Physiology of the Novel: Reading, Neural Science, and the Form of Victorian Fiction* (Oxford: Oxford University Press, 2007).

Danahay, Martin. 'Work', in *Charles Dickens in Context*, ed. by Sally Ledger and Holly Furneaux (Cambridge: Cambridge University Press, 2011), pp. 194–202.

Daston, Lorraine, and Peter Galison. *Objectivity* (New York, NY: Zone Books, 2007).

David, Deirdre. *Fictions of Resolution in Three Victorian Novels: North and South, Our Mutual Friend, Daniel Deronda* (London: Macmillan, 1981).

Davies, William. *The Limits of Neoliberalism: Authority, Sovereignty and the Logic of Competition* (California: Sage, 2014).

Dean, Mitchell. *The Constitution of Poverty: Toward a Genealogy of Liberal Governance* (London: Routledge, 1990).

Delville, Michel, and Andrew Norris. *The Politics of Hunger and Disgust: Perspectives on the Dark Grotesque* (London: Routledge, 2017).

Donnelly, Laura. 'Victorian Diseases have Come Back to Haunt Us', *The Telegraph*, 23 July 2014, https://www.telegraph.co.uk/news/health/news/10985260/Victorian-diseases-have-come-back-to-haunt-us.html [accessed April 2018].

Duchesneau, François. 'Vitalism in Late Eighteenth-Century Physiology: The Cases of Barthez, Blumenbach and John Hunter', in *William Hunter and the Eighteenth-Century Medical World*, ed. by W. F. Bynum and Roy Porter (1985; Cambridge: Cambridge University Press, 2002), pp. 259–95.

Dunnill, Michael, *William Budd: Bristol's Most Famous Physician, Pioneer of Preventative Medicine and Epidemiology* (Bristol: Redcliffe, 2006).

Dzelzainis, Ella. 'Malthus, Women and Fiction', in Robert J. Mayhew (ed.), *New Perspectives on Malthus* (Cambridge: Cambridge University Press, 2016), pp. 155–81.

Eagleton, Terry. *Heathcliff and the Great Hunger: Studies in Irish Culture* (London and New York, NY: Verso, 1995).

Eagleton, Terry. *Materialism* (New Haven and London: Yale University Press, 2016).

Easson, Angus. *Elizabeth Gaskell* (London: Routledge and Kegan Paul, 1979).

Ellmann, Maud. *The Hunger Artists: Starving, Writing, and Imprisonment* (Cambridge, MA: Harvard University Press, 1993).

Eyler, John M. *Victorian Social Medicine: The Ideals and Methods of William Farr* (Baltimore, MD: Johns Hopkins University Press, 1979).

Foster, John Bellamy, and Fred Magdoff. 'Liebig, Marx, and the Depletion of Soil Fertility: Relevance for Today's Agriculture', *Monthly Review*, 50:3 (1998), pp. 43–60.

Foster, Shirley. *Elizabeth Gaskell: A Literary Life* (Basingstoke: Palgrave Macmillan, 2002).

Foster, Shirley. 'We sit and read our time away': Elizabeth Gaskell and the Portico Library', *The Gaskell Society Journal*, 14 (2000), pp. 14–23.

Foucault, Michel. *The Order of Things* (1966; London and New York, NY: Routledge, 2002).

French, Roger, and Andrew Wear (eds). *British Medicine in an Age of Reform* (London: Routledge, 1991).

Frenk, Joachim, and Lena Steveker. *Charles Dickens as an Agent of Change* (New York, NY: AMS Press, 2015).

Fulford, Tim. 'Apocalyptic Economics and Prophetic Politics: Radical and Romantic Responses to Malthus and Burke', *Studies in Romanticism*, 40:3 (2001), pp. 345–68.

Gallagher, Catherine. *The Body Economic: Life, Death, and Sensation in Political Economy and the Victorian Novel* (Princeton, NJ: Princeton University Press, 2006).

Gallagher, Catherine. 'The Body Versus the Social Body in the Works of Thomas Malthus and Henry Mayhew', in The Making of the Modern Body: Sexuality and Society in the Nineteenth Century, ed. by Catherine Gallagher and Thomas Laqueur (Berkeley, Loos Angeles, CA and London: University of California Press, 1987), pp. 83–106.

Gallagher, Catherine. *The Industrial Reformation of English Fiction 1832–1867* (Chicago, IL: Chicago University Press, 1985).

Garrido, Juan Manuel. *On Time, Being and Hunger: Challenging the Traditional Way of Thinking Life* (New York, NY: Fordham University Press, 2012).

Gilbert, Pamela. *Cholera and Nation: Doctoring the Social Body in Victorian England* (New York, NY: State University of New York Press, 2008).

Gilbert, Pamela. *The Citizen's Body: Desire, Health and the Social in Victorian England* (Columbus, OH: Ohio State University Press, 2007).

Gilbert, Pamela. *Mapping the Victorian Social Body* (New York, NY: State University of New York Press, 2004).

Gilbert, Sandra M., and Susan Gubar. *The Madwoman in the Attic: The Woman Writer and the Nineteenth-Century Literary Imagination* (New Haven, CT and London: Yale University Press, 1979).

Gill, Stephen. *Wordsworth's Revisitings* (Oxford: Oxford University Press, 2011).

Glass, D. V. *Numbering the People: The Eighteenth-Century Population Controversy and the Developments of Census and Vital Statistics* (Farnborough: D. C. Heath, 1973).

Goodlad, Lauren. *Victorian Literature and the Victorian State: Character and Governance in a Liberal Society* (Baltimore, MD and London: Johns Hopkins University Press, 2004).

Guerrini, Anita. *Obesity and Depression in the Enlightenment: The Life and Times of George Cheyne* (Norman, OK: University of Oklahoma Press, 2000).

Gurney, Peter J. ' "Rejoicing in Potatoes": The Politics of Consumption in England during the "Hungry Forties" ', *Past and Present*, 203 (2009), 99–136.

Guy, Josephine M. *The Victorian Social-Problem Novel* (Hampshire and London: Macmillan, 1996).

Hall, Donald E. (ed.). *Muscular Christianity: Embodying the Victorian Age* (Cambridge: Cambridge University Press, 1994).

Hamlin, Christopher. 'Charles Kingsley: From Being Green to Green Being', *Victorian Studies*, 54:2 (2012), pp. 255–81.

Hamlin, Christopher. 'Could You Starve to Death in England in 1839? The Chadwick–Farr Controversy and the Loss of "Social" in Public Health', *American Journal of Public Health*, 85:6 (1995), pp. 856–66.

Hamlin, Christopher. 'Providence and Putrefaction: Victorian Sanitarians and the Natural Theology of Health and Disease', *Victorian Studies*, 28: 3 (1985), pp. 381–411.

Hamlin, Christopher. *Public Health and Social Justice in the Age of Chadwick: Britain, 1800–1854* (Cambridge: Cambridge University Press, 1998).

Hardy, Anne. 'Urban Famine or Urban Crisis? Typhus in the Victorian City', *Medical History*, 32 (1998), pp. 401–25.

Harris, Beth (ed.). *Famine and Fashion: Needlewomen in the Nineteenth Century* (2005; London: Routledge, 2016).

Harvey, David. *A Brief History of Neoliberalism* (Oxford: Oxford University Press, 2005).

Henderson, W. O. *The Lancashire Cotton Famine, 1861–1865* (Manchester: Manchester University Press, 1934).

Henson, Louise. 'The "Condition-of-England" Debate and the "Natural History of Man": An Important Scientific Context for the Social-Problem Fiction of Elizabeth Gaskell', *Gaskell Society Journal*, 16 (2002), pp. 30–47.

Heringman, Noah. *Romantic Science: The Literary Forms of Natural History* (New York, NY: State University of New York Press, 2003).

Hilton, Boyd. *The Age of Atonement: The Influence of Evangelicalism on Social and Economic Thought 1785–1865* (Oxford: Oxford University Press, 1988).

Himmelfarb, Gertrude. *The Idea of Poverty: England and the Early Industrial Age* (London and Boston, MS: Faber and Faber, 1984).

Holmes, John, and Sharon Ruston. *The Routledge Companion to Nineteenth-Century British Literature and Science* (London: Routledge, 2017).

Houston, Gail Turley. *Consuming Fictions: Gender, Class, and Hunger in Dickens's Novels* (Carbondale and Edwardsville, IL: Southern Illinois University Press, 1994).

Huneman, Philippe. '"Animal Economy": Anthropology and the Rise of Psychiatry from the "Encyclopédie" to the Alienists', in *The Anthropology of the Enlightenment*, ed. by Larry Wolff and Marco Cipolloni (Standford, CA: Stanford University Press, 2007), pp. 262–76.

Hunt, Lynn. *The New Cultural History* (Berkeley, Los Angeles, CA and London: University of California Press, 1989).

Huzel, James P. *The Popularization of Malthus in Early Nineteenth Century England* (Aldershot: Ashgate, 2006).

Jacyna, L. S. 'Images of John Hunter in the Nineteenth Century', *History of Science*, 21 (1983), pp. 85–108.

John, Juliet. *Dickens and Mass Culture* (Oxford: Oxford University Press, 2010).

Johnson, Patricia E. '*Hard Times* and the Structure of Industrialism: The Novel as Factory', *Studies in the Novel*, 21:2 (1989), pp. 128–37.

Kamminga, Harmke, and Andrew Cunningham (eds.). *The Science and Culture of Nutrition, 1840–1940* (Amsterdam: Rodopi, 1995).

Kamminga, Harmke. 'Nutrition for the People, or the Fate of Jacob Moleschott's Contest for a Humanist Science', in *The Science and Culture of Nutrition, 1840–1940*, ed. by Harmke Kamminga and Andrew Cunningham (Amsterdam: Rodopi, 1995), pp. 15–47.

Kargon, Robert H. *Science in Victorian Manchester: Enterprise and Expertise* (Manchester: Manchester University Press, 1977).

Kennedy, Meegan. *Revising the Clinic: Vision and Representation in Victorian Medical Narrative and the Novel* (Columbus, OH: Ohio State University Press, 2010).

Ker, Ian. *John Henry Newman: A Biography* (1988; Oxford: Oxford University Press, 1990).

Ketabgian, Tamara. '"Melancholy Mad Elephants": Affect and the Animal Machine in *Hard Times*', *Victorian Studies*, 45:4 (2003), pp. 649–76.

King, Amy Mae. 'Taxonomical Cures: The Politics of Natural History and Herbalist Medicine in Elizabeth Gaskell's Mary Barton', in *Romantic Science: The Literary Forms of Natural History*, ed. by Noah Heringman (New York, NY: State University of New York Press, 2003), pp. 255–70.

Klaver, J. M. I. *The Apostle of the Flesh: A Critical Life of Charles Kingsley* (Leiden and Boston, MS: Brill, 2006).

Krueger, Christine L. *The Reader's Repentance: Women Preachers, Women Writers, and Nineteenth-Century Social Discourse* (Chicago, IL and London: Chicago University Press, 1992).

Lansbury, Carol. *Elizabeth Gaskell: The Novel of Social Crisis* (London: Paul Elek, 1975).

Laqueur, Thomas W. 'Bodies, Details and the Humanitarian Narrative', in *The New Cultural History*, ed. by Lynn Hunt (Berkeley, Los Angeles, CA, and London: University of California Press, 1989), pp. 176–204.

Ledger, Sally. *Dickens and the Popular Radical Imagination* (Cambridge: Cambridge University Press, 2009).

Ledger, Sally, and Holly Furneaux (eds.). *Charles Dickens in Context* (Cambridge: Cambridge University Press, 2011).

LeMahieu, D. L. 'Malthus and the Theology of Scarcity', *Journal of the History of Ideas*, 40:3 (1979), pp. 467–74.

Lenard, Mary. *Preaching Pity: Dickens, Gaskell, and Sentimentalism in Victorian Culture* (New York, NY: Peter Lang, 1999).

Lesjak, Carolyn. *Working Fictions: A Genealogy of the Victorian Novel* (Durham, NC and London: Duke University Press, 1997).

Levine, George. *Realism, Ethics and Secularism: Essays on Victorian Literature and Science* (Cambridge: Cambridge University Press, 2008).

Levine, George. *The Realistic Imagination: English Fiction from Frankenstein to Lady Chatterley* (Chicago, IL: Chicago University Press, 1981).

Lewes, Gertrude Hill. *Dr Southwood Smith: A Retrospect* (Edinburgh and London: William Blackwood and Sons, 1898).

Lloyd, David. *Irish Culture and Colonial Modernity 1800–2000* (Cambridge: Cambridge University Press, 2011).

Longmate, Norman. *The Hungry Mills: The Story of the Lancashire Cotton Famine 1861–5* (London: Maurice Temple Smith, 1978).

Mangham, Andrew. *Dickens's Forensic Realism: Truth, Bodies, Evidence* (Columbus, OH: Ohio State University Press, 2016).

Manzini, Francesco. 'Nutrition, Hunger and Fasting: Spiritual and Material Naturalism in Zola and Huysmans', *Forum for Modern Language Studies*, 49:1 (2013), pp. 20–32.

Mathias, Manon, and Alison M. Moore (eds.), *Gut Feeling and Digestive Health in Nineteenth-Century Literature, History and Culture*, ed. by Manon Mathias and Alison M. Moore (Cham, Switzerland: Palgrave Macmillan, 2018).

Mayhew, Henry. 'London and the Poor', *The Morning Chronicle*, 14 December 1849, p. 5.

Mayhew, Robert J. *Malthus: The Life and Legacies of an Untimely Prophet* (Cambridge, MA and London: Belknapp Harvard, 2014).

Mayhew, Robert J. (ed.). *New Perspectives on Malthus* (Cambridge: Cambridge University Press, 2016).

McCausland, Elizabeth D. 'Dirty Little Secrets: Realism and the Real in Victorian Industrial Novels', *American Journal of Semiotics*, 9:2/3 (1992), pp. 149–65.

McLane, Maureen N. *Romanticism and the Human Sciences* (Cambridge: Cambridge University Press, 2000).

Middleton, John. 'Why We Should be Concerned about the Return of Victorian Diseases', *The Guardian*, 8 August 2014, https://www.theguardian.com/healthcare-network/2014/aug/08/return-victorian-diseases-gout-tb-measles-malnutrition [accessed April 2018].

Miller, Ian. *A Modern History of the Stomach: Gastric Illness, Medicine and British Society, 1800–1950* (2011; London: Routledge, 2015).

Miller, Ian. *Reforming Food in Post-Famine Ireland: Medicine, Science and Improvement, 1845–1922* (Manchester: Manchester University Press, 2014).

Mitchell, Robert, *Experimental Life: Vitalism in Romantic Science and Literature* (Baltimore, MD: Johns Hopkins University Press, 2013).

M'Kendrick, John G. *Spallanzani: A Physiologist of the Last Century* (Glasgow: James Maclehose, 1891).

Moore, Tara, 'Starvation in Victorian Christmas Fiction', *Victorian Literature and Culture*, 36 (2008), pp. 489–505.

Morash, Christopher. *Writing the Irish Famine* (Oxford: Oxford University Press, 1995).

Morris, Pam. *Dickens's Class Consciousness: A Marginal View* (London: Macmillan, 1991).

Norman, Edward. *The Victorian Christian Socialists* (Cambridge: Cambridge University Press, 1987).

O'Brien, Mark, and Paul Kyprianou. *Just Managing? What is Means for the Families of Austerity Britain* (Cambridge: Open Book, 2017).

O'Flaherty, Niall. 'Malthus and the "End of Poverty"', in *New Perspectives on Malthus*, ed. by Robert J. Mayhew (Cambridge: Cambridge University Press, 2016), pp. 74–104.

Ó Gráda, Cormac. *Black '47 and Beyond: The Great Irish Famine in History, Economy and Memory* (Princeton, NJ and London: Princeton University Press, 1999).

Ó Gráda, Cormac. *Famine: A Short History* (Princeton, NJ and London: Princeton University Press, 2009).

Ó Gráda, Cormac. *Ireland Before and After the Famine: Explorations in Economic History* (Manchester: Manchester University Press, 1993).

Olmsted, J. M. D. *François Magendie: Pioneer in Experimental Physiology and Scientific Medicine in XIX century France* (New York, NY: Schuman's, 1944).

Packham, Catherine. *Eighteenth-Century Vitalism* (Basingstoke: Palgrave Macmillan, 2012).

Pickstone, John V. 'Dearth, Dirt and Fever Epidemics: Rewriting the History of the British "Public Health", 1780–1850', in *Epidemics and Ideas: Essays on the Historical Perception of Pestilence*, ed. by Terence Ranger and Paul Slack (1992; Cambridge: Cambridge University Press, 1995).

Pickstone, John V. 'Physiology and Experimental Medicine', in *Companion to the History of Modern Science*, ed. by R. C. Olby, G. N. Cantor, J. R. R. Christie, and M. J. S. Hodge (1990; London: Routledge, 1996), pp. 728–42.

Poovey, Mary. 'Disraeli, Gaskell, and the Condition of England', in *The Columbia History of the British Novel*, ed. by John J. Richetti, John Bender, Deirdre David, and Michael Seidel (New York, NY: Columbia University Press, 1994), pp. 508–32.

Poovey, Mary. *A History of the Modern Fact: Problems of Knowledge in the Sciences of Wealth and Society* (Chicago, IL and London: Chicago University Press, 1998).

Poovey, Mary. *Making a Social Body: British Cultural Formation, 1830–1864* (Chicago, IL and London: Chicago University Press, 1995).

Pope-Hennessy, Una. *Charles Dickens* (1945; London: Reprint Society, 1947).

Porter, Roy. *Flesh in the Age of Reason: How the Enlightenment Transformed the Way We See Our Bodies and Souls* (2003; London: Penguin, 2004).

Price, Catherine. 'Probing the Mysteries of Human Digestion', *Distillations*, 4:2 (2018), pp. 27–35.

Pyle, Andrew. *Population: Contemporary Responses to Thomas Malthus* (Bristol: Thoemmes Press, 1994).

Ranger, Terence, and Paul Slack. *Epidemics and Ideas: Essays on the Historical Perception of Pestilence* (1992; Cambridge: Cambridge University Press, 1995).

Raunch Alan. *Useful Knowledge: The Victorians, Morality, and the March of Intellect* (London and Durham, NC: Duke University Press, 2001).

Ross, Eric B. *The Malthus Factor: Poverty, Politics and Population in Capitalist Development* (New York, NY: Zed Books, 1998).

Rothschuh, Karl E. *Gerschichte der Physiologie*, trans. as *History of Physiology* by Guenter B. Risse (1953; New York: Robert E. Krieger, 1973).

Ruston, Sharon. *Shelley and Vitality* (2005; Basingstoke: Palgrave Macmillan, 2012).

Rylance, Rick. *Victorian Psychology and British Culture, 1850–1880* (Oxford: Oxford University Press, 2000).

Sanders, Mike. 'Manufacturing Accident: Industrialism and the Worker's Body in Early Victorian Fiction', *Victorian Literature and Culture*, 28:2 (2000), pp. 313–29.

Schofield, Robert E. *Mechanism and Materialism: British Natural Philosophy in an Age of Reason* (Princeton, NJ: Princeton University Press, 1970).

Scholl, Lesa. *Hunger Movements in Early Victorian Literature: Want, Riots, Migration* (London: Routledge, 2016).

Schor, Hilary M. *Scheherazade in the Marketplace: Elizabeth Gaskell and the Victorian Novel* (Oxford: Oxford University Press, 1992).

Schui, Florian. *Austerity: The Great Failure* (New Haven and London: Yale University Press, 2014).

Sen, Amartya. *Poverty and Famines: An Essay on Entitlement and Deprivation* (Oxford: Oxford University Press, 1981).

Sharps, John Geoffrey. *Mrs. Gaskell's Observation and Invention: A Study of her Non-Biographic Works* (Sussex: Linden Press, 1970).

Shenstone, William Ashwell. *Justus von Liebig: His Life and Work (1803–1873)* (1895; London: Cassell, 1901).

Slater, Michael. 'Carlyle and Jerrold into Dickens: A Study of *The Chimes*', *Nineteenth-Century Fiction*, 24:4 (1970), pp. 506–26.

Slater, Michael. *Charles Dickens* (2009; New Haven and London, 2011).

Slater, Michael. 'Dickens (and Forster) at Work on *The Chimes*', *Dickens Studies*, 2 (1966), pp. 106–40.

Slater, Michael. *The Genius of Charles Dickens: The Ideas and Inspiration of Britain's Greatest Novelist* (London: Duckworth Overlook, 2011).

Sleigh, Charlotte. 'The Novel as Observation and Experiment', in *The Routledge Companion to Nineteenth-Century British Literature and Science*, ed. by John Holmes and Sharon Ruston (London: Routledge, 2017), pp. 71–86.

Smith, Frank. *The Life and Work of Sir James Kay-Shuttleworth* (1926; Bath: Cedric Chivers, 1974).

Smith, Jonathan. *Fact and Feeling: Baconian Science and the Nineteenth-Century Literary Imagination* (Madison, WI: University of Wisconsin Press, 1994).

Smith, Sheila M. *The Other Nation: The Poor in English Novels of the 1840s and 1850s* (Oxford: Clarendon Press, 1980).

Spencer, Jane. *Elizabeth Gaskell* (London: Macmillan, 1993).

Stonehouse, J. H. *Catalogue of the Library of Charles Dickens from Gadshill* (London: Fountain Press, 1935).

Straley, Jessica. 'Of Beasts and Boys: Kingsley, Spencer, and the Theory of Recapitulation', *Victorian Studies*, 49:4 (1997), pp. 583–609.

Tarrant, W. G. *Unitarianism* (Texas: Grindl Press, 2015).

Taylor, Jenny Bourne, and Sally Shuttleworth (eds.). *Embodied Selves: An Anthology of Physiological Texts, 1830–1890* (Oxford: Oxford University Press, 1998).

Taylor, Michael W. *The Philosophy of Herbert Spencer* (London: Continuum, 2007).

Taylor-Brown, Emilie. 'Being "Hangry": Gastrointestinal Health and Emotional Well-Being in the Long Nineteenth Century', in *Gut Feeling and Digestive Health in Nineteenth-Century Literature, History and Culture*, ed. by Manon Mathias and Alison M. Moore (Cham, Switzerland: Palgrave Macmillan, 2018), pp. 109–32.

Thompson, E. P. *The Making of the English Working Class* (New York, NY: Vintage, 1966).

Thompson, Noel E. *The People's Science: The Popular Political Economy of Exploitation and Crisis 1816–1834* (Cambridge: Cambridge University Press, 1984).

Tillotson, Kathleen. *Novels of the Eighteen-Forties* (1954; Oxford: Oxford University Press, 1961).

Tóibín, Colm, and Diarmaid Ferriter. *The Irish Famine*, (London: Profile, 2002).

Tomalin, Claire. *Charles Dickens: A Life* (London: Viking, 2011).

Uffelman, Larry K. *Charles Kingsley* (Boston, MS: Twayne, 1979).

Uglow, Jenny. *Elizabeth Gaskell: A Habit of Stories* (London: Faber and Faber, 1993).

Ulrich, John M. *Signs of their Times: History, Labor, and the Body in Cobbett, Carlyle and Disraeli* (Athens, OH: Ohio University Press, 2002).

Vernon, James. *Hunger: A Modern History* (Cambridge, MS and London: Belknap Press of Harvard University Press, 2007).

Williams, Elizabeth A. 'Food and Feeling: "Digestive Force" and the Nature of Morbidity in Vitalist Medicine' in *Vital Matters: Eighteenth-Century Views of Conception, Life, and Death*, ed. by Helen Deutsch and Mary Terrall (Toronto: University of Toronto Press, 2012), pp. 203–21.

Williams, Raymond. *Culture and Society* (1958; London: Penguin, 1984).

Winch, Donald. *Riches and Poverty: An Intellectual History of Political Economy in Britain, 1750–1834* (Cambridge: Cambridge University Press, 1996).

Wood, Jane. *Passion and Pathology in Victorian Fiction* (Oxford: Oxford University Press, 2001).

Woodham-Smith, Cecil. *The Great Hunger: Ireland 1845–1849* (1962; London: Penguin, 1991).

Index

For the benefit of digital users, indexed terms that span two pages (e.g., 52–53) may, on occasion, appear on only one of those pages.